Where is the Key?

G000136482

To Grenda.

With best wishes

Sheila Gaylor
née
Brook.

Sheila Brook

chipmunkapublishing
the mental health publisher

Published by
Chipmunkapublishing
PO Box 6872
Brentwood
Essex CM13 1ZT
United Kingdom

http://www.chipmunkapublishing.com

Chipmunkapublishing gratefully acknowledge the support of Arts Council England.

I dedicate this book to my late husband who shared in so much of this story
and to all the friends who appear within its pages.

Sheila Brook

Preface

A very long bridge spans the years between the end of my previous book, 'Child of the Thirties', and the year in which I am now writing. My first book encompassed just fourteen years, and I am now attempting to contract a span of over sixty years into a second book. At the end of my first book I had just left school and I am now nearing the end of my eighth decade. Change has been experienced in almost every aspect of life in those years: in the home, in education, career opportunities, medical knowledge, in psychiatric treatment and many other areas. I almost feel that I now live on a different planet.

The thread of my mother's mental illness ran through my first book and she will have a more prominent place in the latter part of this book. In telling her story I feel I have given my mother's life a value to others that she was unable to provide herself. I am sure she would have been thrilled to know that she was 'in a book'. (You can guess what her response might have been as you read of her later on in my story!)

Whilst sometimes deploring change, the world is a better place in many respects. The practice of keeping a child apart from a certified mentally ill parent, and encouraging the child to forget her mother, continued right up until the middle of the twentieth century. My mother 'disappeared' from my life when I was eight years old and I was twenty-eight before I saw her again. What a lot of changes have occurred in this field: in treatment, in care, and I hope, in attitude. The large psychiatric hospitals that existed in the early years of the twentieth century were emptied before the century ended.

It has been difficult to know how to begin this book, how to provide sufficient links with my childhood story without repeating myself.

Now I have broken the ice, I think I feel the urge to continue.

Sheila Brook

Chapter One

WORK AND PLAY

Three years of senior school education came to an end when I reached the age of fourteen in 1945 but, apart from the blissful cessation of V1 and V2 rocket raids, there were few changes in daily life. Six years of the traumas of the war were over - the blitz, the bombs, evacuation and the air raid shelters - but food and clothes rationing continued for many more years. The ending of the war provided a much less fraught existence for everyone, although no improvements or sudden luxuries appeared. Food became even scarcer; frequent power cuts occurred, and there was an increased shortage of fuel during extremely cold post-war winters. There was a lack of everything, from toilet paper to bread and meat, as the almost bankrupt nation helped to feed and restore hope to the starving and homeless in Germany and right across Europe, and then began to pay back its' enormous 'lease lend' loan from the United States, but I am sure I didn't appreciate the reasons behind these continued deprivations in daily life at the time..

Neither did the continued absence of my mother, whom I had not seen for six years, enter my thoughts. She was still in a secure ward in a psychiatric hospital; suffering from what, as a child, I overheard my father saying was 'mania', with consequent long-term deprivation of normal life. I had not seen her since before the war, and had almost forgotten her, and certainly never thought of her as being part of my 'family'. And yet, I didn't really think of 'family' as such – it was just the two of us, my father and me.

One took for granted what life meted out in those days; I don't think I was discontent or even thought about 'what might have been' – it could have been a lot worse. As my mother said to me years' later, "That's your lot; you've got to get on with it". This had been her reaction when her first daughter, Peggy, was born, brain-damaged and epileptic. I think that was the attitude of most people in that period, adult and child alike. My mother accepted that she would have the responsibility for the twenty-four hour care of her first daughter with, I am sure, little advice or support for a baby who nobody would be able to help. Our much-criticised NHS and Social Services would, I hope, provide assistance nowadays. I wonder whether Peggy had suffered from some similar condition to that of David Cameron's little boy? Not much was known then, and epilepsy would be a term that covered more than fits, but a wide variety of the very sad and serious conditions of brain damage, where a short, difficult life both for the little child, and for the parents, was the prognosis.

Thoughts of beginning a commercial course at Hendon Technical College after the end of the summer holidays may have occupied my mind from time to time. I didn't want to learn shorthand and typing and had had ideas of becoming a nurse, so I wasn't looking forward to learning shorthand and typing in September. My father had disapproved of my wish to be a nurse – I guess he didn't fancy the probability of his daughter training to be a nurse in one hospital, perhaps a long distance away from home, whilst his wife was a long-term psychiatric patient in another hospital. I think he had more than enough of medical matters and hospitals, and, understandably, he was also reluctant for me to leave home.

In those days young people had little choice concerning their future. I didn't seriously think about my future, or a career. What was a 'career'? I don't think I had ever heard of the word. One left school and got a job, and part of one's wages went to help with the household expenses. I was lucky to be given the opportunity of further education and office training. In those days one's parents' wishes prevailed, and vocational opportunities were almost unknown if one had not had the privilege of a grammar school education. There was no career guidance or presumption of the idea of further education for anyone; university would have been a dream that would only come true for the brilliant, the very bright – or the very wealthy.

Three years of secondary education seemed a long period at the time, but now they appear to have passed by so quickly. The ending of the war brought almost immediate, though minor, hints of change in the educational field. No more air raids meant that the risks of additional people visiting the school during the day had disappeared, and the only invitation to an 'open afternoon' for parents occurred towards the end of my final term. Sadly, this invitation from my school was not in the evening; fathers didn't have the opportunity of seeing the inside of their children's school, looking at their work or meeting the teacher. Children's education was considered the responsibility of the teachers then, and parents were not at all involved in school life.

I can remember 'auntie' (who was our housekeeper during the war) attending this parents' afternoon and looking through my composition book. She was reading through an essay I had written on the subject of 'friendship', but I had not written about the activities I had shared during the war with my friend Joan. Instead I had written about the constant friendship of David and Jonathon in the Bible. I think we must have had a Sunday school lesson about them! 'Auntie' nudged the mother of the girl who was sharing the narrow bench seat attached to our double desk and showed her my composition. They both seemed to be talking about it, and I could see expressions on their faces that seemed to imply that they were rather impressed, but they said nothing to me. I had received a house mark for my composition together with a good comment from my form teacher, but neither our housekeeper nor her friend commended me! I think praise (like mental illness) was another thing that was kept under cover, not easily expressed in those days.

I now realise that I didn't have a close group of friends when I was young. School did nothing to encourage each pupil to have a group of supportive friends, and Joan had been my sole friend through most of my childhood. My other close friendship developed in my last year at Chandos School, when a member of my class, Beryl, was appointed captain of our school House, 'Brockley', and I was asked to be vice-captain, and this developed into a lasting – though distant - friendship. Sole-mate friendships are rare. (Perhaps this was why I chose to write as I did in my essay on this subject?) But boy friends soon appeared.

Soon after the end of the war my father dug up the Anderson shelter that was half-buried in our garden, and tried to make the ugly area of clay soil that it left behind into a flowerbed, but there weren't many plants to buy and no garden centres existed then. I believe that the shelters had to be returned to Harrow Urban District Council unless local residents had bought them at the beginning of the war. What did the council do with them? What use were they to the public?

Oddly enough I did learn the post-war fate of one Anderson shelter. Some years later I saw a very presentable, neatly painted, corrugated iron Anderson shelter in my fiancé's parents' garden. It was not the one from my garden I am sure, but my future husband had bought an old Anderson shelter from the Council after the war. He had cleaned it up and sandpapered it smooth before painting it green to blend in with his father's well-tended lawn, and made it into a mini-garage to shelter his motorbike. It was discreetly positioned at the bottom of his parents' garden. The old air-raid shelter was now serving a very useful purpose above ground, proudly showing its curves, instead of being half-buried and rusting in the damp ground.

My mother had to return to Shenley Hospital in the summer of 1939, and some months' later my father employed a housekeeper, but not long after the end of the war our peaceful, companionable life was shattered after some big row had occurred over I knew not what. My strongest recollection of mealtimes in those immediate post-war years, was of breakfast in the kitchen, when we sat in stony silence at the kitchen table, together with our ex-housekeeper and her daughter, only speaking to each other when necessary, Rose was now in her late teens, and was at work. Her mother also had an office job, but they were still living in our house and had found nowhere else to live. Accommodation was hard to find in those years and 'auntie' and her daughter, Rose, continued to live in the house for some years. We still had our lady lodger whose bed-sitting room had been my parents' bedroom in earlier years. My father still slept on the 'put-you-up' in the dining room, sharing the small wardrobe in my little bedroom in which to put his clothes

I did the shopping on Saturday morning, the cooking, cleaning, the washing and ironing, and my father bought our weekly rations at a grocer's shop in Ealing. He carried them home in panniers fixed to each side of the back wheel of his bicycle, with our ration of one egg each - when available - carefully wrapped and placed in a cardboard box strapped on to the carrier fixed over the back wheel. Housekeeping was still considered women's work in those days, and I don't remember my father ever attempting to cook a meal, pick up a duster or wash up the dishes. I admire the men who today can cope with, or at least attempt, the weekend shopping, cook a meal, and share in the housework.

I carried on the household duties exactly as our housekeeper had done, although I am sure that I didn't have the time to be as meticulous as she had been. I always laid the table with a white tablecloth for Sunday dinner, setting out the cutlery properly. During the winter we ate our weekday evening meal in the kitchen, where the solid fuel boiler provided some warmth. I have always enjoyed cooking, but I have no recollection of what I managed to put on the table to eat, nor, strangely, can I remember sitting down actually eating a meal with my father. I do remember making mint sauce with fresh mint picked from the garden that must have accompanied roast lamb for a Sunday dinner. During the week we both had our main meal at work or college, and I must have produced something in the way of a meal for our supper in the evening.

The kitchen boiler heated our water, but washing machines had not yet appeared on the domestic scene and I did the weekly washing in the kitchen sink, using a scrubbing board and Sunlight soap to rub the clothes before washing them in Persil soap powder. My father's Van Heusen stiff collars, the sheets and our towels went to the laundry. I neatly wrapped the dirty washing in a brown paper parcel, tied it up with string and placed the package outside on the doorstep, ready for the laundryman to collect. On top of the parcel of clothes I put the money to pay for the previous week's washing. The laundryman collected the money and left the change on top of the parcel of clean washing, also tied up with string and crisp brown paper, which I reused the following week. We recycled years ago. Honesty was taken for granted.

Bed linen was very scarce and required clothing coupons. I can remember accidentally pushing my foot through the thin cotton of a well-worn sheet as I turned over in bed one night. I cut the sheet in two, as I had sometimes watched our housekeeper do in earlier years; we called it 'putting sides to middle'. I machined the two stronger outer edges together on my mother's old Singer sewing machine, making a new strong middle, and then hemmed together the rough, weakened material to become the new edges. There was now a hard but strong double seam down the middle of the sheet that would make it last quite a lot longer. I had obviously learned something useful in my sewing lessons at school. It gave the sheet a new lease of life, saved my father money and saved our coupons. Can one imagine a teenager, or anyone for that matter, doing this tedious work nowadays? I don't think even the Green Party has advocated 'renewing' sheets.

Where is the Key?

I have only begun to think about the past now I am old. I didn't appreciate that anything was unusual when I was young, and believe that I only lived for the day. Surely that first, war-free, summer must have made me feel more carefree?

Early on in that summer holiday I began to be more interested in boys. I didn't know any boys, had no boy cousins, had been to a girls' school and was an only child. The small boys I had known before the war had been evacuated. Our Scottish neighbours had moved and I never saw Roy again, or David who had lived a little further along the road, with whom I had made mud pies in his barren garden. Keith and his parents had moved away from Kenton before the war began, but I discovered that my pre-war friend, Johnny Boughton, had returned from his evacuation abroad. I didn't know he had been evacuated overseas; he had just disappeared at the beginning of the war. He seemed quite different from the gallant little boy who had been invited to my small birthday tea before the war. I didn't recognise this tall gangly youth, and he had to remind me of who he was. He was now called John, no longer Johnny, and was often hanging around down the road during the summer holidays with nothing much to do. I was not very interested in him, but he introduced me to his friend Tony, who lived in the road where I used to spend hours playing ball with Joan, unaware that Tony lived in the same street. I guess that Tony was oblivious of our bouncing balls while he was engrossed in more homework than we were given in our school. Perhaps he spent more time on his violin practice than I did on my piano practice. Probably Tony's mother wouldn't let him play in the street. I doubt whether he would have enjoyed our ball games. Tony was a very gentle, humorous and musical boy and I fancied him more than the post - war John.

I guess that Tony was my first – very innocent – boyfriend. I grew very fond of him, although he was a little younger than me, and was still at his boys' grammar school when I started work two years later. We had a few cycle rides to Stanmore during the summer holidays, with walks around the Common and a cuddle in the grass, but our friendship was very innocent, even by the standards of long ago.

Sometimes Tony and I spent a Saturday afternoon, making music together at my home, with Tony playing his violin and me playing our old piano, but I don't remember going to the swimming pool with him or walking to the park. My father and I were invited to Boxing Day tea with Tony and his parents, and I remember they were also entertaining a German prisoner of war. There was a German POW camp somewhere in the locality, and this young German soldier often spent a Sunday with Tony and his family before he was repatriated to his home country. He must have been only a youth, as my recollection of him is of a boy rather than a man. He accompanied the family to their Presbyterian church and occasionally I joined them too. The church was quite large and lofty; so different from the small black-painted building that we used as a church every Sunday.

We didn't meet very often once he had returned to school and I began my commercial training at the end of the summer holidays. We soon went our separate ways the following year, although we sometimes met on the train two years later. Tony was still travelling in to London to attend Marylebone Grammar School, and we sometimes met on the crowded, morning rush-hour train to Baker Street. There was not much difference in our ages; by then I was 16-going-on-17 and Tony was 17-going-on-18, but a 'working girl' and a 'schoolboy' in the VIth form seemed poles apart. I wonder what became of him. He wanted to be an airline pilot. Did he achieve his ambition? He was a very nice boy, and I hope life has treated him well.

It was during the next summer that I noticed two or three boys – Roger, Stan and Eric - frequently cycling past my house while my father and I were eating our evening meal, giving a loud 'wolf whistle' as they slowly pedalled by. I was smitten with Eric, and as soon as I had finished my meal and done the washing up I dashed off to meet them in the local recreation ground. I sat on the benches at the far end of the park, furthest away from the park-keeper, with a crowd of other girls and boys, having an occasional kiss and a cuddle, the boys joking and chatting - mostly about bikes, as I recall. The boys' non-uniform attire out of school or work was a black 'bomber' jacket and old grey flannel trousers. Neither jeans nor anoraks – and certainly not hoodies! - had as yet appeared. Bicycles were a constant topic of the boys' conversation - the superiority of one type of three-speed gear over another; or the efficiency of Raleigh brakes, and the type of handlebars (drop-head ones were very popular). While the girls sat on and around the park seats at the far end of the recreation ground, or playing on the American swing, a bicycle was dismantled and reassembled, while enthusiastic discussion went on between the boys before they clambered on to the swing, pushing it higher and higher until the girls screamed. What would they have made of present-day multi-geared, lightweight cycles, I wonder?

Stanley was mad about jazz and was forever humming his jazz tunes, and drumming the rhythms with his fingers on the park bench. He also went to my church, and whenever he could get near the piano after our youth fellowship meetings he practised his jazz and entertained us – or drove us to distraction – as we stacked the chairs at either side of the hall at the end of an evening.

On summer evenings our crowd of boys and girls gathered at the far end of the park where we would chat, have a laugh; the girls had to listen to the boys' enthusiastic talk of the latest bicycle development. There was a lot of general banter, a bit of kissing and a cuddle, but we didn't drink, we didn't take drugs, we didn't have sex, we didn't exchange text messages or take embarrassing photos on mobile phones. Neither did we fight, 'throw up', shout obscenities at each other or attack the park-keeper when he told us to go home. I think one of the boys smoked – but cigarettes, not pot or anything worse. We'd never heard of any of these things, let alone had to resist their temptations. We had also never been made aware of teenage pregnancies; how times have changed! We were just ordinary youngsters living in suburbia.

One summer evening Eric cycled slowly along the road towards my house just as I pulled the front door shut behind me. He skidded to a standstill at the kerbt as I stepped on to the pavement. Had he been waiting nearby for this little piece of drama, I wonder, as he casually produced a matchbox from his pocket? He carefully opened the tiny box and nestling inside, like a small trophy, was a shrivelled chunk of flesh. I shuddered as Eric told me casually that he had accidentally chopped the top of his finger off while tinkering with his bicycle. I almost shudder again as I think of this incident. It must have been agony for Eric, but I think he bravely covered up his pain with his dramatic appearance from the end of a side road and arrived outside my house just as I shut the front door; a well planned little scene! But Eric has had to endure the loss of the top of (I think) an index finger for the rest of his life.

Any spare time I had in these mid teenage years was taken up with mild flirtations first with Tony, and then in our local recreation ground with Stan, Eric and Roger – all very nice boys, all of whom I can think back on with affection.

As our ex-housekeeper and her daughter continued to live in our house their bedroom became their bed-sitting room. One day my father and I came home at the end of the day to hear a piano being played upstairs. Auntie's piano had been in storage for years, along with some other pieces of her own furniture. Her piano and a sideboard had been brought in and carried upstairs while we were at work and without my father's knowledge. I remember my father was furious (a very rare state to see him in), worried that the back bedroom floorboards would not be strong enough to withstand the weight of the piano. It was impossible to force tenants to move out of furnished accommodation then and alternative homes were difficult to find. I was nineteen years old before they moved from our house and my father was able to have a bedroom once again (albeit the little bedroom over the hall) and no longer had to sleep on the put-u-up in the dining room. We no longer had to share the little wardrobe in my small bedroom. I returned to my nice bedroom at the back of the house, with its floor-to-ceiling fitted cupboards on either side of my bed, and electric fire with modern tiled surround fitted into one wall. I found the morning sun came streaming through the windows in the summer to wake me up early. I had not slept in this room since I was eight years old.

I didn't appreciate the deprivations my father had suffered for so many years, nor do I think I was disgruntled that I had also been deprived of my own pleasant bedroom for eleven years, but, strangely, I don't remember any outburst of joy at returning to it. My childhood toys had long gone, including my art deco style, white-painted, Triang doll's house with all its miniature furniture that I had loved playing with when I was small. Like so many other collectables, discarded toys were handed on or thrown away, but there was nobody to hand my toys on to and I have no idea where my dolls' house went. I saw an identical doll's house to mine on the Antiques' Road Show a while ago, and it was a highly valued item.

I then did not recognise, but now can see, that we had all lived through a long period of anxiety and strain at home. We had experienced a lot together and had got on well through the war, but the difficulties of the last few years at home had been unpleasant to live through. Our lady lodger still occupied the main bedroom where my parents used to sleep. Our household set up must have been quite a mystery to our neighbours for many years! Auntie Susie, Rose, my father and I all became friends again a few years later, and remained so until Rose's mother died about thirty years later. Rose and I are still in touch, although we live too far away to visit each other. Our lodger continued to make her little home in the main bedroom until I married in 1952, when she exchanged the front first floor room in our house for the front bedroom in my in-laws' home.

We didn't expect or crave for happiness or treats during the period in which I grew up; I had no expectations. Our lives contained little or no indulgence or extravagance, but had far less pressure, demands, or temptations, than young people have nowadays; a time that, without our awareness, inculcated a different set of values and contentment with life. Looking back, I think I was happy, but we didn't look for happiness. A more appropriate description of my life then would be that I was carefree, but without great expectations of my future.

However, my long school holiday was not spent entirely in doing household jobs, swimming, church activities, and boys. My father had a full week's paid (I think) holiday before my new studies began in the Commercial Department of Hendon Technical College. Our only holidays during the war had been a very brief cycling holiday by the River Thames just before D-day in 1944, and few days in the Quantock Hills in the late autumn of that same year, when my father came to see me while I was evacuated in Somerset during the Vl/V2 rocket attacks.

My father had kept up his membership of the Cyclists' Touring Club, and their accommodation listings were helpful in providing us with our next holiday on the outskirts of the village of Winterbourne Abbas in Dorset. He thought that we could attempt something a little more ambitious now that the war in Europe was over. Cycling was quite hard work in Dorset; there was a lot of hard pedalling up hills, and I can still remember the cycle ride from Sherbourn Station to Dorchester and the long drag uphill to our destination on a hot August Sunday afternoon. I can also remember the cooked breakfast we had with freshly cured and salty bacon from a recently slaughtered pig that was shared between two or three families in the village.

It was while visiting Weymouth when we were on this holiday in 1945 that we heard the news that the Second World War was finally over and it really was peacetime. I don't remember any cheering, or celebration of any kind. It was accepted quietly in this rural area and everyone continued as if nothing momentous had happened. Our celebration had been with the ending of the war in Europe, and the Far East seemed so far away to me, like another planet. I was not aware at the time of the enormous importance of this tremendous news, did not understand about the war in the Far East, and knew nothing of the atrocities committed in the Japanese prisoner of war camps and may not even have known of the dropping of the atom bombs on Hiroshima and Nagasaki. I am certain I would have had no understanding of the magnitude of these bombs, or the significance of the bombs' explosion on the Japanese islands. Without the benefit of television, faraway places didn't seem real; they were simply names on newspaper, and my awareness of the continuance of the war in the Far East was remote.

It is curious that I was on holiday in Berkshire in 1944 when my father and I saw the boats along the Thames in readiness for D-Day, and I was again on holiday when we learned of the final ending of World War Two. These two events are my main and almost sole memories of these holidays taken at such momentous times. I knew so little about the detail of the war apart from that which affected me directly, but it was our history that was in the making, and it has now made me keen to fill in the gaps and devour any information about those years.

Chapter Two

PREPARING FOR THE FUTURE

Education has changed unrecognisably since I left school in 1945. The school leaving age was raised to fifteen the term following the end of the war and new grammar schools were soon built in order to begin fulfilling the promises of the 1944 Education Act. It was many years before I realised that the girls in my year at Chandos School who had not moved on with me to do a Commercial Course at a Technical College, or taken a Civil Service examination, had remained at the school for a fourth year, and were actually taught shorthand – although I have been told that they couldn't learn typing as there were, as yet, no typewriters in the school! I am unsure as to what use shorthand would have been if the user couldn't type. Nowadays, it is the other way round; shorthand is now rarely used except in law courts but nearly everyone uses a keyboard for their computer – although I notice that not many have been taught to 'touch-type', which is a great advantage.

An Education Act was one thing; putting it into practice in a war-impoverished nation was quite another, but eventually education became almost a complete reversal from the limited, sound, but formal schooling that I described in my earlier book. The child-centred, broad curriculum, central Government-controlled education of today, with the pressure of frequent tests and exams, followed by abundant opportunities for extended learning of recent years is now being challenged again. An economic crisis of huge proportions is upon us, with more needs than there is money to fulfil, and as I write further changes are promised, with less government intervention, fewer tests and a little more emphasis on job-related further education and apprenticeships.

Many who have benefited from a university education are now finding it difficult to get jobs, but many others seem to miss out on the basic skills that were considered essential years ago. Most of my generation would not have expected our lessons to be interesting and challenging in order to keep our attention and interest, and many of our lessons would appear boring to young students today. We would never have answered back to our teachers or shown them disrespect in any way. Our written work was meticulously marked; we learned from our mistakes and were immediately corrected if we spoke ungrammatically. We had a very limited curriculum, no class discussion or inter-action between pupils, no school outings or visits, few opportunities, and didn't anticipate treats, but when we left school we were numerate and literate, had been cared for and brought up to be law-abiding, honest, polite and considerate; we worked hard, made our mark, small though it might be. Further education was limited, and unlikely for many, but I don't think we feared being unable to get a job.

I began my commercial training in the September of 1945. I have a number of recollections, plus a few 'snapshot' memories of the two years I spent in the Commercial Department of Hendon Technical College. The first of these occurred on my first morning, when I clearly recall the huge *faux pas* I made. I had not wanted to do this commercial course and didn't want to work in an office, and dreaded the thought of shorthand, but I can't think why I forgot to put a pencil into my pencil case alongside my fountain pen and ruler that morning. (Biros? Ballpoint pens? What were they?) Perhaps it had not occurred to me that I would be required to endure a shorthand lesson on my first day, nor had I expected that I would need to use a pencil to write down the first few 'thick' and 'thin' outlines of our Pitman's shorthand course: f/vee; ith/thee; s/zee... and all the rest, requiring a thick or thin outline. Everyone else had a pencil; why had I forgotten mine?

My form mistress was understandably annoyed with me for forgetting to bring a pencil for a shorthand lesson, but to make matters worse, I named her incorrectly when standing up to apologise for my omission. My teacher's name was Miss Vinelott; I innocently called her Miss Vineyard, and she seems in my memory to have become incandescent with rage. I had not meant to be funny or rude, and had just mistaken her name. I grew scarlet with embarrassment as I was severely told off, and consequently felt cowed and kept my head down for the rest of the day. How different is the attitude with some young people today – we had no attitude then, were always respectful to our teachers, and those older than ourselves. I did not dare to explain my mistake, but I had not been used to such vehement rebuke, even though my beloved form mistress at Chandos School, Miss Oyston, could be quite sharp and was very strict. I don't think she ever actually lost her cool. Perhaps she did, but never with me. I can't remember ever being the recipient of her reproof – apart from a glance, a frown and a firm 'Sheila!' in my direction for talking in class; I *was* a chatterbox!

However, after this unpleasant start, Miss Vinelott and I soon got on well, and she found that I was actually a conscientious student. She must have been having a bad first day of term, may have had personal worries, or just couldn't cope with her new workload. Maybe she was a newly qualified teacher, lately discharged from the Forces. Who can tell? She married shortly after this and became Mrs. Roberts. I guess her fiancé had probably recently returned home from the War, but strangely these possibilities never occurred to me at the time. I had no relatives who had been in the Forces; my father was, thankfully, too old to be called up, and I never thought of the possibility that some of the college staff had served in the war.

The limited education most of my generation had received was extended a little at Hendon Tech., and we began to learn French as well as our secretarial subjects of shorthand, typing and bookkeeping. Our general education continued, with geography, history, maths, English and P.T. lessons. Although my old reports indicate that I did well in these subjects, I have little memory of what I studied. I have always enjoyed reading, but I can't remember any of the books we studied in literature. However, I do remember the class being asked to write a composition describing our ambitions for the future. It is the only time I think the word 'career' might have been mentioned in my youth, although I honestly believe that I had not heard of the word then. I wrote about my desire to become a nurse, and presumably described as best I knew (which was very little) about what I would have to learn, what I would do on a hospital ward and what the prospects were for my future.

When our essays had been marked and were handed back to us, Mrs. Roberts asked me to come and speak to her at the end of the lesson. I wondered what I had done wrong this time! However, she kindly told me she was concerned that I had written about nursing, but had not mentioned the training I was now being given to prepare me to become a shorthand-typist, and then, hopefully, a secretary. Why was I in the commercial department of the college when there was a pre-nursing course in the same building, she wondered? She said she had spoken to the head of the commercial department about a transfer. Mr. Smith had agreed that I had been misplaced, and I was called to his office to discuss this. He told me that the pre-nursing department had consented to my transfer from the commercial department, but I had to tell him that mine would be an unfulfilled ambition, as my father did not want me to become a nurse. So I remained on the commercial course. One obeyed one's parents' wishes in those days.

I can understand now why my father didn't want me to train as a nurse, not only would he have his wife in one hospital and his daughter in another, but I would have left him with no companionship at all, and no-one to do the various duties of housekeeping. The thought of being a shorthand typist was a poor substitute for nursing as far as I was concerned at the time, and I hated the next few weeks as I struggled with my Pitman's shorthand outlines.

However, after a while I found I quite enjoyed learning shorthand and I practised the outlines, memorised the ever-lengthening list of short-forms and did quite a lot of homework in the evenings. Eventually I came to tolerate writing shorthand at speed, although I found my left-handedness seemed an impediment to very high speed. Pushing the pencil in front of the left hand rather than allowing it to follow the right hand naturally, seemed, and still seems, a much harder exercise. You can also see what you are writing when the pen follows the hand, whilst the poor left-hander covers up what has just been written. Children had to hold their pen or pencil in a particular way when I was young and do a particular style of forward-sloping handwriting with loops to certain letters.

Typing became a skill that has been extremely useful all my life, and made me much less dependent on my wobbly handwriting. I have kept up and possibly increased my typing speed over the years. Touch-typing on a computer keyboard is a delight compared with banging on the keys of an old-fashioned typewriter and is extremely useful in my present task. Among the memories I have of my two years at Hendon Tech. is the sound of the harsh metallic clatter of keys on our old pre-war typewriters in our first few typing lessons, as my class of about thirty girls tapped away in unison to the music of a gramophone record. I can still remember the tune that accompanied our early typing lessons, teaching our fingers to move rhythmically on our keyboards.

I was very busy after I arrived home from College, and often fell asleep in the evenings while doing my homework at the dining room table. My father was worried, and we paid – literally; this was pre NHS - a very rare visit to the doctor. Practising my shorthand outlines must have had a soporific effect on me, as nothing appeared to be wrong with me. However, suddenly becoming very sleepy and lifeless seems to have remained with me throughout my life, and still occurs.

Holidays had been important in my parents' lives between my mother's episodes of mental illness before the war, and my father made every effort to make a holiday possible now the war was over. At the end of my first year of office training we set off on another cycling holiday in August 1946. My father had studied his Cycling Tourist Club handbook once again and thought that we could travel further afield, and revisit some of the beautiful spots in Devonshire that he had driven to with my mother in their old Austin 7 in the 1920s. He had sold its' replacement at the beginning of the war, a Ford 8 that I can vaguely remember, and I know he missed it a lot. A limited amount of petrol was becoming available, and a few people were driving their cars again, and he must have remembered all the holidays he had had prior to 1939. All we now had in our garage were our second-hand bicycles. He had arranged for us to stay in a boarding house at a small resort on the North Devon coast.

We cycled from our home in Kenton, near Harrow, to Paddington Station and watched our bikes being placed in the luggage van before we caught the early morning fast train to Taunton. We waited impatiently for the local train to arrive and take us on to the coast at Minehead in Somerset, when our long cycle ride would begin. Our bicycles were once more put in the luggage compartment for the brief journey. Minehead Station was closed by Dr. Beeching in the 1960s and no longer exists. My last holiday with both my parents had been to Minehead in 1938, and I have a memory of donkey rides on the beach, and watching a Punch and Judy show. Sadly, my mother was readmitted to a mental hospital the following summer.

Sadly there was no time to sit on the beach on our arrival at Minehad, and we set off immediately for our long cycle ride to Combe Martin in North

Devon, way along the coast on the western edge of Exmoor. My father hadn't learnt the lesson that miles on a bike soon appear much longer than miles in a car when actually being pedalled. I had no idea what lay ahead of me and I don't think my father had appreciated the gradient of the hills we were to encounter on our bikes. We had a fairly gentle cycle ride to Porlock, but now faced the ascent of the famous Porlock Hill. (I can remember my father telling me the story of driving up Porlock Hill backwards in reverse gear in his first Austin Seven. Can this be true? I think I remember him telling me that the reverse gear was more powerful than the first forward gear! I am sure I saw an old sepia photo when I was a child of the old car at the top of the hill, with my father standing at the side.) The present road that replaced the steep old road had not yet been constructed in 1946, and I think we had to climb up the very same hill that my father had driven up in the 1920s. I had no idea of what was still ahead of me. It took us over an hour to walk up Porlock Hill step by step, slowly pushing our bicycles, which were nothing like the light-weight machines available today, and were extra weighty because of our fully packed saddlebags plus the panniers my father had attached to each side of his back wheel. His bike must have weighed a ton. Was this supposed to be a holiday?

However, the view was wonderful when we reached the top of the hill, with a viewing point of the coastline and the sea just a little further along the road. I would guess that the present large car park with similar views is over almost the same spot. As we cycled on we had views of Exmoor all the way, and it was bliss to cycle along the top of the moor, until it began to drizzle. We were soon in a mist, but after a while the rain ceased, the mist cleared, and we stopped to look at the wide expanse of Exmoor to our left, whilst being aware of the sea almost immediately beneath us on our right. The views were breathtaking. But it was even more breathtaking a few minutes later when I saw the long steep slope of another hill in front, this time dropping away beneath me. The amazingly long, steep slope of Countisbury Hill confronted us, and we had to cycle down it. My three-speed gears which helped me a little to get up some hills at home were not much good on Exmoor hills, which had to be walked up, but this was a massive *downhill*, and my brakes would be needed. I hoped they would be strong enough to slow me down and control my descent; it was very scary.

I gripped the brakes as firmly as I could, but the handlebars were juddering as I held them tight whilst hurtling downwards, bending low over my semi-dropped handlebars, but with my head up as I stared fixedly in front of me. I can still remember the sensation of fear and excitement. My heart was in my mouth. Suddenly the little town of Lynmouth came into view, but it was still a long way down. I was relieved when I felt more in control of my bike. I soon saw a little hump-backed bridge over the River Lyn. I was able to slow down a little more before I reached the bottom of the hill, and had firm control of my brakes before I cycled across the narrow bridge and then turned into the little main street. My father was tailing me, making sure he could see me and that I was OK. I don't think he could have remembered how steep these hills were when he decided to arrange a cycling holiday in North Devon. We gradually came to a standstill, got off our bikes and stood at the kerbside breathing heavily. I was shaking all over. I looked back at the long steep hill, snaking up to the top of the moor. Phew! Was I glad to be safe! Whenever I have visited North Devon since then I have looked at Countisbury Hill, winding down from the edge of Exmoor to the very edge of the sea. It always brings back very mixed memories. Even nowadays it is quite exciting to drive down it in a *car*.

We had safely reached the little harbour town of Lynmouth, but we were by no means at the end of our journey. It was now early evening, and we still had a long way to go. It had begun to rain. My father considered trying to find accommodation for the night, but feared that the time might be wasted with a fruitless search in August, the height of the holiday season. It was imperative for us to get moving if we were to reach our destination before it was really dark, so we pressed on. It was raining quite hard, and was very gloomy as we began our journey once again, with another hour-long climb up Lynton Hill on foot, feeling tired, and wheeling our heavy bikes in the rain. I can't remember the last part of the journey after we reached the top of the hill, but only know that we reached our destination very late in the evening, and had missed dinner. Our landlady had given up on us, and thought we would not arrive until the following day. What a start to a holiday!

To make matters worse, my late developing and unprepared-for, evidence of the arrival of puberty, probably already experienced by most of my friends, descended on me a day or two later. I had quite obviously not fully understood the chapter our housekeeper had given me to read in her medical book the previous summer. No one had explained to me the necessities of life required by teenage girls every month. One didn't talk about such intimate matters in those days, even to one's friends – it was just like mental illness – unspoken, shameful and hidden.

I was so uncomfortable and had found it so embarrassing trying to explain and ask for my father's assistance. I don't know whether either of us knew what I needed but he got me to a chemist's shop. I found it all immensely embarrassing and the experience has stayed with me all my life.

Without being blatant about it, I do think that the openness of society nowadays is better; we are all human. I don't think any difficult or personal matters were ever mentioned. Everything was quietly assumed or kept hidden 'underneath the carpet'. However, I wonder whether we are becoming less civilised in our open society in the use of language. The present-day coarseness and crudeness about personal and intimate matters, the swearing and obscene language used by so many - from the well educated or well-born, down to young children - seems to be a retrograde evolutionary move. Newspapers blank out the vulgar words with asterisks or dots, but one cannot help but read in the erased words. Does this make us more civilised? I doubt it; I think it possibly leads on to the violent, boorish, uncouth behaviour that we see today, which was unheard of in my youth. My father used to say that if a person swore or used vulgar language, it showed his ignorance and his lack of proper education. This wise comment came from a man who was brought up in a very poor one-parent family, and who left school at thirteen, but who became well read, well spoken, literate and moderate in his use of language; who surmounted immense difficulties with no assistance, no credit, no praise – from government, bank, relatives or society.

But I would never have contemplated talking to him over anything I might be worried about, and he never shared with me about any of the worries he may have had. There was a common saying in those days 'least said; soonest mended'. I am not convinced that this saying is true, and believe that the very opposite is often more likely to be helpful.

However – back to my summer holiday. There was no swimming in the sea for me that August. I remember sitting on a deck chair on the beach at Combe Martin, looking enviously at the other bathers in the sea. I didn't even wear my bathing costume. We cycled to Ilfracombe one day and to Woolacombe with its wonderful sandy beaches on another, but I fear I was a rather gloomy and grumpy adolescent, resentful at being unable to go swimming. I remember paddling at the water's edge, still wearing my summer dress. My father came up to me and said he didn't think I should be standing in cold water for a few days! It was altogether too much for me.

I don't think I've ever had a tantrum in my life, but I don't think I was very good company that week – I was at the seaside and I wanted to swim. I guess my father would have liked a swim too but felt unable to because he knew it would have upset me. I didn't know anything about possible teen-age tantrums, or hormones that might excuse bad behaviour, but I know I was not my cheerful self, and my main memories of that holiday were the tiresome hills, the frightening, but exciting, descents, and my personal 'miseries'.

At the end of the week we made the journey in reverse, walking wearily in the August heat up the very long, steep Countisbury Hill, then having an easy ride down Lynmouth Hill, then freewheeling down Porlock Hill in fine weather, before the comparatively easy cycle ride back to Minehead Station. After our train journey on the main line from Taunton to Paddington we had another cycle ride of about nine miles, mainly up the Edgware Road before, a few miles later, we could at last say we were back home. I have no idea how many miles we cycled on that holiday. I would like to know. Despite the beautiful scenery and the fine weather, I think that was the worst holiday in my life. I was quite pleased to get back to my shorthand and typing.

Chapter Three

NEW EXPERIENCES

A new maths teacher appeared in our classroom at the beginning of my second year at Hendon Tech. who immediately became very popular amongst a class of fifteen-year-old girls. He was only the second male teacher I had throughout my entire education. The first one had been my class teacher at junior school at the beginning of the war. As a nine-year-old I had idolised him, but he suddenly disappeared in the middle of term when he was called up into the RAF. Our new maths teacher looked very young, and it is highly likely that he had been demobbed from the Forces immediately after the war had ended, had completed a one-year teacher-training course, and that Hendon Tech. was providing his first teaching experience. A friend of mine, Joy, sat in the desk behind me, and whenever he entered the classroom to take a lesson I heard a big sigh as she swooned at the sight of him! I think most of the class of girls experienced a flutter of the heart too. We hadn't seen many young men and not many boys of around our own age.

It was during our second year that some of the post-war attempts to widen our horizons began. This young maths teacher told us that he and his wife were starting a weekly evening madrigal group at his home in Edgware, and invited any students who were interested in singing to come along. Several girls in my class decided to join, including me and my group of friends, Beryl, Margaret, Joan and Joy. It was quite an adventure to go out in the evening once a week, take a bus ride to Edgware, and visit our teacher's house. Our sessions singing madrigals became the highlight of my week. I think all the girls in the group enjoyed it – particularly Joy, who had a lovely singing voice and was overwhelmed to see her heart-throb at home. We learned to sing in harmony, and this was my only experience of choral singing throughout my education. . I don't remember what he taught us in maths, but I do remember our weekly attempts to sing madrigals.

There was no choir during the war in my previous school, nor did we have one in our commercial college. I have loved singing all my life and regret being unable to follow up this brief experience of singing in a madrigal group. This was the first of the few optional cultural activities that were introduced soon after the war at Hendon Tech, endeavouring to enlarge our outlook, but without the facilities to do so. It was a successful attempt to give us some cultural experience, but would certainly not be allowed to take place in a teacher's home nowadays. For us, it was part of the excitement.

This teacher's wife was German; she spoke very broken English, which I found interesting and attractive to listen to. At the time it did not enter my head that our teacher may have met this lady in Germany whilst he was in the army, and was able to marry her after the war and bring her to England when he was demobbed. I don't think I was aware of anything to do with post-war politics, and took no interest in the news. We had not been taught to 'think', and our ability to understand national, or local situations or politics was very restricted at best, but almost non-existent as far I was concerned. I think I was too busy and don't even remember reading the newspaper; as yet there was no television to bring the world into our homes, and we listened to the radio at home for our entertainment and always listened to the nine o'clock news.

Although the sense of community and school loyalty we had at my senior school, Chandos, seemed to be missing from Hendon Tech., we had a little more social involvement. There were quite a few boys doing a commercial course in a separate class in my year group. I think their course differed in some way from the girls' course, perhaps with a little less emphasis on typing and more on what was then called bookkeeping, probably with a view to the boys getting a job in a bank. A few lessons in ballroom dancing were organised by another member of staff immediately after college hours, where the two sexes met. Quite a few boys were brave enough to come to the weekly dancing class, and they were taught the proper way to approach a girl and ask her to dance. This sense of politeness and respect soon disappeared with the advent of modern dancing. These classes were not very successful as there were too many people crowded into too small a room, with atrocious sound reproduction from a record player and I soon lost interest. It was too crowded, too noisy and we couldn't hear or understand the instructions of the teacher for the sound of scuffling feet. We shuffled about on the floor for a while, but it was all more off-putting than appealing.

However, I suppose I must give the staff full marks for effort. I have for many years wished I had had the opportunity to learn to dance. It was a pursuit that I feel sure I would have enjoyed if I had learned the steps properly at college. I feel quite envious when I see people ballroom dancing, even though ballroom dancing soon went out of favour, until 'Strictly Come Dancing' came along on BBC TV, and that's quite a bit different from how we were taught sixty years ago.

Our form teacher arranged to take a group of interested pupils on one or two visits to the opera. I wonder whether a special price was offered to young students? I don't believe that either my father or the parents of any of my friends could have afforded the normal cost of a seat at the opera nowadays. I remember going to the old Sadler's Wells theatre to see Tosca one evening. The theatre seemed very dingy, shabby and old-fashioned, and was in their previous, very old theatre somewhere in Islington, before the Sadler's Wells Opera Company moved to Covent Garden. I can't remember how I got there by bus, but I do remember seeing Tosca, and recognising one or two of the arias from hearing my father singing them, or playing them on his old 78rpm HMV gramophone records at home.

I made a long unsuccessful bus journey to go to second school opera visit on another occasion; I missed the bus connection where I should have met with my classmates, and continued the journey to somewhere in north London – I think it was near The Angel, Islington, but I didn't know exactly where I should get off when I reached this area, hadn't got the courage to ask, got completely lost and never turned up. There were two other very memorable occasions when a group of girls from school went to the Royal Opera House in Covent Garden soon after the end of the war to hear, I think, the first of Sir Malcolm Sargent's concerts for children. On another occasion we went to the Royal Opera House to see the Magic Flute – a magical memory. That was certainly the most memorable musical experience of my youth. The Royal Opera House looked very drab and war-torn then, and it was a long time before it was partially rebuilt to become the present stunningly beautiful home of the Royal Opera and Ballet. Several members of staff were putting themselves out to provide us with some of the extra-curricular activities that are expected in today's secondary education, but which were initial, immediate post-war, implementations of the all-important 1944 Education Act.

My long-standing friend Beryl and I started the Christian Union in the college, with the initiative coming from one of the teachers, Miss Marianne Cross. She taught us office practice (another subject the content of which I have totally forgotten). She seemed rather a stern lady when she first took our class, wearing her hair in two long plaits, which were wound round to the top of her head, rather like a crown. It made her appear very formidable, but she was very kind when you got to know her, and we became – and remained – friends after I left college. At the start of her first lesson she asked if there was a girl named Sheila Brook in the class. I wondered what I had done wrong, but she simply asked me to speak with her outside the classroom when the lesson was over. I couldn't understand why this unknown teacher could want to speak to me, but I followed her into the corridor after the lesson and she just said that she had been given my name and she would like to have a chat with me in the refectory over a cup of tea at the end of the afternoon.

This all seemed very mysterious and I was rather bewildered at this apparently social invitation from a member of staff. Students didn't mix socially with the staff, but I was sure that I hadn't done anything wrong when, at 4 p.m., I went into the empty refectory and sat waiting at a table for a few minutes before Miss Cross bustled in. She bought me a cup of tea, then sat down and told me that the person who took the older boys' Bible class at my church had given her my name. She would like me, together with any friends who were interested, to start a Christian Union at the college. This was all quite a shock, a bit beyond my aspirations. However, I told her I would speak to my friend Beryl and we would see what we could do.

Within a few weeks we had got the CU under way between us, and quite a number of interested students met each week. We had different speakers, most of whom were supplied by Miss Cross, as at the age of fifteen Beryl and I had no contacts. I guess that we did the publicity! It seems strange that I have no other memories of how we organised the CU, or in what room we met, or what we did. Memory is so fickle! I do remember that we had an outing to Buckinghamshire in the summer holidays, with a ramble along the Chess Valley, followed by tea in a teashop. The only speaker I can remember is Flight Lieutenant Branse Burbridge, DFC and Bar, who had been an ace fighter pilot during the Battle of Britain and who was invited to address us at our last meeting before we left college. Hendon Tech. became part of Middlesex University many years later. I wonder whether they still have a Christian Union. If so it is probably the one my friend Beryl, Miss Cross and I started in 1946.

I met my next boy friend in the Christian Union. Although only about sixteen, we became quite fond of each other for a long while. Our activities were very simple, but he always seemed to have ideas of places to visit on Saturdays and we had a lot of fun. John and I went to Kew Gardens one cold Saturday in early spring, and I can remember us snuggling up to each other on a seat in the palm house, with John's arm around me as we ate our sandwiches. I thought this the height of sophistication – to be 'going out' with a boy friend, although the closeness of contact may have had as much to do with the fact that we were cold and the palm house was heated. Ours was not a sex-obsessed friendship – the word was never mentioned, probably not even known! Our friendship continued for some time after we both started work. Nobody had to warn me in those days to 'be careful', to 'say no', or to 'be prepared'; it wasn't necessary. But I had nobody who could have advised me, and there was no close female relative to whom I could have talked about my relationships or other personal matters if I had had a problem (but who would have talked to their mothers about their boy friends in those days anyway?).

At the beginning of my second year at Hendon my father said that I could have my bus fare as extra pocket money if I felt like cycling to college. I weighed this up in my mind and decided that I would prefer a little extra money to spend, so I 'got on my bike', and traded fun and company for extra money! I can't remember exactly how much it was, but I don't think my ordinary pocket money would have been more than a shilling (5p.). With my holiday cycling experience and, I hoped, stronger leg muscles, I began cycling to Hendon every day, taking a more direct route than the bus. But it was a long ride each morning and afternoon, with a lot of hills to pedal up (without the compensation of beautiful scenery) although the suburban hills of north London were nothing when compared with the steep gradients on the edge of beautiful, remote Exmoor. However, those West Country hills had to be walked up, and the long gradual climb up Colindeep

Lane in north London had to be pedalled up each and every morning before lessons began.

I had enjoyed the companionship and fun with my friends and the larking about on the top of the bus on the morning and evening bus journeys to and from Hendon, the thrill of jumping off the moving No. 183 bus from Kenton if we saw the No. 83 bus from Ealing appearing at the Kingsbury Green road junction. Oh the dismay, if we missed it! The No. 83 bus saved us the long walk up the hill from Hendon Central Station. I soon realised that the companionship of my friends was worth more to me than the extra cash I had for a few weeks in the summer term, and it was not long before I gave up my morning and afternoon exertions on my cycle. It was quite a long journey on an old second-hand bike, and had excluded me from the companionship of my friends and classmates.

After we had been given the results of our exams near the end of our final term, the top few students from each of the classes in our year were given the opportunity of staying on at college for a further year in order to prepare for the General Matriculation examination the following summer. This was another new opportunity for which we had to thank the 1944 Education Act and before 0 levels and subsequently GCSE's were introduced. Mr. Smith, my head teacher, had put a very favourable comment on my last report; all my grades were good, and I was in third position among three classes that comprised my year group of 87 girls, so I was one of the students to be given this opportunity. I thought I would like to stay on another year in order to take my Matric, and finish my education with a *real* qualification, but my father was not so enthusiastic when I eagerly told him about it, and so he was invited to come to the college and discuss it with the head teacher.

An evening interview with Mr. Smith was offered, which gave my father the only opportunity he had throughout my entire education to visit any of my schools. He had never met any of my teachers; neither did he see any of my work or enter any of the classrooms in which I had spent so many hours. I don't even know whether the college or my previous schools knew that my mother was in a mental hospital, and I am sure they were not aware that I was caring doing the housekeeping when I was at Hendon Tech. I don't think my dad ever recognised from my reports what good grades and positions in class I had attained. Parents were not involved in their children's education then and just left it to the teachers.

I waited expectantly for my father to come home late that evening, and to learn how he had got on with Mr. Smith, but was deeply disappointed when he said that he couldn't see the point of my studying for another year. He thought it would be better for me to start work. He didn't really see how it would benefit me to stay on at college until I was seventeen in order to take an examination that would be of no value to me. He was probably right. I doubt if it would have made much difference to my prospects or my immediate future, but I was really very upset at the time, although I didn't show it. (Just as I had been shocked and upset when I learned that I hadn't passed what used to be called the scholarship exam. in order to get a place at the local County Grammar School. I had been very upset when I learned that I had failed the entrance examination, but I didn't show it. My headmistress felt there had been some mistake and had told me to urge my father to ask the local authority why I had not been offered a place, but he didn't query it. But − 'there you go' as they say!) I don't think my father thought that a good education was necessary for girls. So with these two years of further education I would soon be launched into the world of work.

I still have all my six-monthly reports from Hendon Tech, which have a number of facts in addition to our exam marks that I was interested to read again after so many years. They indicated age, height and weight, as well as exam results, shorthand and typing speeds and position in form and in year. I notice that my weight increased from 7st.3lb when I was fourteen-and-a-half, to 8st.11lbs. just before I left two years later. (Girls were 'lean beans' in those days; we never had to consider dieting!) I had grown one-and-a-half inches in that period too. I don't think anybody had a weight problem in the 1940s, and I was surprised to read that I had managed to put on 22lb. in two teenage years. I feel quite ashamed of my present weight when I compare it with the slight figure I must have presented then. I knew of nobody who was fat in those days.

I was in either second or third place in my form in my four six-monthly reports, and varied between second and fourth position in my three-form-entry year group, so I don't think Mrs. Roberts had any further need to reprimand me, but I had had a bad start, and one that I have remembered clearly. I had consistently good marks and grades for arithmetic (still not called maths) bookkeeping, English, French, geography, history, shorthand and typewriting, but only received a 'B' for physical training (as it was then called) until a wonderful 'A' appeared on my last report. I have no recollection whatsoever of where our P.T. lessons occurred or what they consisted of but I know I was highly delighted at the time to get at 'A' for my physical training at last. I don't think I would qualify for an 'A' grade in the weekly exercise and movement classes in which I have taken part since I gave up playing tennis some years ago, although I haven't done too badly until very recently. Although I can remember my history teacher, her lessons, together with our geography lessons are also complete blanks in my mind, although I had 'A's or 'B+'s for both these subjects. I can still recall some of my shorthand outlines, but my typing lessons have been a lifetime's resource, particularly in typing the manuscripts of my books.

My two years at Hendon Tech. passed by very quickly and I didn't have the attachment that I had to my old senior school. I think I had so much to do both at home, at college, at my church and youth organisation (in addition to my various boy friends) that most of my further education was, hopefully, just absorbed. We must have had regular college assemblies, yet I can only remember the one at which I was asked to read the lesson. I had to arrive early at college that morning in order to practice reading from Isaiah, chapter 6. I rehearsed the passage in a small stock room (Room B7?) with my history teacher, on how to project my voice and to say the words clearly. I felt very nervous, when, a little later, I walked up the steps, and on the stage of the assembly hall, stood at the lectern and read, 'For unto us a child is born, unto us a son is given, and his name shall be called Wonderful, Counsellor, the Mighty God, the Everlasting King...' so this must have been the end of Christmas term College assembly in my second year. The assembly hall was vast when compared with my old school hall. When I first stood at the lectern I was over-awed by the size of the hall, and the number of faces below me. However as soon as I had got started I enjoyed doing the reading and can remember the occasion vividly.

Towards the end of my final term I was once again told that my head teacher wished to see me in his office. Again I wondered what I had done wrong, but soon discovered that he had kindly remembered my interest in nursing, and had thought a job in the medical field would be an interesting substitute. He had obtained an interview for me at a pre-National Health Service, private clinic in London that specialised in the treatment of rheumatic diseases. I was delighted with this prospect and a week or two later I went up to London for an interview with Major Forbes the secretary of the Clinic. Was he another ex-soldier now in a peacetime career? I was given the job, but before I started work at the beginning of September in 1947 I had another summer holiday.

My second year at Hendon Tech. had passed by so quickly and in the summer of 1947 my father had planned another holiday. We were going to the West Country once again, and of course making use of our bicycles, but this summer our holiday was in South Devon. Although I had moaned a bit during our previous year's holiday, I was quite proud of the high hills I had walked up and cycled down, and the distances we had covered – and indeed I still am. I did enjoy our 'adventures' together. I think I was more able to be a companion to my father as I grew older, and we were 'good mates'.

This year we were to stay in the little village of Bigbury in South Devon. This time the train took us much nearer to our destination. We had a long railway journey from Paddington to Kingsbridge and a much shorter, but still hilly, cycle ride to our destination. I visited Bigbury again many years later, and saw nothing in the village that looked familiar or reminded me in the least of where we had stayed many years ago. It brought back not a single memory, although I know that we stayed at another of the little boarding houses recommended in my father's Cyclists' Touring Club handbook.

However I do remember freewheeling down the long hill from the village to the coast, with the sudden amazing view of Burgh Island, a tiny islet just off the mainland almost surrounded by deep blue sea, with two little frills of waves meeting each other across a spit of golden sand as the tide receded. I remember the 'terrapin' that drove across to the island at low tide, and floated back to the shore when the tide was in. We were told that it was an old landing craft that was used in the Normandy landings and had been converted into this strange vehicle. Was this true, I wonder? The weather was fine, and we cycled to various places, but mainly we swam, sunbathed and sat on the beach reading our library books. Each morning I propped my shorthand notepad up against a long, flat, low-lying rock, almost like a table, at the foot of the cliffs, and my father gave me some shorthand dictation from his newspaper. I was afraid that I would lose my speed, or forget my outlines and wanted to be well prepared for my new job. I think this was a more restful holiday than in previous years, and was a good preparation for the job I was about to begin, but I have so few memories of it. Maybe my new job was on my mind, and the very uneventfulness of this holiday was a good thing, a calm preparation for what was to come, and is the very reason why I have so few memories of it. It was the last holiday we had from the accommodation list of the Cyclists' Touring Club

Tourism was beginning to develop again and holiday accommodation would become more available and more widely advertised in the coming years

Chapter Four

A WORKING LIFE

In September I began work at the Charterhouse Rheumatism Clinic in Marylebone, a walkable distance from Baker Street station. This was a pre-HNS Clinic, which, although considered a private clinic was very different from present-day BUPA Hospital. There was a semi-private, fee-paying department on the ground floor, where patients paid slightly lower fees than those who took the lift up to the second floor to the Private Patients' Department, whose surroundings were presumably plusher. The private patients paid a full consultant's fee for their treatment and were also charged the full cost of any blood tests or x-rays and for any physiotherapy that was required, but the actual quality of treatment was the same for every patient, and a large proportion of patients only paid low fees for consultation and treatment, others were able to get grants from provident societies or, if they were really poor, had their treatment free. These patients were all seen in what was called the Hospital Department, which was in the basement of the clinic.

I was to be secretary to the almoner in this department. Almoner is a title that is unknown now, a name and a job that has become redundant. In those pre-NHS days, the almoner interviewed each new patient in order to assess their ability to pay the full fee of six shillings (30p) for each consultation and treatment or to enquire whether they belonged to one of the many provident societies who might pay for their treatment. The Hospital Savings Association, Prudential and the Liverpool Victoria Provident Societies were the most frequently used societies and many of the patients were funded by grants from one or another of these provident societies. The almoner also enquired as to whether there were any associated problems, or to find out if hospital transport was needed, which we requested from the Hospital Car Service. It was a very busy department before the arrival of the NHS.

Those who had paid into one of these medical insurance funds, or friendly associations, could qualify for a grant to pay their fees. Patients without medical insurance were assessed as to whether they could afford to pay the full fee for their consultation and treatment. If the almoner found that they were too poor they were seen for a reduced fee or no fee at all if she considered they needed treatment but could not possibly afford it.

I can well remember two such patients; one was a poor man, very crippled with arthritis, with a bald crown to his head, but with long hair at one side which he brushed over his bald pate. If it was a windy day he hobbled in, leaning on his walking stick, with his long hair blowing all over the place, and certainly not plastered across the top of his head. Another disabled man used to make plaster brooches of ladies wearing crinoline dresses, holding a basket of tiny flowers. He painted these brooches very delicately and used to sell them for 5 shillings (25p.). They were beautifully decorated and carefully executed, but would have brought him in a very small income. One day he came in and after booking in at the reception desk, he came over to my desk and presented me with one of his pretty brooches. I felt very honoured. He was not an elderly man, but I think this was his only way of earning a little money, and yet he had generously given a brooch to me. Many of these patients must have had very small incomes and difficult lives to cope with alongside their arthritis or rheumatic disease, with untold sad stories locked up inside their heads.

If the consultant recommended a further course of treatment the almoner had to send a report to the appropriate society of the doctor's opinion regarding improvement or why there was a need of a further course. Treatment normally meant weekly injections, and physiotherapy was often recommended. As they improved the period between injections was lengthened. Very occasionally patients were recommended to have a course of treatment at a spa, which would be arranged by the almoner. Requests from various Hospital Car Service centres were made for those who were too disabled to come to the clinic by public transport.

In between taking dictation and typing out reports and letters I was sometimes required to escort a disabled patient in the lift to the x-ray department on the first floor, where Dr. Seth Smith was our radiologist, or take someone who required a blood test to the lab. on the third floor. I quite enjoyed these little excursions away from my life in the basement, with the opportunity to have a little chat with a patient on the way up in the lift, and sometimes have a peep at what was going on in the x-ray department, or more excitingly, in the lab where I saw blood samples being whirled around as if fitted into a washing machine (although I had never seen a washing machine in those days). It was a busy, varied and interesting environment for a sixteen-year-old just starting work, one who was a little bit worried about her shorthand capability, and not used to dealing with people, although it was the people who interested me.

I was paid £3 a week, with an additional five shillings towards the cost of my season ticket to Baker Street station. I was offered a midday meal for which five shillings (25p) a week was deducted from my wages. This was a real bonus in those days of acute food shortages, and as my father had a midday meal in a café in Ealing, it also saved me having to cook a dinner at home in the evening, and I accepted this low-cost, no trouble, mid-day meal with alacrity. I discovered that a nice meal was provided each day, which was eaten in a pleasant atmosphere in the basement refectory of the large physiotherapy department that was situated in an adjacent road. I met with all the staff, and sat at tables together with the physiotherapists, laboratory technicians, nurses, some of the doctors, receptionists and secretaries, although I recall that the medics were often seated together and talking shop (or was it politics - with the imminent arrival of the NHS?) animatedly, but on the whole everyone was very sociable.

I believe that a Dr. Warren Crowe started the Charterhouse Rheumatism Clinic as a charity in the heart of London, when he set up a clinic in The Borough after the First World War. So many people suffered then, and still suffer today, from various rheumatic diseases, and Dr. Warren Crowe's work increased until there were clinics in London, Surrey, Essex and Sussex. He still had an afternoon clinic in the basement when I was working there, and was much revered, although he frightened the life out of me on the rare occasions I had to take dictation from him. He was a somewhat formidable old gentleman.

A Nurse Hodges had assisted him in the Borough Clinic, and she was still working in the Weymouth Street Clinic during the time I was there, and was known affectionately as 'Hodgie', although she had a tricky temper. The treatment was unconventional, and consisted mainly of injections of minute doses of streptococcal and staphylococcal vaccine, the dose being reduced to the lowest that the patient found gave the most benefit. All the consultants were well qualified; some had consulting rooms in Harley Street, but a few were in general practice, and drove in to London from quite long distances to see patients in their half-day clinic. Other treatments were used too, including 'manipulation' by Dr. Guy Beauchamp, a Harley Street consultant, which was in effect osteopathy performed by a qualified doctor, in the days when osteopathy was very much frowned upon. There was also a gynaecologist who had an occasional clinic, and a foot specialist, a Dr. Meyer, a very kind man who helped me with a painful ganglion I had on the top of my foot at one time, probably caused through walking quite long distances each day in ill-fitting high heeled shoes, which I have never been able to wear since.

A lot of physiotherapy treatment was provided at the clinic that is now sometimes difficult to obtain on the NHS. A charitable trust gave a lot of help to poor people in those days, and much first class treatment was given.

Barbara was the medical secretary and she and I had no office of our own; our desks and typewriters were situated in a corner of the large waiting room in the basement. There were no timed appointments, and the patients usually arrived before 10a.m. and sat patiently in rows, often waiting for a long time before their name was called by one of the two nurses to see one of the consultants – it's no wonder those sitting in hospital or our G.P. waiting rooms are called 'patients'! I enjoyed the jolly atmosphere of my first job, the banter and gossip among the staff, and I especially enjoyed meeting the patients.

There was a friendly atmosphere in our department between the office and nursing staff, but we all treated the consultants with immense respect. Three doctors held a clinic each morning, and another three in the afternoon.

Patients always saw the same consultant. Barbara usually dealt with the consultants' dictation of reports at the end of each session, although I sometimes had to fill in for her. If she was with one doctor and another was clamouring for a secretary at the end of his clinic, finger pressing on his buzzer, impatient to dictate reports and letters to GPs and get off to his own consulting rooms, I had to answer the call. For a while I dreaded this happening, as I had not acquired the knowledge to form outlines of all the medical terms that were rattled off. My pocket nurse's dictionary was well used, and I think I made a few clangers at first, but the doctors all read their letters before signing them, and a mistake would be noticed and corrected before it was signed.

I got on well with Mrs. Ricketts, the almoner; she didn't dictate too quickly, her reports were not too long and didn't contain too many complicated medical terms, and in time I began to feel quite excited if the doctor's bell rang and Barbara was with another doctor. I had to respond quickly, take dictation from an impatient doctor and manage his rapid speech. I learned quite a lot of correct medical vocabulary along the way. I think most of the consultants were understanding and tried to speak a little more slowly for this inexperienced new girl.

However, I still remember one call to take dictation from our visiting gynaecological consultant who always wore a floral buttonhole. I had picked up some of the medical terms used by the doctors, but did not understand a gynaecological term used by this particular consultant, and typed some totally inappropriate word. I can recall my embarrassment as he brought my typed letter out to the reception area and showed it to our elderly, rather formidable receptionist, and they both burst out laughing. I knew they were laughing at something I had typed. I still remember the incident, but the incorrect term I used, and also the correct medical word I should have used, are now long forgotten. Dr. – handed me the letter to be retyped, with the correct term handwritten over the top of my unfortunate mistake.

All the staff – but not the consultants - used to have our coffee and tea breaks in a tiny room where all the patients' records were filed. If we were informed that a patient had died, Hodgie always hastened to remove their medical notes from one of the old-fashioned filing boxes during our coffee break, almost reverently write 'RIP' on it, and return them to another box – the 'dead file'. Fifi had served in some way in the Red Cross during the war, but she never spoke to us of her experiences, and I didn't like to ask her what she had done in the war. Although it had only ended two years previously, nobody seemed to talk about any wartime experiences.

As soon as all the patients had arrived and the morning clinic was under way, the staff coffee break was taken, when we all crowded into our little sanctuary, away from the buzz of conversation in the waiting room. One of the nurses stayed on duty in the waiting area, ready to call out the next patient's name, and to be on the spot in case any crisis developed – usually a harassed doctor. Whenever possible one of us would bring in something edible to share with everyone over our coffee. We were always delighted when Mrs. Ricketts produced squares of homemade gingerbread spread with butter (or, more probably, margarine). I walked past a baker's shop just off Marylebone High Street on my way to work, and I noticed that on Friday mornings some trays of little iced sponge cakes were on display. I ordered a dozen of these when it was my turn to supply the 'eats' and carried them very carefully to the office. They were freshly baked, very light and enjoyed by us all. If there were any cakes left over at the end of the day I took them home and it made a little treat for my dad. Treats did not occur very often – they were real, occasional luxuries in those days of austerity.

The consultants didn't get a coffee or tea break, nor did they receive a cup of coffee to drink while 'on the job'. There were also no facilities for the patients to buy a cup of tea or coffee either - there was actually no spare room in the department for a coffee bar. They just sat and waited to see their doctor, and then sometimes had to wait a long time after their consultation for the Hospital Car Service to come and collect them. Quite a tough day out for very unwell, mainly elderly people.

There was a particular hierarchy in the way we were all addressed; the two nurses were known by contractions of their surnames – 'Hodgie (Hodges) and 'Fifi' (Fifield); the almoner and the receptionist by their surnames, Mrs. Ricketts and Mrs. Manders, the two secretaries were known by their first names and, of course, all the doctors were addressed formally.

Barbara, the medical secretary, and I were given time off by Mrs. Ricketts to go and watch the then Princess Elizabeth's wedding procession in November 1947. On a very dull, grey day we stood among the crowd lining the roadside in Whitehall. We cheered as the procession passed, waving and cheering enthusiastically as the various members of the royal family drove by, and especially when Princess Elizabeth passed us in her beautiful golden coach. We had never seen such splendour. The surrounding buildings looked drab and dirty, the day was dull and drizzly, but it was the first bit of brilliance since the war, and certainly the first bit of luxury and romance that I had experienced. We had been told we could take a taxi back to our office afterwards; it was the first time I had ever been in a taxi. What a thrill!

The buildings in Whitehall now look fabulous, gleaming white on a sunny day, and Westminster Abbey is absolutely breathtaking, both inside and out. It is almost impossible to believe how dingy London remained for many years after the war. The wedding procession, the coaches, the horses, the glimpses of the bride and groom and the royal family were the only splendorous memories in 1947. The buildings looked so dirty with a post-war-weary air and were greyish brown in colour. Today the brilliant white buildings in that area look as if newly built, and have much more grace and architectural beauty than many of the new, post-war constructions.

I went to my first (and only) office Christmas party that December, held in the familiar basement department, which was the most spacious, when all the staff mingled together, including many of the consultants. Everyone was dressed up in party clothes. I felt a bit of a fish out of water without a party dress amongst all these grandees, but found a companion in Marie from the semi-private department on the ground floor, and we sat in a corner of the almoner's waiting area, chatting about this and that, and the good and bad things about our boy friends. I don't think her experience was any more serious or any less innocent than mine had been. I think we both felt a bit out of our depth at this 'grown up' office party, which was a little merry, but nobody was drunk. Neither of us had been to parties, and felt ill equipped to enjoy all the hilarity and jocular conversation.

In reading about the early post-war years, I find that the winter of 1947, my first winter at work, was an exceedingly bitter one and was considered to be the most severe for a hundred years. There were power cuts, fuel shortages and food was in extremely short supply. The already small meat ration had been reduced; newsprint and petrol were very scarce. Although bread and potatoes were not rationed during the whole of the war, rationing for both of these staple foods was apparently imposed in 1946, but I remember none of this. I think I always lived for each day, and didn't consider whether it was bad or good; it was just life. But I must have had difficulties in that severe winter in getting to and from work and problems in finding enough food for our evening meal.

I took the crush on the Metropolitan line train to Baker Street every morning as part of life – no better, but no worse than expected! Passengers lined the station platform, pushing up one behind another and crowding the platform as the delay went on and on in the bitter weather until eventually a train arrived. It was my first experience of winter rush hour travelling, but, again, I didn't consider that it was worse than usual because of the extreme weather. It was winter, and it was cold and the trains didn't arrive – what's new?

Passengers waited so long for a train on those icy, often foggy, mornings. Sometimes it was so crowded when it did arrive that only a few of those waiting near the platform edge at Northwick Park managed to squeeze in and the rest of us would-be passengers stood, stamping our feet, waiting for another train to arrive; but nobody grew angry or made a scene. There were no empty seats on the train when I did manage to get on, and it was standing room only all the way, as more people forced their way on at each stop. We were frequently packed like sardines in a tin. There were often very lengthy delays between stations due to fog or ice, with passengers squashed close together, unable to move, but waiting, patiently and silently, for the train to start once more. The silence of the passengers during these delays was made more acute by the silence of the stationary train. It was sometimes quite eerie. I envied the people who were seated and able to read their newspapers, many of them smoking, and the fug added to the discomfort. There were not many non-smoking carriages as I stood waiting on the platform, trying to judge where one would be likely to stop. Not many women smoked in public, but a cigarette almost seemed to be an integral part of most men. This was my first winter travelling into London, and I didn't see any of this as unusual; I just accepted it as the norm – but have remembered it very clearly, and now realise how awful it was.

We suffered long weeks of snow that winter, and it was difficult to walk to the bus stop, with the icy pavements and piles of dirty snow swept up in the gutters along either side of the roads. Women usually wore short fur boots, not for fashion, but for comfort and a greater feeling of security on icy pavements. My boss often arrived very late in the mornings during those icy-cold weeks. She lived in Rickmansworth in Hertfordshire, now recognised by meteorologists to be one of the very coldest spots to the northwest of London, and she had a much longer journey in to work, and consequently must have had longer delays with trains. Some of the staff felt that she was a late riser, or had an early date elsewhere, but I think she really did have more delays on her journey and had a valid reason to arrive late for work. We didn't hear detailed weather forecasts and knew nothing about cold spots caused by low areas in surrounding hills then.

There were no Saturday morning clinics and a five-day week was a bonus, making it easier to get the house cleaning done, the washing and the weekend shopping for our food. There were no supermarkets, and all our food was purchased in small, local shops. Even with some queuing, it probably didn't take any longer than the present day drive to the favoured supermarket, the long trail up and down the endless aisles and the wait at the checkout. Our simple food essentials didn't take long to buy, but it was the queuing before you reached the counter that took the time. There was no choice in the shops – if you were lucky you were able to buy one toilet roll, and that would have a horrible, greaseproof-paper feel. You didn't make a choice between almost limitless brands of any products. A loaf of bread from the baker's was either a 'national' loaf (whitish) or a brown; tin or farmhouse, but the bread was *real bread*, not adulterated with chemicals or extra raising agents to make it keep fresh longer or rise higher. There was little choice, and so fewer decisions to make, but quality, even then, was sometimes better than now.

I sometimes managed to fit in a game of tennis with my friend Janet on a Saturday morning during the summer. We had to book a court and cycle to some poorly maintained Harrow Council tennis courts that had probably not had any attention since before the war. They were very gritty, with areas of broken, crumbling tarmac – somewhat like many of our present-day roads! I spent some of my precious clothing coupons on my first tennis dress around this period, feeling that I had been very extravagant and wasteful. At first I was almost ashamed to wear such non-utilitarian clothing, but I can still remember the dress fondly, how it swished as I moved on the court, and I wore it for some years. I'm sure it improved my play! I just felt good in it.

I still used my mother's old 1920s racquet. (My first tennis racquet of my own was a gift on my twenty-first birthday.) I wonder whether my mother was told that her daughter was playing tennis with her old racquet. There was little my father could have told her in the way of news when he visited her. I suppose he would have had to weigh up in his mind whether a bit of chat about me playing tennis with her racquet might have upset my mother, or made her angry, or generally unsettled her. She may have been totally disinterested, but it's possible that it might have been of interest to her, and it could have pleased her.

Janet and I didn't shop for clothes together. We never went retail shopping, 'therapy' shopping or even window shopping; there was not much to buy in those austere days when clothing coupons were still needed, and yet things were beginning to change and new styles were beginning to appear. Coffee bars first appeared in the late 1940s and Janet and I really thought we were living it up when we met up one evening for a coffee at a new coffee bar that had opened in Marylebone High Street! I believe it was among the first to appear.

My father was a quiet man with no friends, no social life or outside activity, but I don't think people did have social lives or outside activities in those days. I can't imagine him or any of our neighbours going to the pub in the evening after work. It would have been about twenty minutes walk to the nearest one. Few people would have gone out in the evening after a day's work, so I don't think my father's life was any different from any of our neighbours, except that they had their partners – wives or husbands. All our immediate neighbours must have been past the call-up age during the war, or were in reserved occupations. I knew little about them. We never visited each other or went into their homes. My father's only opportunity for light conversation was with his staff or with customers at work. Apart from the friends/relatives we visited in Mill Hill, he lost contact with the friends my parents' used to have before the war because of the difficulty with transport or communication.

Holidays were coming round again at the end of my first year at work, and my father and I were going to have a 'proper' holiday - or so we hoped. For the first time in my life I had my own money - £3 a week - to spend on myself, and I had bought a wonderful, delphinium blue, New Look-style dress with a long, full skirt and a narrow waistband, with my own money. I gave my father some of my wages each week for my keep at home, but the rest was mine to spend or save. Clothes were still rationed, but more material was becoming available, and the skimped wartime clothes were slowly being replaced by new styles and fashions. At last life was beginning to brighten up a little in those harsh post-war years. I was delighted with my first grown up new dress.

My father had abandoned his CTC handbook, and we were going to stay at a guesthouse on the Isle of Wight. This almost felt like going abroad, although at that time we would never have dreamed of leaving the country for a holiday. That would indeed have been 'out of this world'. My father was looking forward to using his well-loved Kodak camera once again and had been able to buy one reel of film with eight exposures. His last pictures had been taken eight years previously, when he had used up the last few frames of film in his camera early in 1940, taking three snaps in our back garden; sadly my mother could not appear in any of these pictures.

A week before the start of our holiday we packed our clothes into an old leather suitcase that had been in the loft since our last family holiday in 1937. In went the essentials, and then my new blue dress, my bathing costume, my father's sport's jacket and grey flannel trousers for casual wear, his treasured pre-war camera, plus the film, and his bathing costume - yes a one-piece, gents' black bathing costume. It was a pre-war model, as men's bathing trunks were not yet familiar swimwear in the late 1940s. The case went off by rail and ferry as 'Luggage in Advance' to our holiday address. A few days later we took the train to Southampton at the start of our holiday. We had to queue a long time for the ferry to Ryde, and as we watched all the luggage being transferred by a crane from the port side to the boat, my father jokingly said, "What if someone 'lifted' a case before it was taken from the portside to the boat?"

"It would be very easy," I giggled in return. "Supposing one dropped off the crane and fell into the sea?" It was all very light-hearted.

We reached our guesthouse that evening, only to discover that our luggage had not arrived. In view of our observation while waiting at the dockside in Southampton, seeing the ease with which luggage could be stolen, and our light-hearted jokes on the subject of luggage, we were immediately alarmed. So, straight after breakfast the next morning, instead of going to the beach, we walked up the hill to Ventnor Station, hoping to find the old suitcase sitting on a platform, or dumped in the left-luggage office, or even deposited in the stationmaster's office, with someone waiting to hand it over to us with an apology. Nobody knew anything about our holiday luggage, or even seemed concerned. It would turn up, we were told.

We walked away rather dismally, and went on to the beach, where we sat, my father in his business suit, and I, longing to don my bathing costume (in the case) and go for a swim, and wear my new blue dress (in the case) for dinner that evening. We were actually staying in Bonchurch on the outskirts of Ventnor and at the bottom of a hill, so our trudge to the station on two further mornings was uphill each day. We gave up eventually and came to the conclusion that our luggage was lost, sunk or stolen.

We had only the clothes we stood up in to wear for a week's holiday. Had someone stolen our case? Had it fallen into the sea? We shall never know. We never saw it again. My father had lost his treasured camera; I had lost my beautiful dress; we had both lost our bathing costumes. Clothes rationing was still in place. How could we buy some suitable holiday clothing when we had no coupons? What were we to do? I felt very miserable to be at the seaside once again, and once more unable to swim or even sunbathe. My bathing costume was my most essential item, together with my new, blue dress – nothing to wear for dinner except the dress I had made myself and had travelled in, and worn each day while sitting on the beach, looking longingly at the sea. My father wore his navy-blue business suit (always navy-blue in those days; black was only for funerals) while sitting in his deck chair, also looking longingly at the sea, as he too loved swimming. I remember him feeling embarrassed, and so out of place, when all the men around us were wearing their bathing costumes or casual clothes - grey flannel trousers, sports jackets and ties in those days – how times have indeed changed.

Fortunately, a branch of the menswear firm my father worked for had a shop in Shanklin. We went in to Shanklin on the bus and found Meaker's Men's Outfitters, and my father explained our situation. He and the manager had a quiet little talk; a 'phone call was made to the head office in London, and after some discussion we were unofficially loaned sufficient clothing coupons from those the manager had received from customers. My father was able to buy himself some essential and informal clothes from this shop. We then had to find a shop that would accept our explanation for the loose clothing coupons, where I could make some essential purchases, a bathing costume and another dress.

My lost dress was the first one that I had bought with my own money since I had started work and I had been so looking forward to wearing it on holiday. It is now just a faded memory - or perhaps I should say, an *unfaded* memory, as I can remember the beautiful delphinium blue quite vividly. It was impossible to replace it in the Shanklin of 1948, which had small, rather dowdy, old-fashioned shops. I couldn't find anything that had the style of that New Look dress that I had bought in Marylebone High Street, and the bathing costume I bought was very frumpish. But it was good enough to bathe in, and swim I did!

We had spent several days of our holiday trudging back and forth to the station, getting the authority from Meaker's head office to use substitute coupons, and then buying the essential items of clothing. It was a memorable holiday, but for all the wrong reasons; the luggage was never found. We claimed the coupons, and when they were issued my father returned them to Meaker's shop in Shanklin. We were insured and were recompensed in money, but nothing could replace my father's camera, and the snaps he could have taken for the first time in eight years. He never bought another camera. Nothing could restore the days when we sat on the beach in inappropriate clothing, or the swimming in the sea that we had missed – or my beautiful blue dress.

I was soon back at work, and life went on as usual through the autumn, until November, when to my surprise one of the doctors called me into his little consulting room, and after dictating some letters to me concerning patients, he asked if I would consider becoming his private secretary. I was not sure that my shorthand speed was up to the daily task of taking down his very rapid dictation, and I had not considered changing my job, but I found the opportunity of becoming secretary to a Harley Street consultant difficult to resist. My father thought it would be a lonely job without the social contacts I enjoyed at the clinic and he was reluctant for me to accept the position, (he was possibly right) but I think I felt flattered to have been asked to work for a Harley Street consultant and was keen to accept this post. He was one of the most popular doctors at the clinic, and I decided to take on this more important position, and accepted the offer. I left the clinic, with very happy memories, plus a little trepidation about my new post. I realise that I must have left the Clinic staff feeling that the help and friendship they had offered had been unappreciated and suddenly thrown back at them, but they had initiated me very kindly into the world of work and encouraged me to advance my career. My old school friend, Beryl, wanted a change from her first job in the City, and I was able to recommend her to the Clinic secretary. She was interviewed by Major Forbes, and was appointed to replace me on the staff, so I didn't actually leave them in the lurch. I left with happy memories.

Chapter Five

NEW RESPONSIBILITIES

With the start of my new job in November 1948 I discovered that my comparatively easy journey to work was drastically changed. Although my new boss had his main practice in Harley Street, his secretary had always worked from an office at his private address. However, a large fire had occurred some months previously at his home, and he and his family were living temporarily in a large, furnished house near Hampstead Heath. Not only had I moved from the convivial atmosphere of the Clinic, but I had also given up the straightforward journey on the Metropolitan line to Baker Street and then an easy walk to work. I now had a complicated journey to Hampstead, with a bus ride and then two trains before reaching Hampstead Station. The deep lifts from the underground to street-level only held a comparatively few passengers. I waited impatiently each morning for the lift to descend, then surged forward with the crowd when the lift gates opened, hoping to be one of the passengers who crammed into the first 'cage' before being raised in mysterious silence to ground level. The lifts are still in use at Hampstead Station, the deepest station on the London Underground system.

A draught of cold, fresh, November air greeted me as I reached the exit, becoming ever stronger and chillier as I climbed up the hill from the station towards the White Stone Pond at the top of Hampstead Heath. I used up a lot of calories in my rush to be on time, but it was essential that I arrived promptly each morning. My new boss was waiting after his breakfast to deal with the morning's work before leaving for Harley Street to start his private patient list of appointments. He was always in a hurry, always busy, but always good-humoured.

My temporary office was in the bay of the spacious sitting room of a large house, and as I sat at my desk I looked out on to the garden. A grand piano took up most of the space of an even larger bay – surely built specifically to house a grand piano. During the morning an elderly aunt was assisted into the spacious sitting room by my boss's wife and settled into a high-backed chair by the fireside. Coffee was soon brought in for her by May, the maid, and another cup of coffee was passed over to me as I sat at my desk. During the rest of the morning this dear old lady sat reading the daily paper, while engaging me in light conversation from time to time as I tried to get on with my work.

I explored Hampstead High Street in my lunch hour, venturing into various cafés for my mid-day meal, eating very cheaply in what are now very smart restaurants. In 1948 Hampstead was not the up-market area it is today – certainly not in the daytime. The streets were almost empty at midday; the little town seemed rather bleak during the winter months with few shops and only one or two little restaurants open for lunch, serving a basic mid-day meal for two or three shillings (10 or 15p.). My starting wage was £5 a week, so I was not what you might call flush with money, but it was an increase from the £3.5s. I was earning when I left the Clinic. Massed produced sandwiches, fresh and packed ready to eat had not yet appeared, and was an industry waiting to happen. On sunny wintry days I sometimes found time after my meal to have a short walk around the top of Hampstead Heath, but it was very exposed to the wind and the weather in the winter.

On my first day I discovered that my boss employed a resident maid and also had a cook. He had a full-time chauffeur, and was the owner of several cars. I soon learned that he had a dairy farm in Berkshire and at the end of my first month I was asked to deal with the farm accounts. I had never written a cheque in my life nor even seen a chequebook. In those days most people were paid a weekly wage in cash; we didn't have credit and only rich people had bank accounts and chequebooks. My boss had a herd of pedigree tuberculin-tested, Ayrshire cows at his farm, and I had to renew each individually-named cow's annual insurance when it became due. I had never even heard of pedigree Ayrshire cows, or ever seen an insurance policy of any description. What had I taken on?

' Doctor', as I always addressed my boss, was usually driven to Harley Street by his chauffeur, who was known to everyone as 'Bean', never Mr. Bean or even George, for I knew from his insurance card that his first name was George. Not only was Bean always smart in his uniform and wore his peaked cap for the drive, but my boss also wore his Homburg hat, (colloquially known as an 'Anthony Eden' because the politician and former Prime Minister, Anthony Eden, always wore one and thus it became famous) as he hurried out to the car carrying his large medical bag. Gentlemen never went out bareheaded in those days, not even if they were sitting in a car, but this didn't seem odd to me at the time. Workmen wore caps, middle class men wore a trilby hat, city bankers wore bowler hats, and professional men wore Anthony Eden hats.

Bean was soon back at the house and busy during the morning, driving the doctor's wife to the shops, or washing, polishing, or servicing one of the three cars. Car engines were much less complicated than today and were often serviced at home by their owners – or, for the wealthy, by their chauffeurs. At 12.30p.m. he drove back to town to bring his boss home for lunch. Doctor sometimes drove himself to work if Bean was required elsewhere, or was busy servicing one of the other cars. Parking was not a problem in Harley Street in those days; there was no congestion charge to pay, and not even a parking meter at the kerbside.

After a quick lunch at home my new boss sat at the writing bureau that served as his desk in this furnished rented house, and dictated to me any letters and reports, before reading out the prescriptions resulting from the morning's clinic. I had a fairly small desk for my typewriter with not much room for my shorthand notepad, but we both managed. The house wasn't designed for an office and also could not be used for consultations. After Doctor had returned to Harley Street I dictated the long list of prescriptions together with the names and addresses of each patient over the phone to Nelson's Homoeopathic Pharmacy in Mayfair, and to Downing's the allopathic chemist (as it was called then) in Highgate. The two pharmacies made up the prescriptions, packed them safely and posted them to the patients, who would expect to receive their medications the following day. Mr.Downing's medicines were sometimes liquid and I often wondered how he managed to pack these bottles of medicine for safe delivery. I don't ever remember having to deal with an angry patient complaining about undelivered or damaged medicine. A number of these patients' names and addresses are still imprinted on my memory after repeating them so frequently so long ago. When driving through many towns over many years, I often used to say to my husband, "Ah...I remember Mrs. So-and-so lived here" and would reel off a patient's name and address – and yet nowadays I can't even remember the name of the book I have recently finished reading!

After lunch the elderly aunt departed to her room for her afternoon rest, and I was able to get on with my work without interruption. At about 4 o'clock she was again assisted into the room and made comfortable in her armchair, and soon afterwards the maid brought in afternoon tea. My boss's wife always invited me to join them for my tea break. I came to the fireside, where I was made welcome and sat chatting, sharing in their (very nice) afternoon tea, before returning to my desk. I am sure I stayed chatting for longer than I should have done. I wasn't part of the family but I was made so welcome, and I think the elderly aunt enjoyed having someone to talk to. As a consequence I still had to fit in the rest my work, and often left late. Looking back on it, it was all rather surreal, but I enjoyed the cosiness, the nice food, the atmosphere of this very pleasant home and the kindness of my boss and his wife.

Doctor used to supervise the execution of the quarterly accounts and this was done after dinner over a period of two evenings. I was invited to join the family for dinner on these two evenings, and when I had finished my day's work I sat around the fire, making polite conversation until Doctor arrived home. There was quite a long period of time with nothing to do and I felt a bit awkward, and was relieved when May, the maid, banged the gong in the hall to announce that dinner was ready. At the end of each course Doctor pressed his foot on to a concealed bell on the floor somewhere beneath the table, then May appeared to clear the plates and bring in our dessert. I don't remember what we ate, but I think it was very homely, not anything very special, but in those days everyone's meals were pretty ordinary. But I remember the big gong and was fascinated by the secret bell.

The table was cleared as soon as the meal was over and Doctor and I got down to work. I carried my heavy old pre-war typewriter to the table and placed it in front of me before I sat down. Doctor was at my side with one of the huge, heavy, leather-bound ledgers in front of him. He read each patient's name, followed by some detail of what services had been rendered. While I was typing these details out, he totted up the bill, called out the total, which I typed in. It was quite a performance, and it was about 11 o'clock when I arrived home on the first night, and my father was wondering whatever had happened to me. It had been a long day. The next morning I typed the envelopes, enclosed the accounts, stamped the huge pile and posted the lot. It was quite a weight off my mind. The second half of the quarterly accounts were dictated and typed the next evening, with another late night's work.

Doctor handed me a chilly parcel as I was leaving for home on my last day's work before Christmas at this strange 'office'. He told me it had come straight out of the refrigerator, and to open it as soon as I arrived home, then keep it cool. Together with this parcel was a £5 note, a 'Christmas box', as a gift of money from one's boss at this festival used to be called. On arriving home I opened the package and found a bird, trussed ready for the oven. My father and I were not sure what type of bird it was. It wasn't a chicken, we didn't think it was a duck, and came to the conclusion that it was a goose, a bird that had obviously been reared on the farm. We had not seen much poultry during or since the war, and were not quite sure what to do with something that wasn't a chicken. I had no fridge to put it in, so it went into the larder until Christmas morning. I was given a similar gift of money and a bird each Christmas until I left work – and indeed I was given a bird from his farm each Christmas until my ex-boss died in 1960.

Sadly, I had just about got used to my new surroundings when my boss's wife died quite suddenly at this temporary home before that winter was over. I was confronted for the first time with a death of someone I knew. I was very stunned by this tragic event, but I don't think I understood the awful, sudden bereavement that my boss, whom I liked and respected, had suffered. I was only a little younger than his daughter, but I was unable to enter into how she must have felt at suddenly losing her mother. (I can't remember how I felt at losing my own mother in an entirely different way when I was a little girl. I suppose I didn't know I was losing her, but it must have been something like a bereavement, one, I think, that I didn't understand at the time.) I remember all the floral tributes that covered the hall floor of the rented house in Hampstead on the day of the funeral; I had never seen so many flowers in my life.

I am amazed as I look back at how unmoved I think I must have appeared. I don't remember expressing sympathy; I didn't know what to say. I just got on with my job. I don't think I knew how to handle such an event, or understand my place in it, but I think that my mother's absence in my life may have led me to be unable to understand the family's loss. (Maybe emotion I should have expressed when I was a child had been bottled up; my mother's frequent, sudden hospital admissions in my very early life surely should have upset me, but they didn't as far as I can remember. In those days the phrase 'least said, soonest mended' prevailed; people were not encouraged – or perhaps not even allowed – to express their feelings, and were far more stoical than today. Children were not told the reason why a parent disappeared from their lives, whether this was through illness, death, or a marriage break-up.) I think I was shocked, almost disbelieving, at this sudden death of this caring doctor's wife. Maybe my calmness helped when my boss got back to the practice work a day or two later.

I can remember the day of the funeral very clearly even now, and have the same sensation of disbelief, sorrow, of not knowing my place in this family bereavement, not knowing what to say. It was the first time I had been, even in the slightest way, involved with death. But I think that even today people do not know how to handle someone else's bereavement. They don't know what to say, when often all that is needed is, 'I'm so sorry,' and to offer help or company if that is needed.

When day-to-day life was resumed the maid now escorted the aunt to her chair. She still brought us both a cup of coffee in the morning and a nice tea in the afternoon, when I left my desk and came to the fireside to make conversation with this elderly lady over our afternoon tea before getting back to my work. This was easier said than done as the aunt wanted someone to talk to and didn't appreciate that I had a lot of work to get through. It all sounds quite bizarre as I recall it now.

Doctor and I had formed a good working relationship, and I dealt with all the secretarial aspects of his professional, domestic, and personal life. Letters and reports were typed on the smallest pieces of notepaper possible. I used 'octavo' size (a quarter of an A4, and the same size as my wartime Junior School reports) to type out the quarterly accounts to patients, and also for any very brief letters; the other headed notepaper was only half the present A4 size, and I would type on both sides. Paper was still in very short supply. (Perhaps these wartime restrictions should reappear; we could all help to save the forests, and thus the planet, by using much less paper. Printers should be adapted to easily take smaller sheets of paper; at the moment everything appears on A4 sheets, usually printed on one side only.)

Taking shorthand dictation for medical reports and private letters, ordering patients' medicines from our two chemists were among my daily duties. Attending a Saturday afternoon Medical Missionary Conference, with my notepad and pencil ready to take notes and summarise the speakers' addresses and reports from mission hospitals overseas for the magazine my boss edited, thankfully occurred only once. The latter was a most stressful undertaking, as I feared my shorthand speed was not fast enough to take down lengthy addresses accurately. My boss's dictation speed was very fast, and at first my shorthand speed didn't always pick up entire sentences, but I had a good memory, and hastily scribbled down in longhand after dictation the bits I had been unable to write in shorthand outline. I soon found that my speed increased, and I was able to cope with his rapid dictation, but long speeches by an array of different doctors at a conference were a different matter.

A few months after his wife's death, Doctor had to make a further household move. The lease on the house in Hampstead was at an end, but the work on the restoration of his family home had scarcely begun. I think there had been some delay because of a bit of a conflict with the insurance company. The house was still uninhabitable, and before the end of the summer, only a few months after his bereavement, my boss had to find other accommodation for himself, his family and his staff. It was decided that I should move temporarily to Harley Street, so I found myself once more in my old location, not far away from the Charterhouse Clinic. My office was once again in a basement.

The nine months in my new job had passed by so quickly; so much had happened, including two different office locations and a death, but soon my annual holiday was due in the summer. I now had a steady boy friend. My father obviously approved of him, as he had invited him to join us on a two-centre holiday, with a week in South Devon and a second week in Cornwall. It would have been unthinkable for me to share a room with Maurice, so I had the single room, and my father and my boy friend shared the twin-bedded room in the guesthouse where we stayed in Torquay. It may seem strange to write this with today's vast changes in acceptable behaviour, but at the time it would have been thought most improper for us to share a room before we were married – or even engaged - and it didn't enter my head that the arrangement might appear at all odd.

I have very few memories of the week in Torquay apart from bathing or walking along the promenade. We sat on the beach in deck chairs, and my father and I enjoyed a swim. Maurice could not swim; swimming instruction was not in the school curriculum in our day, and he had not had the benefit of seaside holidays with his parents when he was growing up, nor the advantage I had of day trips to the sea in my father's car when I was little and my mother was well and at home. His father was an electrician and, along with most of the workforce at that time, he did not have a paid summer holiday.

My father and I tried to teach Maurice to float, but he seemed unable to breathe while he was in the water, his cheeks puffed out as he held his breath out of sheer panic, and he kept sinking. It was such a pity, because he learned to swim about thirty years later, taking swimming lessons for adults with professional teaching at our local indoor swimming pool. From then on until well after his retirement he remained a competent, but never entirely confident, swimmer. Who said he couldn't swim? It was quite an achievement for an 'over 50' in the 1970s.

After our week in Devon we took the train from Torquay to Looe on the south coast of Cornwall. Maurice and I didn't think that 'two's company' and three might be a crowd! We were glad that my father had suggested that we should all have a holiday. After all, we wouldn't have gone away at all as a 'twosome'. My dad arranged it; it would not have occurred to us to go on holiday together, and I don't think my father would have relished a holiday on his own. It didn't cross my mind that he might think of the times when he would have been on holiday with my mother as well as me. He must have thought of my mother at times, shut away in a psychiatric hospital while we were enjoying ourselves, but he never spoke about her, and I didn't think of her at all. I had forgotten all about her; forgotten her voice, forgotten what she looked like.

After my father had retired many years later, I sometimes urged him to have a holiday, he commented, 'How can I go off enjoying myself with your mother 'in there''? It was one of the few occasions when he mentioned my mother or showed a little of his concealed anguish at her absence. Mental illness was thought such a disgrace, almost a crime, or possibly the relative's fault. He hid all his feelings; he had no one to share them with. I think he still felt unable to talk to me about my mother because she had been a taboo subject throughout my childhood. He was very reluctant to go on holiday on his own, but eventually he did. He commented once on his return from the Lake District that there were beautiful views, but 'What is a view if you can't share it?' (I can deeply appreciate his comments since the loss of my husband three years ago.)

The strongest and happiest memory of our holiday in Looe is of an afternoon spent rowing up the River Looe. It was very peaceful, and my father began singing the Barcarolle from Tales of Hoffman as he and Maurice rowed while I sat in the stern. We joined in with the singing and I always associate that melody with our holiday in 1949. The gentle splash of the oars matched the rhythm of the music as we sang together, with Maurice, with his natural sense of harmony, putting in the bass part. The memory of my father's habit of singing while doing a job when I was a child is now reinforced by this holiday memory.

I remember very little else about either holiday centre; it was not that long after the war and I guess that the tourist industry and local coach tours had not yet got underway, although I vaguely remember that we went to Mousehole one day, but my strongest recollection is that it poured with rain. I have no memory of our long train journey home from Cornwall, and can't imagine how my father managed to arrange such a complicated holiday. Trains were the usual way of getting around then; there were many different lines, many reaching directly to seaside destinations, that were subsequently closed by Dr. Beeching, and nowadays a two-centre holiday at two seaside resorts in two different counties using public transport would, I think, be well nigh impossible.

Chapter Six

BACK IN THE BASEMENT

When I left my first job I didn't appreciate that there was little glamour involved in putting myself into a lonely work situation in another basement office in nearby Harley Street. Apart from my boss and the secretaries to the two other consultants in the house I met very few people during the course of my day. The secretary to the consultant who owned the house sat at her typewriter in a small space on the ground floor, beneath the bend in the wide staircase leading up to her boss's consulting room, who was quite a well-known cancer surgeon at the time. Mary's office was not much more than a large cupboard space under the stairs – just a cubbyhole - with a small desk, a typewriter and a few shelves built in beneath the staircase. She saw everyone who passed through the hall, was on view to anyone, and had no privacy at all. The other secretary worked for a pathologist and shared her galley-like office in the basement with jars of specimens of human organs ranged along the walls. I think the room must originally have been the butler's pantry when the house was a wealthy Regency family residence but I trust that human specimens weren't to be found on his shelves!

My office was also downstairs and was huge when compared with Mary's or Winnie's. I occupied only about a quarter of a very large room that encompassed the width of the house, and I sat at a huge old desk in the corner nearest to the limited natural light. The typist's chair was merely an old dining chair to which I added two thick London area telephone directories to bring it up to a suitable height that allowed my hands to be level with the keyboard of the heavy, old-fashioned, pre-war typewriter. Electric light was needed all day. When the telephone rang, and the caller wished to speak to my boss, I had to rest the receiver on my desk, rush up the flight of what were once the servants' back stairs to a small telephone room in the hall. Several pre-war telephones were ranged along a shelf inside, one for each consultant, and each had a very old-fashioned tall column with a speaker at the top. I would lift the receiver off the pillar; wind a little wheel, which rang in the consulting room. My boss picked up his telephone while I bent down in order to speak to him through a mouthpiece attached to the top of the pillar. I told him who the caller was and listened at the earpiece receiver to learn whether he wished to interrupt his consultation to speak to the caller. After the call was passed on, I quickly replaced the earpiece before rushing back along the corridor, and down the narrow staircase again to replace the receiver on the 'phone on my desk enabling doctor's conversation to be private. What a performance, just for one telephone call. It was all pretty primitive! My boss didn't own the house, but rented the consulting room, a cloakroom and my office, and had his share of the telephone room. There was little glamour in being a Harley Street Consultant's secretary in those days.

Modernisation of property and equipment did not begin until some years later when the country began to recover from the immediate effects of the war. The telephone in my father's shop was exactly the same style as the one in the telephone room in Harley Street, where one spoke into a mouthpiece at the top of a Bakelite stem and listened with a separate earpiece. At least there were far better toilet facilities in Harley Street than in Meakers shop at Ealing Broadway, but I had to rush up the back staircase to reach the cloakroom that was part of my boss's consultancy suite whenever I needed the loo (another word, a colloquial term that didn't exist in those days). Central heating, health and safety laws, up-to-date equipment and properly designed office furniture were still dreams – not even that - of the future.

I shared my office with some physiotherapy equipment, plus a physiotherapist's treatment bed. I never took the opportunity to lie on this bed on occasions when I felt unwell at work, but I can remember curling up on the floor in front of the electric fire with certain occasional pains. Perhaps it was warmth I needed more than a cold, hard, physio table. Sometimes a physiotherapist came in to treat a patient. I felt invisible on most of these occasions; the therapist and her (it was usually a lady) patient chatted amiably away on one side of the room, while I sat in my small corner tapping away at my noisy typewriter or did some quiet filing – with one ear on the adjacent conversation, which was sometimes very interesting.

There was plenty of available space in this huge, cold, sunless room, and I placed the two-kilowatt electric fire very close to my desk in the winter. Nevertheless I preferred this environment in central London to the strange, but very pleasant, environment in Hampstead. I wasn't aware of the solitary nature of my job; I was too busy. I must have been a much 'hardier' specimen than I am now, for where would I be nowadays without the warmth from my centrally heated home?

At mid-day on sunny summer days I carried my typist's chair outside my rather gloomy basement office to a spot of sunshine in the area outside my office. There was no garden in this large house in the heart of the West End; the French doors in my office opened out on to a square, concreted space surrounded by the solid walls of other basement rooms in neighbouring Regency houses. Instead of going to a café for my midday meal in the summer, I often preferred to sit in the corner that caught the midday sun, eating a sandwich while reading a library book (or sometimes preparing my Sunday school lesson) in my lunch hour. The house is now transformed into offices. I saw inside my late boss's old consulting room some while ago, and the lovely, high-ceilinged, well-proportioned room was crammed full of desks and computers.

Most of my lunch hours were spent wandering around the old streets tucked away behind Oxford Street and around Marylebone High Street where I found little cafés that produced a good, cheap, midday meal. They offered much better fare than Hampstead High Street. The hour passed quickly if I had walked along to Oxford Street and had a quick look around Selfridges and D H Evans. On another day I might browse in a bookshop or stroll up Marylebone High Street, which was not nearly so up-market and interesting as it is today, although it did have a small department store. It was a very old-fashioned store with long overhead tramlines that whizzed the customer's bill and payment from the assistant to a cashier sitting at a desk hidden away somewhere. The cashier dealt with the money, put the change back into the appropriate container, hung it on the line above her head, pulled a handle, and it was whizzed back again. The store was alive with the sound of these little contraptions being pulled up, whizzed overhead then shot back to the appropriate counter and customer. No plastic cards were used then; it was cash or no deal, unless you were a wealthy customer in one of the West End stores, when a chequebook might appear.

I made my mid-morning coffee and afternoon tea by turning the electric fire on to its' back and boiling a kettle on the wire guard covering the electric element. I don't think tea bags had appeared, but instant coffee, although not yet freeze-dried, had. Coffee and tea breaks were usually taken whilst still at my typewriter, unless I had a visitor. Sometimes Winnie, secretary to the pathologist, left her specimen-lined office a few yards along the corridor from me and joined me for a cup of tea, leaving her door ajar so that she could hear her office phone. My door was left wide-open too, and we also kept our ears open, half-expecting to hear the heavy footsteps of her boss coming down the back staircase. Then she would rush back to her office, hopefully reaching it before he had reached the bottom of the stairs. He usually had the day's post-mortem or autopsy reports to dictate and often required them typed out that afternoon. He didn't have a consulting room in the house, but was consultant pathologist to several London hospitals, - sadly, his 'patients' did not require a consultation - so her workload appeared at the end of the day. Electric light was required all day in both our offices.

My boss usually brought sandwiches for his lunch; he probably didn't enjoy going home to lunch alone after the death of his wife. When his morning clinic was over he would go to the telephone room in the hall and twirl the little wheel in order to ask me to come upstairs. As I sat at the other side of his large desk he would produce a tidy little packet from his traditional, large, brown leather medical bag before settling down to deal with the business resulting from his morning's work. Doctor unwrapped his greaseproof-paper wrapped lunch, and then opened up the little packages inside. He seemed quite boyish as he said, with a twinkle in his eye, 'Now what have we in here today?' before beginning to munch his way through his sandwiches, sometimes finding some little extra that the cook had included – a small cold sausage, or a twist of greaseproof paper containing a couple of chocolates. I don't remember any kind of salad accompanying his meal. Food was still in very short supply, even for comparatively wealthy consultants, and little treats were extremely modest by today's standards.

He dictated his letters or reports as he ate, and dictated the prescriptions between bites. He sometimes handed me one of his chocolates at the end of the session, which I placed on top my shorthand pad, together with a pile of patients' record cards as I walked along the corridor and down the stairs to my office.

Small bottles, carefully wrapped in brown paper bags, were sometimes discreetly passed to me after my boss had finished his dictation. These contained urine samples, and it was another of my little tasks to test them over a Bunsen burner situated in a large cupboard/tiny room in another corner of my office, where I also procured and re-filed the patients' record cards each morning and evening.

Each Thursday I went to the bank, travelling on the underground to Highgate, buying a Woman's Own magazine to read on the train. After leaving the station I crossed Archway Road and went into the Westminster Bank, to pay in all the cheques and the small mount of cash (from a few patients who paid immediately for their consultation in real money) that had come in during the week, and withdrew money for the household expenses in the following week, plus my wages and those of the maid, the cook and the chauffeur. Those were the days of pound notes, fivers if you were lucky, not cheques, monthly salaries, direct debits, debit or credit cards. The bank had a quiet, almost reverent atmosphere, with mahogany counters and pillars, and I was always attended to by the same cashier who stood behind the solid, mahogany, polished counter, and greeted me with, 'Good morning, Miss Brook'. I replied, 'Good morning, Mr. Webb'. We were not on first-name terms, and it was all very quiet, respectful and dignified in a bank in those days. Banks have changed completely and have no atmosphere at all nowadays, but as I write there is talk of the need for the bank manager to return to the local bank.

After I had finished the banking I walked up to Highgate village, found a little café where I had my lunch, then took the bus along to Kenwood. A short walk before I met up with my boss in his partly refurbished house. The house was as yet uninhabitable, but the consulting room was now usable, as was what would have been my office; both rooms were in the front of the house. I still didn't appreciate the traumas Doctor had suffered – the fire in his beautiful home, then the death of his wife. (I feel that the fire must have been a terrific shock that may have contributed to her death less than a year after its occurrence.) To return to what was almost the shell of his home each Thursday must have been extremely distressing for him, and yet he was always even-tempered, with a kindly twinkle in his eye. I realise now that he was rather like my father, who remained buoyant through all his distresses.

I passed over all the cash I had withdrawn, and he handed back my £5 wages across the desk. I had a rise from time to time when my wage was increased by 10 shillings (50p) on each occasion. Like most people in those days I was paid weekly, in cash, in £1 notes and 10-shilling notes. Many years passed before I saw a £5 note and many more before I owned a chequebook. It is difficult to realise how comparatively recent is the use of debit or credit cards and all the automation of salaries and household bills, with the consequent reduced need for real money or a chequebook.

After dealing with the business resulting from the morning's work, Doctor dropped me off at an underground station before setting out on his afternoon visits. Back to Harley Street I went, with a lot of work to be accomplished and half the afternoon gone, but the Thursday duties away from my solitary office were almost like an excursion for me. As I write I realise that my eldest son is now about the same age as my boss was when I was his secretary, but in those days I thought of him as 'getting on', almost an elderly man. (I must now apologise to my son!)

Doctor was always away from the practice for the month of August, so I always took my fortnight's holiday (all that one expected at that time) during that month. This year, 1950, my father, Maurice and I had another long train journey before we reached our holiday destination of Barmouth in West Wales. Our guesthouse was facing the sea, and after breakfast on the morning following our arrival we stepped eagerly across the road to the promenade and the beach. We could smell the ozone on this windy, sunny morning. Maurice ran across the pavement to take a leap over the little wall along the promenade, but skidded on some loose sand and instead of jumping over the wall he fell on to it, and badly injured his shin and calf. He was in a lot of pain as we helped him to limp back to our guesthouse, and he rested it for the rest of that day, and then tried to walk about a bit and enjoy his holiday. After a day or two the injury was still very painful and the leg had swollen, so he had to see a doctor who recommended that he exercised it. We went out and bought a walking stick, after which we took a few fairly gentle walks, attempting one or two of the lower hills in the area, hoping that the exercise that had been suggested would help. But it was clear that he was in a lot of pain. On his return home his own doctor told him that he should have rested his leg, and the exercise had made the injury more serious. He was laid up, resting in bed and away from work for quite a while.

We were unable to do any real walking in that beautiful area, so one afternoon we thought we would hire a rowing boat. My father was a little concerned as he stepped into the rather shallow boat; he felt it didn't appear at all suitable for a tidal river. My two men-folk rowed up-river for a while on a rather dull afternoon and all too soon it was time to return. In our enjoyment of the scenery and the rhythmic lapping of the oars in the water, we had not noticed the ease, or the speed, at which we were now moving back down the River Mawdacch, until we realised that the tide had changed and was now going out. There was a cross wind blowing, and together with the strong river current and the ebbing tide, we were being drawn out towards the wide estuary and the open sea. Water began to splash into the boat as the two men endeavoured to row across the river to our boat station.

There was no gentle singing that afternoon. Instead there was silence in the boat, with Maurice and my father rowing for dear life, while I pulled the rope at the back of my seat hard over to the port side (I don't know if *port/starboard* applies to a river) trying to reach the riverbank before we were swept out to sea. We were really very frightened. The strong wind that came with the change of tide, together with the force of the river flowing downstream, and what we were later told were very strong cross currents, were combining to push us towards the open sea. I was especially frightened for Maurice, as he couldn't swim and he had a leg injury. No one seemed to have noticed us on the riverbank, or was at all bothered when we eventually moored the boat. I don't know what would have happened to us in the strongly running tidal waters if our shallow-sided craft had taken in much water, but I think we all felt we had been in great danger, and nobody on either bank of the river was looking out for us. There was not a single notice board warning visitors of these risks; those shallow boats would not be allowed in tidal waters nowadays. We were pretty subdued as we walked back to our guesthouse for dinner.

It was soon back to the office. I was now entrusted with the preparation of the patients' accounts each quarter without the supervision of my boss, and was able to do them in the daytime. These were made up (no calculators, but lots of addition) and sent out with the appropriate traditional heading for each season - Easter, Midsummer, Michaelmas and Christmas; the cheques rolled in over the following weeks. Receipts were posted back with a 2d stamp stuck on the bottom of each account, with the words "Received with thanks, pp *my boss's full name*" handwritten by me across the stamp. The monthly personal, practice, domestic and farm accounts involved writing out many cheques from four different chequebooks. There were no standing orders or direct debits, and no credit cards eased the process of payment for goods or services. Chequebooks *always* had their stubs on the left-hand side in those days, and this made writing cheques very uncomfortable for someone who is left-handed. Oh dear, how awkward it was to write legibly with my hand held over the top of the stubs, but how difficult it is for me to write legibly at all nowadays!

My boss edited a small quarterly medical missionary magazine, and most of the articles that appeared then were extracts from airmail letters from doctors or nurses in charge of the Christian medical work overseas, in hospitals, treatment centres, as well as in schools and local churches. It was a very small production in those days, which my boss had helped to restart after the war. The magazine is still produced every quarter, and now contains succinct accounts and excellent pictures of much enlarged Christian medical work that continues, some of it now in centres with modernised schools and hospitals, some with their own hydro-electric water systems, built with the aid of experienced personnel, and partially funded by readers of Medical Missionary News.

Some of these centres were in existence when I was typing out items of news from the Belgian Congo, Rhodesia and other long-forgotten names of countries in Africa - same hospitals, different names of countries, but much better equipment, and more modern treatments for more needy people. Many ambitious schemes to bring aid to the local people have since been completed, some in very remote areas. However, there are now more physical and political dangers that hinder the work in some places and leave the population, together with the Christian medical, nursing and teaching staff who serve them, in great need and greater danger.

I remember being asked to order a new operating table from a surgical supplier to be sent out to a hospital in Africa, and having to understand and use new technical medical terms when ordering it. I think it was the first large bit of surgical equipment exported after the war that was paid for by the readers of this magazine.

It was a very busy, varied but (as my father had predicted) a somewhat lonely job, and my contact with patients, pharmacists, or other doctors, was almost entirely via the telephone. I came to know many of our patients through this medium, however, and sometimes had little chats with them, and also with the pharmacists when ordering medicines or homoeopathic remedies over the phone. I also picked up quite a lot of general medical terms and homoeopathic knowledge during the course of my work.

I got engaged in 1949, and my boss was very dismayed when I told him, because in those days girls left work when they married. I guess he could see the day coming when he would have to find another secretary. Almost immediately after my engagement he said to me on the day before I went to the bank, 'Oh, Sheila, I think you should withdraw an extra ten shillings for yourself now you are engaged. It will help towards your wedding day'. This brought my weekly earnings up to £7.10s (£7.50), which was quite a good wage in those days. Ten shillings a week extra would help in providing us with a home.

Where is the Key?

Early in the following year, he handed me a slip of paper one morning, and with the usual twinkle in his eye, casually said, 'Will you put this notice in The Telegraph and The Times for tomorrow? We'll beat you to it!' Although I knew that he had a lady friend I didn't quite understand what he meant until I read the notice, which announced his own engagement. So, boss and secretary were both engaged to be married, but doctor's engagement was quite brief and he did beat me to it - he didn't have to save up to provide a home for his new wife! Maurice and I were invited to his wedding service, and my boss and his wife both kindly came to our marriage some time later.

The extensive fire damage to Doctor's house had by then been rectified and he was able to move back into his own home before his wedding, but he had come to appreciate the convenience of having his secretary at his place of work and there was no mention of me changing my work place.

Maurice and I were invited to a party at his house soon after his marriage, when he was back in his repaired and restored home with his new wife. The house interior looked really lovely and I am sure he was relieved to be back in his own home. We were also invited to spend a day 'down on the farm' with doctor and his wife one Saturday before we were married. We took the Metropolitan line train to Finchley Road Station, and it was arranged that they would pick us up outside the station in their new car (the old pre-war Humber had served its' time.) the 2.5 litre Riley. My husband would have remembered clearly, being a classic car buff, but I remember the very stylish post-war, sporty green Riley. We waited outside the station for a few minutes before this lovely car appeared and we had a most enjoyable drive to their farm in Sussex, had lunch, met the farm manager and were taken round the farm. Strangely, and sadly too, I have no memory of the farmhouse, or the cows whose insurance I cared for, but can remember that it was an enjoyable day. It is really strange that some impressions of events can be so distinct but the details are completely lost. I can picture the drive in the car, but can't bring to mind any details of the farm, or how we spent the day – not even what we had for lunch!

The last holiday before I was married was *almost* abroad, when, in the summer of 1951, my fiancé and I once again went on holiday with my father, who had thought that Guernsey might be a good idea. He was really very good at thinking of these interesting resorts, finding accommodation and making all the travel arrangements. We made a threesome once again and shared the cost of our holiday as usual, but I rather think Maurice and I took all my dad's preparation for granted at the time. It was only a few years after the war and the Channel Islands seemed very adventurous; we almost felt we were going abroad even though we didn't fly. We got on very well together and I think my father appreciated having Maurice's male company in his lonely life. We had a wonderful fortnight in Guernsey, no accidents, no dangers, good weather and beautiful scenery. I can't remember the bathing, but do remember the fantastic walks we had along the cliff paths around Moulin Huet Bay. We weren't aware of the horrors of the German Occupation of the Channel Islands that had occurred only a few years before. I don't think the general public in England knew until many years later how extreme had been the Channel Islanders' suffering: the severe food shortages, the deprivation, and the fear of the ruthlessness of their captors. (Having visited Guernsey again recently and been round some of the museums showing various aspects of the war years on the Channel Islands I realised more of what it really means to have your country occupied by an enemy.)

I bought a linen tablecloth in St. Peter Port to embroider when I got home and put in my bottom drawer. Purchases had to be declared on return to England even though the Channel Islands are part of the United Kingdom. I was really upset to find that I was made to pay customs duty on just a plain linen tablecloth, when it was well known that people were bringing in jewellery and expensive items without declaring them. Embroidery was another of the pastimes that many girls enjoyed in those days. Embroidering chair backs, fire screens, numerous tablecloths, and dressing-table sets occupied many of my evenings before television came into our home.

On my return to Harley Street I began to think about my marriage the following year, and I guess that doctor was beginning to think about who would replace me. Although my husband-to-be was not earning a large wage, it was taken for granted that I would leave work when we married. It was a custom that was soon to change, but I was caught up in the tradition of pre-war years. Maurice thought that we should not get married until he was able to provide for me. Days that will never come again!

I realise that my late boss had a very sunny, sympathetic, kind disposition, and although he demanded a lot of work from his secretary he was always very pleasant to work with. In the present sex-saturated world, it is good to look back on those years to my good relationship with this friendly, even-tempered, polite doctor with his old-world gentlemanliness and kindliness. In those days when one didn't think of personal happiness, I think my secretarial career, although it was rather solitary, was a very happy period in my life.

Chapter Seven

FREE TIME

My life away from work during these and later years was centred on my church, as was the experience of many young people of my generation. Many churches had large Sunday Schools in the first half of the last century and from these developed viable or very successful youth groups after the war. Methodist Youth Groups were very strong, with a wide range of activities and amateur drama groups, and the uniformed organisations such as Boys' Brigade and Girls' Life Brigade were popular in many Baptist churches. I remember the local Boys' Brigade in Kenton marching along the road I lived in after their monthly Sunday morning Parade Service. They looked and sounded very professional with their smart uniforms, their skilled marching and impressive band. I must quite unknowingly, have seen my future husband marching along as I watched from the window of my house! His years in the Boys' Brigade before the war certainly made a good preparation for when he went into the RAF in 1945. As a quiet, only child, he had learned to mix amongst other young people, acquired a number of skills, and the discipline of the marching gave him a real boost when it came to 'square bashing' in the Air Force - as well as some valuable physical training for an otherwise non-sports person! Scouts and Girl Guide groups were mainly based in Anglican churches and, together with the Cubs and the Brownies, they all gave children and young people plenty of interest, activity and opportunity to stretch their abilities and make many friends.

There were many thriving youth organisations with a Christian ethos years ago that kept young people off the streets (or, probably, brought them out of their homes; there was not so much 'hanging around with nothing to do so let's get drunk and make mischief' when I was young). Therefore I have no hesitation in including my church-connected experiences as a personal account of generally unrecognised and an undervalued part of 'teenage' life during the middle-twentieth century. The Church seems to get more brickbats that bouquets nowadays, and for all its' limitations the following is, on the whole, a bouquet! It covers a long period from my early teens until several years after my marriage, so the first paragraphs relate to the period I have already written about, and the latter are memories of incidents that occurred after I was married. It is probably an aspect of social history that has not been well recorded.

Not long after the war ended a series of Youth Rallies was held in the Royal Albert Hall on Saturday evenings. A group of young people from my church joined the crowds gathering outside the doors in the early evening, hoping to get a good seat for the big Rally when the doors were opened. These huge gatherings of young people were led by Revd. Tom Rees, an

Anglican vicar who was subsequently responsible for organising the Billy Graham Crusades in England in the early 1950s. The Albert Hall was packed as Tom Rees led the singing, and we nearly raised the roof as we sang a lot of choruses, most of which would appear very old-fashioned today. We sang them with enthusiasm and great fervour; they had a good rhythm and a memorable tune, and there was no slowing down with Tom Rees conducting vigorously from the front. They also often came with challenging words, and to my old ears they were much more musical than many of the repetitive words sung in chant-like worship songs nowadays, with their irregular phrasing of both the words and music, and noisy backing groups. I have no doubt that the Albert Hall organ and organist did well enough in my generation to accompany our singing.

We had fun on the train coming home from Kensington after the rally and it was late in the evening when we reached Northwick Park station. We shunned the bus and walked home arm in arm, often in the middle of the road if my memory serves me right – not much traffic in those days - illuminated by the light from the streetlights, still singing the choruses we had learned that evening. After the dark, unlit streets and the restrictions of wartime, it was great to be out in the evening, exciting to have gone up to London, thrilling to have been in the Albert Hall with this great crowd of young people, thought-provoking and challenging to hear the address. To be able to walk home from the station in safety late at night, with streetlights to light our way was a great way to end the evening. We had walked in the dark for too many years.

The era of worship groups playing in services or meetings had not yet arrived. There would have been very few young musicians before instrumental teaching was given in schools, although it was quite common for parents to pay to have their children taught to play the piano was when I was young. A piano was seen in many more homes than nowadays. My maternal grandmother had to go into her 'yard' where a cold tap provided all the water required for her household, and yet there was a piano in her drawing room on which my mother must have learned to play. What a contrast with today when we have hot and cold running water, bathrooms, showers, toilets, en-suite bathrooms and wet rooms, but not many households own a piano. A piano was popular in pre-radio days when family entertainment was homemade. The old ballads and romantic songs my father used to sing were the pop songs of the early twentieth century, and someone would be needed to accompany them on the piano. The era of piano lessons continued with the next generation but has now declined and been replaced by guitars, percussion, wind and brass. Guitars were unknown when I was young and pianists or organists were essential.

It may be that the Young People's Fellowship was started in our church after these Rallies in London. I believe it began fairly soon after the war, not long before I joined, but it soon became a very important part of my life. My future social activities were mostly contained within this small youth group, which was not among the nationally known organisations. We usually had a speaker at our weekly YPF meetings when one of our members took the chair, welcomed the person who had come to talk to us, and led the meeting, but occasionally one of our small group was asked to arrange the whole evening. He or she would sit in the Chair – literally the head teacher's chair when the hall was part of the private prep school during the day. Another member was asked to prepare a short talk, another led the informal prayers, and perhaps a solo or a duet would be performed – and we had a pianist amongst us! Sometimes we took meetings at other church youth groups, where someone might sing a solo or a couple (often Maurice and I) sang a duet; somebody else gave a talk. We prepared well, and this small youth fellowship of not very well educated teenagers performed very passably. It all appears very formal and rather boring to me now, but doing all this must have developed our self-confidence, helped us undertake a bit of study and made us proficient in speaking semi-publicly and prepared to sing, pray and perform in front of people. I think everyone spoke much more clearly years ago. We were taught to speak clearly when we read aloud, or recited, at school. I find I am often unable to understand what is being said nowadays, as nearly everybody – especially weather-forecasters - speaks so rapidly; the spoken word on TV seems gabbled, the words in plays are not enunciated properly and to me the speech is so fast that it often just appears a jumble of sound (although I admit I am a little deaf).

We went carol singing in the days leading up to Christmas. We sang in harmony, often with a descant, and visited the elderly and many of the church members' homes. It was often freezing cold on those bitter evenings in the second half of the 1940s, and the painful chilblains that developed on my toes often occurred after carol-singing evenings. I am sure I strained my voice trying to reach the very high notes necessary in the descant one or two of us attempted. We had a lamp held up on a pole and everyone had an electric torch to help them see the words of the carols, as we sang our hearts out 'in the bleak mid-winter', hoping the households would hear us and enjoy.

Socials, outings, rambles in the country and 'squashes' were regular activities in the years after the war. Early on every Bank Holiday Monday – Easter, Whitsun and the first Monday in August (August Bank Holiday then) – we met at Northwick Park station, and caught a Metropolitan Line train out to one of the Buckinghamshire towns. After a country footpath walk of several miles we had a break to eat our sandwiches and perhaps played a game of rounders before completing the route our YPF leader had previously planned - simple food, no loud music, no mobile phones, but all good fun. We had enjoyed ourselves without recourse to binge drinking or even having cans of Cola. I recall several wet rambles; Bank Holiday weekend weather does not seem to have changed much over the years. Even then it often heralded a cold and wet weekend, but our planned ramble would always take place whatever the weather.

Just before I reached my sixteenth birthday I was baptised by immersion as a sign of my commitment to my Christian faith. The service took place in another local church that had a baptistry suitable for full immersion, as the little church I grew up in was a rented building without a baptistery. My father, my school friends and many members of the YPF (some of whom were also being baptised) joined the congregation for the baptismal service. We each had to give a testimony addressed to the congregation before we stepped down into the water in the baptistry, where the minister was already standing, wearing his ministerial robes. These must have become soaking wet as he supported each individual's body as we were briefly immersed in the water. This service is customary in all Baptist churches, and in many other non-conformist churches. I understand some Anglican churches now perform baptism of adults by immersion. It was a memorable and meaningful occasion for me, but was somewhat daunting when it actually occurred. The baptistery was not very long. Would I bang my head as I was immersed? Would the minister be able to take my weight as he dipped my body into the water? All went well, and I can still recall the hymn that was sung as I came up out of the water.

Now on a lighter note, I think it was the Boys' Bible Class leader who suggested that we might like to go ice-skating at the Wembley Ice Rink. I must have started work by this time, as I wouldn't have been able to afford the entrance to Wembley Ice Rink and the cost of hiring skates until I had some of my own money to spend. I remember Stanley, Peter and Val, but am sure that there were others too who donned their hired ice skates - which were very uncomfortable, made from very hard leather and not a very good fit - and slowly ventured on to the rink. Loud music was being played as I cautiously stepped on the ice, skating slowly around the edge of the rink, learning to keep my balance. Every time I ventured towards the middle I think I fell over. I wobbled around, and eventually managed to keep my feet – or rather my blades – on the ice for a while, but I was never confident. We went skating for several weeks but I don't think any of us became very proficient. We realised we were spending our money only to feel uncomfortable, and then come home with bruises, or sprained ankles and aching muscles. Skating gradually slipped out of our diaries. Good skating boots would undoubtedly have made quite a difference to our skill and success at this sport. I now have difficultly in keeping my balance if I try standing on one foot – but keep trying as this is supposed to be a very good exercise in helping to maintain balance in old age.

The Boys' Bible Class leader also provided another bit of social activity by inviting the young people (sorry – teenagers!) to his home on Friday evenings to play billiards. He lived with his elderly mother, and it was a very cold house. I am not sure that we were particularly welcomed by his mother, who used to bring in a tray holding glasses of cold water for our refreshment towards the end of the evening. It was the signal that it was time for us to go home. I know we were still suffering great shortages of food, but cold water, in a cold house, after playing a slow, quiet, thoughtful, cool game of billiards didn't make for a very sociable evening. I think we had more fun when we joined arms as we strode homewards, singing at the tops of our voices – not the latest pop songs but our Christian choruses. (What was pop music? I had never heard the word, and many of us, apart from Stanley, knew nothing about jazz or the music of this period.) Our linked arms and our singing soon warmed us up as we stomped down the wide pavement along Kenton Road and we ended up having a good evening. As I write, I realise that the leader of the Boys' Bible Class had quite an influence on my life – Christian Union, skating, billiards - although I didn't really know him well personally. Mr. Jahn was a very quiet man and very reserved.

We began to have occasional Saturday evening socials in the little wooden prep school hall that served as our church, when an evening of games was arranged, with some refreshments provided within the restrictions of post-war food shortages. Homemade cakes, sandwiches, orange squash or tea were consumed, and we all went home sober, but we had all enjoyed ourselves. I remember one social that was arranged by Val, which ended with us all dancing around in a circle, as we sang the Hokey Cokey while putting our 'left arms in' or our 'right legs out'. The Church Council heard of it, and I believe some deacons disapproved. As I look back I can see that our very narrow church life restricted our experience and social development to a considerable degree; we were subtly expected to live *in* the world, but not *of* it, but I was not aware of feeling deprived at the time. I am not at all sure that there was anything more interesting or stimulating organised in our suburban neighbourhood if we did want to step out of line, but my church was rather strict and I knew of no other social life. The young people whose parents were church members were, no doubt, warned more vocally or forcefully about the worldliness of dancing. Others who wanted to dance found somewhere to do so (or someone to dance with) and left the church.

Church attitudes have changed almost indescribably since those days, but dancing, popular music and the post-war London shows were considered very worldly then, and although disapproval was unspoken, these were somehow accepted as improper, and most of the young people in the church abided by this expectation. However I know I would have loved ballroom dancing, and still wish I had learned to dance. I wish I had been able to go to the new musicals that were produced then – Oklahoma and South Pacific for example. Sadly I didn't go to the theatre either; I missed out on many of the wonderful shows of that post-war period, and a lot of plays and films with unrepeatable performances by the actors of that period.

My father never suggested that I had a wider social life. Although he didn't attend the church services, perhaps he felt I was happy and secure in our little church. He had no social life of his own after my mother became a resident patient in psychiatric hospital. I know my parents used to go out in the early years of their marriage, and I am so sad that my father, who was so good at arranging holidays, didn't suggest that we went to the theatre or a show together. He was probably too tired after a day standing in the shop, and certainly too weary after an extra long day on Saturdays when the shop closed much later in the evening. The price of theatre tickets was probably another disincentive.

Soon after I reached the age of sixteen I had left the girls' Bible class to become a helper in the beginners' section of the Sunday school. I was asked to play a very small portable organ to accompany their little choruses, and can remember the tiny children singing, 'Here the pennies dropping, Listen as they fall…' as the bag was handed round for them to drop their collection pennies in. Later on I became a Sunday school teacher at a little Sunday school that was held in one of the church deacon's homes. He lived quite a long way away from the church and held a branch Sunday school in his own home. I played the piano (a great improvement on the little harmonium) to accompany the hymns and choruses, and then told the Bible story and taught the lesson to the youngest children in the drawing room. Mr. E. taught the older boys in the kitchen, and his wife had the older girls in the dining room. It was a nice, homely, little Sunday school

I remember one almost uncontrollable little boy, a very hyperactive youngster, who insisted on crawling all round the room while I was telling a Bible story from the Old Testament. As all the other children listened attentively, Lindsey suddenly popped out from behind the settee, held up his fingers in the form of a gun, then shouted, "And along came Elijah with a gun, and said, 'Bang, bang, bang, you're all dead'". I don't know how I coped with that dramatic distraction. I think we all just burst out laughing, but nevertheless it seemed outrageous – but amusing nonetheless – at the time. Lindsey must have been listening as he had picked up the name of Elijah, but preferred his own version of the story and produced a very dramatic ending. At the end of each Sunday afternoon I walked home, had my tea and then walked a good mile to church for the evening service, where I met up with my boy friend. We certainly didn't need gyms, or exercise classes or diets to keep us slim in those days. Walking took up quite a lot of everybody's time.

We occasionally had an interesting visiting speaker at the church, the most memorable being a visit from Gladys Aylward. She was the heroine in the old film 'The Inn of the Sixth Happiness' in which Ingrid Bergman played the part of Gladys, a parlour maid who felt sure that God was calling her to be a missionary in China, a country about which she knew virtually nothing. We met the real Gladys Aylward, who was invited to tell us her story one Sunday evening.

She was a tiny little woman, who told us that although her lack of education had meant that she was not accepted for training as a missionary, she was sure of her calling. She continued her work as a parlour maid, saving all her wages until she had enough money to pay for a ticket to China in 1930, not by ship (too expensive) but on the Trans Siberian Railway. She took with her little more than an over-night bag, her passport, her Bible and about £2 in her purse. When she reached Vladivostock she discovered that a war was raging between Russia and China, and she had to leave the train and get a ship to take her to Japan.

She then travelled by bus and mule to an inland province in China and eventually reached the city of Yanchen, which she found was an overnight stopping place for many muleteers. She had no organisation behind her, had paid her way and found that in Yanchen there was an elderly lady missionary living with the poor people in this city. She stayed with her and helped her, and although they had no financial backing or support from a missionary society they decided to open an inn. They gradually won the confidence, the trade and the respect of many of the traders, who were grateful to have a good bed for the night, good food for an honest price, safety, and free entertainment of 'story-telling' in the evenings. The men would settle down after their meal, and the two English ladies told them Bible stories, which these tough men in turn retold to their families – no doubt together with tales of these two strange white women who had provided them with their B and B.

Sadly her elderly companion died not long after this, and Gladys became the sole innkeeper, aided by a Chinese Christian cook. The binding of feet was still happening to many young girls to make them appear beautiful and desirable in traditional Chinese culture, but crippled them for life. The Chinese Government had made a law forbidding foot-binding, but it still occurred. The Mandarin in charge of the district heard of the work that Gladys was doing. He visited her little inn and she earned his respect for what she was doing for the tradesmen. The Mandarin asked her to be his foot-binding Inspector, which gave her another opportunity to serve the people and simply live out her Christian faith. She was certainly fulfilling her call to missionary work in amazing ways.

The district later became embroiled in the Japanese advance in the Chino-Japanese War and she had to flee from her home in Yanchen, leaving everything behind, but taking with her a large group of orphaned children she had rescued, or bought, from people who were abusing them. She led about a hundred children to safety, walking for twelve days over the mountains; they slept rough and had hardly anything to eat. Eventually they reached the massive Yellow River which Gladys realised it was impossible to cross without a boat. But still she didn't give up; she and the children prayed together, and then sang. An army officer happened to hear them singing, and when he saw one small woman in charge of the huge crowd of starving children he ordered a Service boat to take them to safety across the strongly flowing river.

She was a real 'superwoman', tiny in stature but strong, physically, mentally and spiritually. She had to return to England in 1947 and her health had been permanently damaged after this ordeal. She was never able to return to China, but once her health was sufficiently recovered she told her story in many church venues, including ours, all around the country.

I heard her tell this story so simply but so vividly almost sixty years ago and I remember it in most of its detail. It is such a compelling story that I felt I had to relate it fully. It became so well known that eventually the famous film was made about her.

I have remembered almost every detail that she told us that evening, but looked up on Google in case I had misrepresented anything, and so have been able to add a few details to my memories, as I felt it was a story that was worth retelling.

From time to time missionaries who were back in England on furlough gave a midweek lanternslide lecture at church about their work, illustrated with black and white, often hazy, pictures. These slides gave us a vague insight into life in parts of Africa and South America, but were eye-openers to a pre-TV generation who had never seen pictures from abroad. I remember looking with wonderment at faint, somewhat blurred pictures of poverty-stricken villages in 'regions beyond' in Africa, and of the people in Bolivia, with their hard, round, black hats. How poor these people seemed to me then - but how primitive some of my memories must appear to a modern generation. But the poverty in so many parts of the world remains the same, and in many areas it is worse and the governments are so unstable.

As soon as post-war conditions improved coach outings were sometimes arranged, with invitations extended to members of the church, who helped to fill up the coach. I remember our first coach outing was to Oxford on a predictably dull August Bank Holiday Monday. How impressed I was as we peered into various college precincts and walked around some of the colleges. Our generation had had little opportunity to see any of our country's heritage, and as yet little had been done to provide beautiful flowerbeds or floral decorations to attract visitors to historical places. Several August Bank Holiday trips to the coast were arranged in the following years. We went to Bognor one year, sat on the beach on a sunny day; we swam and paddled in the sea at Brighton the following year. These were real treats after the limitations on travel during the war when coach outings were impossible and most of the coastline in the south was forbidden territory, protected with huge rolls of barbed wire against possible invasion. They were a real change from our usual rambles.

Church attendance was all-important, and throughout the rest of my youth and early adulthood I attended the morning and evening services as well as afternoon Sunday school. Our Sunday services were quite solemn, a little heavy, with very lengthy sermons and prayers. I didn't appreciate then how very long the sermon was, and listened seriously to all the points in the address, but wonder how much of these lengthy sermons could possibly have been remembered by anyone in the congregation. I was aware, even then, of the very long, extempore prayers, which often seemed more suitable for the preacher's personal, private intercession than in public worship.

The slow singing of the hymns is another contrast with today. A Welsh lady in the congregation had a very strong voice, and she slowed everyone down, including the organist, with her vocal emphasis on the words of the hymn, and also led the congregation to follow her own *rallentando* towards the end of each verse. A hymn would grow slower and slower as the congregation influenced the organist, who then accompanied us instead of leading. At one period a few of us more rebellious YPF members tried to speed up the hymn singing a little. We sat in the back row and tried to gently quicken the tempo by singing loudly, emphasising the beat of the hymns, and endeavoured to prevent the congregation from slowing down at the end of each line. One Sunday we had a rather important visiting preacher, none other than the President of the Fellowship of Independent Evangelical Churches, who interrupted the congregational singing to reprimand 'those individuals who were spoiling the worship'. We were so shamed by this public rebuke that we ceased our endeavours to *improve* the worship, not *spoil* it, and sank down into our seats with our heads lowered to hide our faces, which I am sure were red with embarrassment

In time our elderly organist retired and I was asked to play the organ for the Sunday services, so I had to find time to practice the hymns and learn a voluntary or two. I couldn't improvise very well but often found a suitable hymn tune that I played around with on the keyboard before and at the end of the morning and evening services, but I bought a book of organ voluntaries with simple arrangements and quite enjoyed practising them up to performance level. The old-fashioned American organ required a lot of quite vigorous exercise in order to produce any sound. To work the bellows one had to pedal continuously with both feet, and when increased volume was required for special emphasis I pressed my thighs against the two swells set at knee height on either side of the organ. When I felt competent enough to do all this while keeping my eyes on the music, and my fingers were playing familiar notes, I might 'give it a go' and select, then quickly pull out, one or another of the small array of knobs set just above the keyboard to produce a different sound. What with bellows, and swells and organ stops I think my mind must have been in a whirl at the end of each service, but the experience made me appreciate the vast number of things which have to done simultaneously by a real organist.

After a while a new, younger YPF leader was appointed whose enthusiasm led to our preparation and performing of what was called an 'Easter Anthology'. This was quite ambitious for our small group of young people. Few of us had been stretched academically at school during the war years or had experience of singing in a school choir and only one or two had received the benefit of a grammar school education. Mr. Fortnam trained the YPF members into a choir, rehearsing us in a number of hymns and songs, which we rehearsed in four-part harmony, with one or two tenors and basses, and a few altos to support the stronger sopranos. Maurice had a good singing voice and was able to put in a strong bass part. Our vocal efforts were interspersed with Bible or other appropriate readings surrounding Passion Week. The readings were done by different people, and were accompanied by suitable recorded music played quietly in the background. It sounds very simple when describing it now, but it was very effective at the time. I always remember part of Vaughan Williams Variations on a Theme by Thomas Tallis as being a piece of music that seemed especially suitable for one of the readings. We were also being subconsciously introduced to some classical music.

Mr Fortnam (we never called him Les; formal titles were always used) had a talent for stage design. He arranged a bank of spring flowers and pot plants in front of the little stage, and scrolled huge, tall rolls of pastel-coloured, corrugated card behind the choir to form a background. Mr. Fortnam played the appropriate music quietly on his record player to accompany the readings while hidden behind the scrolls of card. The needle was placed on each record at just the right moment before the reading began, when he volume on the record player was very slightly raised. It sounded very effective when we performed it in front of a crowded church audience on Good Friday. With the musical items sung between the spoken words I believe we gave quite a moving recital of the Passion of Christ.

These details sound very amateurish in the twenty-first century, but considering the limitations of the period, the available talent and the small, bare, rented hall that was our church, they were quite commendable. The audience was appreciative, and someone was so impressed that we were asked to perform this Anthology at a church in Surrey the following year. There was great excitement in the coach as we drove to Godstone Baptist Church the following Easter Monday, eating our sandwiches in the church on arrival, fitting in time for a short afternoon ramble, and an even briefer rehearsal, before sitting down to a sumptuous tea provided by the ladies of the church. A little time passed - when we all grew nervous - before we presented our Anthology.

Most of us had no experience of performing in musical or drama productions in our schooldays, but some of the younger members may have had the opportunities as the 1950s dawned, but I have not heard or seen anything performed by a church youth group that approaches the standard of singing, or the clear, expressive and unrushed speaking, than that well rehearsed, simple production by our YPF so long ago.

Our singing was really quite good, our diction was clear, our harmony was apparent – if a little off-key here and there – and in 1951 Mr Fortnam had somehow arranged for us to make a recording at the HMV studios in Oxford Street. He would soon be leaving us, and I think he wanted to take a tangible memory of our combined efforts to his new home. I can't imagine what the recording staff thought of this little group of amateurs as we trooped into a recording studio. I have no idea what it must have cost Mr. Fortnam. After our recording session most of the YPF spent the afternoon at the1951 Festival of Britain. It was a memorable day. In due course we each received a gift of a 78rpm record of our performance. It was quite a thrill to listen to our recorded voices, but I don't think we considered ourselves to be stars. I wonder whether anyone still possesses his or her record. Our leader was an unassuming, quietly spoken, charming man. He had four young children, and his wife had been one of my Sunday school teachers a few years earlier.

We were sorry when he and his family moved to Devon, but Miss Jones took over the YPF Leadership for a short period before she retired and moved away from Kenton. Gwen (but still Miss Jones to us) had an evening YPF garden party before she moved, with the usual refreshments accompanied by outdoor games and races. No alcohol was drunk and nobody smoked; and no boy smooched off into a bedroom or a corner of the garden with another girl. It wasn't forbidden; it just didn't happen. The garden was full of laughter.

Maybe our life would be considered extremely boring today, but it was interesting and satisfying to us at that period; it kept us occupied in our free time, and we appreciated our occasional excursions. I wonder which society actually has, or had, the greatest pleasure or lasting satisfaction when they were young. Any spare time I might have had seems to have been very fully occupied. On looking back I can see that although our life was rather humdrum and very narrow, (it certainly wasn't the frenetic affair that it seems to be for so many nowadays) but neither was it the boring existence that many experience in inner cities where they have nothing to do - we could have been as equally unoccupied and bored as the present generation. We did a number of interesting things that cost very little, extended our own talents and capabilities and we were all happy together. There were no fights, quarrels or spats of anger.

Chapter Eight

LIFE GETS SERIOUS

I was still at Hendon Tech when I began to attend the Friday evening meetings of the local branch of the Young Life Campaign, mostly I guess, because my Hendon Tech. boyfriend, John, was a member and I knew I would meet up with him there. In the summer of 1948 the YLC organised a week's holiday at the seaside. I had never been on holiday on my own until I joined around a hundred other young people from all parts of the country on this holiday. We were accommodated in, and used the facilities of, a private boarding school in Sussex. I met people from places in England that I didn't know existed. I had never heard a Midland or a Northern accent before. I slept in a dormitory with girls I didn't know at all. I felt a little shy. I didn't have the confidence of some of these other girls and I had never shared a bedroom with anybody else before. There was quite a bit of larking around, which was quite new to me, and I think I stayed quietly in my bed and watched, and listened, but neither the girls, nor the boys in their dormitories, made contact with each other after lights out and eventually everyone settled down.

We had fun at the large open-air, unheated swimming pool at St. Leonard's, near Hastings. We spent time on the beach, played tennis on the school courts; on other days there were organised rambles, followed by a lot of singing before a thought-provoking talk after supper. I enjoyed all these activities and the companionship immensely. It was the first of only two independent holidays I had before I was married, or indeed for many years after that.

John was never asked to tea in our house, although I remember once being invited to Sunday tea with his family. I don't think my father encouraged my friendship with him, although he was a very nice young man, who grew up to have a successful career in banking. My dad was much more in favour of the young man from my church who had started 'walking me home' after our Youth Fellowship meeting on a Monday evening, and then accompanying me home after the Sunday evening service at church. He had just been de-mobbed from the RAF, and later became my husband. I was seeing both John and my new boyfriend, Maurice, for some while, until I eventually realised that perhaps it was not a good idea to be two-timing and I gradually ceased to see John.

I think my father encouraged my blossoming friendship with Maurice, and I can remember an aunt leaning across the table at my cousin Daphne's wedding, quietly whispering to my father, 'Is there another wedding in the offing?' My father with eyes twinkling, replied, 'I think so'. I hadn't as yet thought of my new boyfriend in terms of a serious relationship. All my previous romances had been mainly friendships; we enjoyed the companionship and just had a kiss and a cuddle. However, I think others might have considered me a bit of a flirt at that time, as I seem to have had quite a number of boy friends by the time I was eighteen.

Perhaps my father thought I should settle down. He had the sole care of his flighty daughter, and was possibly worried about things that had not occurred to me. He always insisted that I was indoors by 10.30 p.m., and if I still happened to be at the front gate saying goodnight after this hour, even after I was engaged, he stood at the open door, with the hall light switched on, twiddling his spectacles around in his hand until I came in. Light flooding out from the hall made any embrace very noticeable, and curtailed our farewell kisses. He must have taken his responsibilities as the only parent very seriously, and a lone parent today would have similar, or perhaps greater, concern, but I don't think that many would intervene so obviously nowadays!

My succession of boyfriends came to an end some time after I began 'going out' with this young man from my church. I was six years younger than Maurice, and during his month's demobilisation leave from the Royal Air Force in 1948 he began to meet me at Northwick Park Station after my day's work, and we would walk home together rather than my getting the bus. I could remember him as a young Sunday school teacher when I was a pupil in his mother's Sunday school class some years previously, and thinking it was rather odd to see this young man teaching a group of young boys. All the other young men in the church were away in the Forces, but Maurice had been in a reserved occupation in the aircraft industry throughout the war, and was called up to do his two years' National Service immediately after the war was over. When he was demobbed and returned home he joined the YPF, and was a little older than most of the members, but the age difference between us soon disappeared once we got to know each other. Once a fellow and his girl friend sat together in church in those days they were considered to be 'courting' and it was 'serious'.

Maurice returned to his old job at de Havillands in Edgware after his month's demobilisation leave from the RAF, but it was not long before he was transferred to their engine test and development site in Hertfordshire. With no public transport available from Kenton to Hatfield he got a bus to Mill Hill every morning and thumbed a lift along the Barnet-by-pass, to arrive at work at 8 a.m. This road is now called the AIM, but it wasn't even a dual carriageway in those days. Getting to work wasn't easy. There was no rail access or bus route going from Harrow to Hatfield and thumbing a lift from someone driving along the road was quite acceptable then. There is still no direct public transport linked to Hatfield.

Maurice had a life-long, almost fanatical, interest in engines of every kind, and was in the forefront of the comparatively short history of the development of the small jet engine by de Havillands in their production of helicopter engines.

As soon as he had saved enough money Maurice bought himself a motorbike, which enabled him to get to work far more easily. He was very proud of his AJS British-made motorbike and it made his journey to work much easier. He didn't allow me to ride pillion on his bike at weekends, so we didn't zoom around the countryside together. I am sure I would have enjoyed this very much, and think I should have been much more persuasive. Before we began 'going out' together regularly Maurice had spoken with my father, asking his permission to 'court' me. How old-fashioned this sounds today, and I think it was quite an unusual thing to occur even towards the end of the 1940s.

A bicycle, the bus, or the train were the usual means of transport in the late 1940s and early 50s. We both had bicycles when we first met, but we didn't go on cycle rides at weekends. Perhaps I had had enough of bicycle rides after the strenuous cycling holidays I had with my father, and Maurice may have had enough of travelling on two wheels after his daily motorbike journey throughout the week. We needed more companionable transport to get us into the countryside, and the faithful Metropolitan Line enabled us to get into Buckinghamshire very easily. We often went for long walks around Chesham, Chenies, Rickmansworth, the Chess Valley and Chorley Wood on Saturday afternoons in the summer. Then it was usually home for tea with Maurice's parents; I think his mum tried to entice me into the family by making a special tea on Saturdays. A cake stand full of assorted fancy cakes was always in the centre of the table. Occasionally we had a melon for tea, and that seemed extremely special. I had never eaten melon before. A jar of ginger in syrup sometimes appeared on the tea table, and we ate a small piece of this with bread and butter, cutting the ginger into tiny slices with a small tea knife and pastry fork. The ginger was so hot!

We did our courting in the drawing room, as we listened to records on Maurice's record player in the evenings. Perhaps that all seems very dull to today's partygoers, but I think we were tired out after our long walks in the afternoons, especially on the days when I had to work at the office in the morning. I also think that 'entertainment' was very restricted by the church, and also by my boy friend's upbringing.

We didn't go to dances and I don't think the delights of dancing entered our heads. I had never thought of going to a dance, had no idea of where a dance might have occurred and with my solitary workplace I didn't have the experience or knowledge of other young people to enlighten me. The only time I attempted to dance was at Christmastime during the war, when my father put on his old records, and I tried to waltz and do the fox trot with him in our home. This music must have given him bitter-sweet memories of the times before my mother was ill, but in order to cope with day to day life he must have put the past firmly out of his mind in order to give me a happy upbringing. Perhaps he thought of my mother as he danced with me in those old days, but I wish that he had talked about her too. There was such a taboo about mental illness with the public in general, but also for those most closely concerned. I think this taboo affected my father and made him feel unable to mention my mother, or anything about her. I think that in those early days it was not thought that she would ever recover and that it would be better for me to forget her. There were no photos in the house to remind me of what she looked like. How did he keep so outwardly cheerful in the face of such a difficult life?

In June 1949 I prepared a small tea party at home for my eighteenth birthday, for four girl friends, my father and my boy friend, Maurice. There was no sumptuous meal or huge family party; there were no fabulous restaurants around locally and I had no relatives who lived near to make my birthday a family celebration. So it was a very simple, low-key affair. My friends were those who had been at school with me and with whom I had kept in touch – Beryl, Margaret, Joan and Jean. We posed in the garden for a snapshot I still possess. I subsequently lost touch with Margaret and Joan, and we didn't meet again for over forty years, and that's another story, but Beryl and I have remained friends throughout all our lives, although we rarely meet. Sadly, Jean died while still quite a young woman.

--------- ---

One Sunday the following year Maurice told me that he couldn't get to our youth fellowship the following evening. I thought he had to work late. He didn't give me a reason, but unbeknown to me he intended visiting my father while I was out of the house to ask his consent to our engagement. I guess that my father was relieved to think that I was going to settle down with a sensible, kind and thoughtful young man. I wonder whether he wished my mother was with him to consider the engagement of their only daughter. It must have been quite a responsibility for one parent to carry. I knew nothing about this conversation until a few days later, when... the following Saturday Maurice and I went on one of our country walks, and as we sat at the edge of a field, in the peace of the warm autumn countryside, he proposed to me and I accepted his proposal.

I had no idea that he had had a talk with my father before I received this proposal; they were both very good at keeping a secret. My father had given his consent to my engagement in 1949 on the condition that my fiancé was earning £7 a week before our marriage.

An aircraft engineer's enthusiasm in the development of the jet engine was assumed to make up for a low pay packet, and my new fiancé's job was not well paid. Development of a new jet engine was extremely costly, but enthusiasm was free. He often had to work in the evenings and occasionally he was required to be present on the engine test bed on a Sunday, which was totally misunderstood and disapproved of by our minister. The aircraft industry at this period, and for the next few years, was almost frenetic with the stress and exhilaration of the development of the small jet engine. Maurice was working on the engine test beds, and they frequently had twenty-four-hour testing during the development of a new engine. Overtime was expected, even on a Sunday, without consideration for staff – or their families or their church! This overtime wasn't voluntary, to get extra money, as our minister had wrongly assumed, but was insisted on by the boss, in order to maintain the continuity of work, or the assessment of a one hundred hour test, or a seven-day continuous test, on a developing engine. Sundays were quiet in those days, with closed shops, and most people having the day off.

Our engagement was announced soon after my nineteenth birthday, and we were married a few weeks before I was twenty-one. I was young, possibly not really ready for a serious boy friend or for marriage, but couples often became engaged when they were younger in those days, and usually saved for a long time before they got married. Once married they usually delayed considering starting a family until they had the means to provide for a baby, but thoughts of babies didn't enter my mind when I got engaged. Like many in those times, we didn't make marriage plans, or even talk about our future, but…we *saved* until we had got a home together.

We both saved as much as we could from our wages and I very gradually filled my 'bottom drawer'. I embroidered the tablecloth I had purchased in Guernsey in a very pretty willow pattern using different shades of blue thread, and had embroidered a pair of chair backs. I began buying useful household items for our future home, which were literally all placed in the bottom drawer of the chest of drawers on the landing. (In former years when I was a schoolgirl, this drawer had contained my collection of shrapnel, picked up on my way to school after a heavy air raid. These relics of used shells or exploded bombs were treasured 'souvenirs' during the war, but discarded long after as rubbish. Also thrown out when I began to fill my bottom drawer in preparation for marriage were my old school tie, the braided blue and purple girdle that was tied round the waist of my gym slip and my house badges.)

I was now earning £7.10 shillings (£7.50) a week. My father had offered us the two main upstairs rooms in my existing home for our first home, so we didn't really think of looking elsewhere. Accommodation was very difficult to find at the time and I had cared for my dad for so long I didn't like to leave him alone after my marriage. He thought that young people should be responsible, (but also because he was hard up, and would lose the rent from our lodger) so after we married we paid him £1 a week for our accommodation, which he recorded in a little rent book.

I would have been financially compelled to keep my job if we had had to find a flat or accommodation elsewhere. Perhaps, in the long run, that would have been a good thing, but there would still have been the problem of *finding* the accommodation in that period, plus the reluctance to leave my father to manage on his own. It didn't seem the right thing to do.

As the time of my wedding drew near, and we had fixed the date, I chose the material for my wedding dress in my lunch hour from the large fabric department of John Lewis in Oxford Street, feeling a bit out of my depth as I hesitated for a long time over which material and what dress pattern I should buy. I rushed down to Bourne and Hollingsworth in New Oxford Street in another lunch hour to buy a mock orange blossom headdress. One Saturday my two bridesmaids and I chose the material for their very pretty, pale lilac bridesmaids' dresses. Nylon nightdresses were just becoming available, and I extravagantly bought three in the lingerie department of the small, old-fashioned, family owned department store in Marylebone High Street, called, oddly enough, Gaylor and Pope. My nightdresses were not at all glamorous by today's standards, but I thought they were very sophisticated at the time – *nylon* nighties!

Preparations were made for the wedding. My father sent out the invitations, and my fiancé and I booked the caterers and reception hall, ordered the cake, arranged the date and time of the wedding at the church, and met with our minister. I don't remember any pre-nuptial course on married life! I think I was the first bride in our church for many years and my wedding would be only the third I had attended in my life. I had been a bridesmaid once, along with Winnie, my fellow-occupant in the basement, at the wedding of Mary, the secretary to the cancer specialist in the house where I worked in Harley Street,. Her boss gave the bride away, and my boss and his wife were guests, so it was an unusual wedding. We never met the bride again!

It didn't enter my mind that my mother was absent from the preparations for my wedding. Did she even know that her daughter was about to be married? I wonder whether my father thought it wise to tell her when he visited. Perhaps I was the cause of her illness? I never asked. It might have unsettled her to know I was getting married. But it might have enabled her to understand that the young mum named Sheila, who she met seven years later, was, in fact, her daughter! I think I must have been omitted from his conversation with my mother over all these years, just as she have been omitted from any conversation with me as I grew up.

Shortly before our wedding day our lady lodger moved out of my father's house and into my in-laws' home, to live in my future husband's old bedroom, which had been transformed into a bed-sitting room for Miss Rich. She was much relieved to find alternative furnished accommodation so easily, and the two ladies, the lodger and my mother-in-law, became good friends. All parties were well satisfied, although my father still only had the small room above the hall as his bedroom.

My fiancé and I set about making our first home. The front bedroom that had been the lodger's bed-sit for about ten years became our living room, and the back bedroom that had been occupied by our ex-housekeeper and her daughter in previous years became 'our' bedroom instead of 'my' bedroom.

The tiny pre-war fireplace was removed from what had, thirteen years earlier, been my parents' bedroom, and was replaced by a smart modern tiled fireplace, which Maurice and I had chosen. This immediately transformed the look of the room from being a bedroom into that of a sitting room. A fireplace was a necessity for the living room then; coal was the only source of heating.

Maurice had passed my father's stipulated '£7 a week before marriage', so we were able to prepare a home for our future life together. We fixed the date of our wedding and began to furnish our two rooms. It was exciting to walk around the furniture shops in the early fifties, when a lot more goods and furniture were becoming available, and some stores had better quality goods, with different styles and prices. We bought a good, firm mattress for £7 in a small furniture shop in Harrow to put on the bed that was bought separately from Maples in London. Our bedroom suite had a lovely, maple-veneered surface, and consisted of a very attractively designed dressing table, a chest of drawers, a wardrobe and a bed with a maple-veneered headboard and bottom board and a coiled spring base. We bought a delicately patterned floral carpet with a beautiful cloud effect background for our bedroom, and shortly before our marriage the furniture was delivered and placed upon the new carpet. I thought our new bedroom looked delightful. Bedroom suites have almost disappeared with the advent of fitted wall-length wardrobes, but to me a bedroom seems to lack some essential element when minus a dressing table, which seems to have completely disappeared from the shops nowadays. Nobody would have had enough clothes to fill a fitted wall-length wardrobe in those days, but a dressing table was an essential part of bedroom furniture.

Our dining room suite also came from Maples, a wonderful furniture shop that used to be in Tottenham Court Road. The dining table was in veneered mahogany, which could be extended when we had visitors, six very comfortable upholstered dining chairs and a delightfully styled sideboard, which had a capacious cupboard on either side of a set of four drawers. Dining room suites have also largely gone out of fashion with the advent of the kitchen/diner. Two Parker Knoll fireside chairs costing £7.10s each, good quality but quite compact, completed our first home. All of this furniture was well made and designed to fit into an ordinary semi-detached house and was moderately priced.

After redecorating the rooms our furniture was delivered shortly before the wedding. It was very exciting to be making our first home as we arranged it all; it's a very enjoyable memory to recall.

Where is the Key?

Wedding presents began to appear, and they provided us with cutlery (from Maurice's parents) a handsome Bush radio (from my father), an eiderdown (from Maurice's grandmother). My boss gave us a beautiful Copeland Spode dinner service. I still have it and take pleasure in using it whenever I have visitors. Its' pattern is timeless and quite delightful. Charterhouse Clinic staff were so generous and gave us a Phoenix glass dinner service for four, and it had a very practical everyday use in our home for many years. It was a very kind and unexpected gift, as I had left the Clinic four years previously. It was a strange coincidence that I had a dinner service from each of my two employers. A number of   patients very kindly gave us wedding gifts, (one, a Mrs. Richardson - whose name and address I have remembered for over sixty years - had hand embroidered a most beautiful pair of chair backs, which were very popular then, as most men put oil on their hair!) Maurice's work colleagues gave us a Morphy Richards toaster. An aunt gave us a prettily decorated china tea service, which we used for 'best' for many years. We were overwhelmed with the kindness shown by such useful gifts from relatives, friends and patients.

I was sad to leave my job but I guess that the excitement of my forthcoming marriage overcame my sadness at giving up my interesting work. It is an extraordinary thought now, but in those days most men still felt that they should earn enough to support a wife, who then gave up her employment. Many businesses insisted that female staff left their workplace when they married. Not many parents in my suburban area would have had spare capital in that period to help their sons and daughters to get a mortgage. We may not have lived from hand to mouth, but I believe that most people I knew lived from week to week. 'Wealth' was an unfamiliar word.

Our own church did not have a licence to perform marriage ceremonies because it was only a rented building, so we were married in Harrow Baptist church, a building that has now been replaced by a modern church centre. On the afternoon before the wedding my fiancé and I bought some nice flowers, took them by bus to the church and placed them in three vases on the Communion table. Flower arranging had not yet come into vogue; flowers were simply placed into suitable vases of water.

All was ready; the presents were on display on our new dining table in our newly transformed upstairs living room. We had nothing more to do before the great day, and so we went to our respective homes for the last time as singles. There were no pre-wedding parties or celebrations then, and I don't think stag nights or hen nights had been thought of. They wouldn't have been our scenes even if they did exist. I have no memory of how I spent my wedding eve – writing 'thank you' letters probably!

My wedding day dawned, with my father bringing me a cup of tea in bed. Soon telegrams began to arrive. As the busy morning began it didn't occur to me that most brides had their mother to help with the preparations for the big day, maybe to organise, supervise or calm their daughter. I am sure that most mothers would also be adding some excitement to the event. My bridesmaids and I quietly attended to each other's appearance as we put on our finery in my, soon to be 'our', bedroom. I think we were having a bit of a nervous giggle together when my Auntie Ada arrived, possibly showing a little well-controlled nervous excitement herself.

My aunt handed to me an old lace wedding veil and told me that she had worn it at her own wedding. My aunt was a lot older than my mother and had no children of her own. I had lived with her and my uncle for some months before the war when my mother had the nervous breakdown that had led to her permanent residence in hospital. It didn't cross my mind that maybe this veil was not just 'something old', but it was very likely that my aunt had been keeping her veil for me because my mother had also worn it, and may have been dropping a hint to that effect, but could not bring herself to talk explicitly of my mother. Perhaps, with the reticence of the period, or the stigma of even mentioning my ill and absent mother, my aunt couldn't bring herself to simply say that this had also been my mother's wedding veil. She had told me some time previously that I could use this wedding veil, but I had not seen it until my wedding day. I wore the lovely, delicate lace veil, thinking of it simply as the traditional 'something old' that brides should wear, without giving a thought that my mother was not present, nor that she may have worn the same veil in 1920. I still have it, but it is not likely to be worn again and I still don't know for certain whether it was my mother's. It is now over one hundred years old.

Although I have just written that flower arranging was not yet popular, professional florists made me a beautiful wedding bouquet, with lovely pale golden roses and freesia that blended with the ivory damask of my dress and the cream of my veil. My two bridesmaids' bouquets of mauve sweet-smelling Brompton stocks and cream carnations matched their pretty mauve dresses to perfection.

I wish I had given a thought to my mother on my wedding day, but her personality had been so thoroughly wiped from my memory, and nobody mentioned her name or talked about her in my presence. But my relatives, especially my aunts, her two much older sisters, Ada and Alice, must have been so aware of her absence as the service proceeded. Did my father think of her? She must have been in his thoughts, and probably crossed the mind of most of the guests as they saw my father sitting alone on the bride's side at the front of the church, with my new in-laws on the right. When I think of my wedding day now, so many years on, my mother's absence must have been so noticeable to all our guests as they sat behind the wedding group, looking at all the figures, noticing the gap next to my father, and everyone must have thought about her – except me.

I have since wondered whether my birth was the cause of her subsequent life-long mental illness. She may have suffered from post-natal depression, which would not have been recognised in those days. If this was not understood and could not be treated, she may have grown worse when detained in hospital. I feel that her subsequent schizophrenia and psychotic illness might have developed through her own anguish at the lack of understanding or treatment of her symptoms. Perhaps she had resented her pregnancy and my subsequent my birth nine years after the loss of Peggy. My presence at home as a small child, may have caused her frequent breakdowns. Perhaps there was concern that if she saw me she would have become more acutely ill. These thoughts didn't occur to me until long after my mother's death and may not be true.

If she had suffered from some untreatable physical illness I think that I would have been told about it; she would have been mentioned in conversation, and as far as possible, she would have been a part of my life, or at least aware of, and present at, her daughter's wedding. Why could not the same response be given to someone who had a mental illness? The probable answer is that if the modern antipsychotic drugs were available at that time my mother would have been at my wedding.

Maurice's grandmother, his parents and relatives, and my two aunts and uncles arrived at the church, along with my one dear cousin Daphne and her husband, her parents, my father's cousins, together with my boss, his wife, and a number of friends. My long-standing friend, Janet, was my bridesmaid, and Audrey, another friend from church, took the place of my old school friend Beryl, whose Commissioning as a Salvation Army officer took place on the same day as my wedding. We had shared so much in earlier years, and if I had known sooner that her special event clashed with my wedding I would have chosen another day. However, Audrey and I have now shared a lot over most of the rest of our lives and, together with her husband Stanley, they have both been long-standing good friends.

The one bit of the wedding service that I can remember was that our minister took the analogy of a 'boat' as the symbol of the 'marriage', and that Maurice and I, as the two rowers, should row together through the, sometimes rough, waters of our life. I think it could be said that we did just that.

The wedding reception was a formal lunch of roast chicken and roast potatoes, but I think it was the first time that I had tasted frozen peas. I hardly had time to greet my boss and his wife, to meet my new husband's relations, or speak to my own relatives, some of whom I never saw again; it seems such a shame it was all over so soon. When the cake was cut, the speeches were over and the telegrams read, there was so little time for a few words with our guests before I had to change into my going away outfit - a two-piece costume (as a suit was called then), together with a navy blue straw hat, handbag and shoes. It all passed so quickly and seems very formal and serious as I look back on it now. There was no time to relax and really enjoy myself, and the few hours in my wedding dress were over by 4 o'clock. I envy the bride of today who wears her wedding dress for the entire day, with a party or dance after the reception. My beautiful ivory brocade dress was no sooner on than it was off, never to be seen in public or worn again. However my going-away suit, smart but much less glamorous, was worn every Sunday in spring and autumn for many years afterwards.

The wedding had been at 12 noon, and we left the reception at 4.30 p.m. to catch the evening train to our honeymoon destination. Looking back I realise that I had few personal friends at my wedding, and can only remember Janet, Audrey, Stanley and Winnie.

Maurice had arranged the luxury of a taxi to Paddington Station (a great indulgence in those days) but May 3rd 1952 happened to be Cup Final day at Wembley, so the driver had to find a route through the back streets to get us to the station on time. We had to catch the evening train to the long-since-closed railway station at Sidmouth in South Devon. We arrived in thick mist, which we have discovered over the years is a common occurrence in Sidmouth. After breakfast the following morning we were asked to hand over our ration books. I felt embarrassed about handing in my ration book in my maiden name, and Maurice suddenly remembered he had left his at home. Neither of our homes had a telephone. He had to write home asking his mother to post his ration book to Meadhurst Private Hotel, Sidmouth immediately. Our honeymoon destination was no longer a secret! The hotel had to cater for him without any evidence to their suppliers of an extra mouth to feed until his mum posted his ration book back. Food was still rationed seven years after the war had ended and meals at the hotel were rather sparse and very uninteresting by today's standards; the import of luxury and out-of season-food did not get underway until many years later.

The hotel charged six-and-a-half guineas a week (just under the £7 that my father had insisted should be Maurice's income before we could marry!) I remember very little about this small hotel in which we stayed, apart from the profuse blossoms of the wisteria that clung to the attractive building, and the convoluted twisting of its branches. I had never seen wisteria before. (By a strange coincidence, the family house that my husband and I bought many years later, and is still my home, has a large, now old, wisteria that spreads its twisted branches over supports and extends right across the width of the garden. Its beautiful bloom and exquisite perfume are much admired, and much enjoyed during the month of May.) There was a hand basin in our bedroom, but there were no en-suite rooms and the toilet was across a large landing. You had to listen carefully at your bedroom door for any sound that would indicate that a guest was vacating it, and then rush across the landing, with lino covering the floor, in as casual a manner as possible, to claim possession of the loo. On a subsequent visit to Sidmouth many years later we found that the attractive old hotel had been demolished and replaced by a large, plain block of apartments.

Chapter Nine

NEWLY WEDS

After we returned from our honeymoon I finished writing all the 'thank you' letters for our wedding presents but when all the excitement of my new life had died down I began to feel a little lonely during the day. There was nobody else of my age living in the immediate neighbourhood. I vacuumed and dusted, polished the lino surrounds to all our carpets, scrubbed the kitchen floor, shopped and cooked for my two menfolk. My father joined us as we ate our evening meal together in our living room upstairs, sitting at the new dining table, using our new cutlery, and china. We ate our Sunday dinner together upstairs, and if we had visitors for Sunday tea, all the food was carried up from the kitchen, and we carried all the used china etc. downstairs to the kitchen afterwards. When Maurice was working late, which was very often, my father and I ate our dinner in his dining room. There seemed to be a lot more housework to be done in those days, but I missed my job, and found it very solitary at home. I did some occasional work on my portable typewriter at the dining table for a surveyor. and later was asked to do some temporary work in London for a solicitor.

I was given a new, modern tennis racquet for my twenty-first birthday, which occurred only six week after I was married but we didn't have a party – we had only just had our wedding reception. I learned that my father had taken out an annuity for me some years previously, which terminated when I reached twenty-one. It amounted to £25 – quite a sum then – and I bought myself a modern Singer sewing machine with the money. I have never been a particularly adept or enthusiastic seamstress, but found it very useful for many years.

Kenton library continued to be a good companion, as it had been throughout the war, and I remember enjoying reading the popular authors of the day – Warwick Deeping, Naomi Jacob, Philip Gibbs – authors whose stories I have long forgotten, but I can still recall with pleasure the Herries Chronicles by Hugh Walpole, John Galsworthy's Forsyte Saga, and the absorbing tales and descriptive writing of Howard Spring. I also recall a novel called 'The Hill' based on the history of Harrow on the Hill, by an author named Horace Vachell that I much enjoyed. On a recent visit, I found that Kenton Library is still open on the corner of the now, very busy, traffic-light controlled crossroads and is exactly as I remembered it as a child, with its *art moderne* style of architecture. The original interior has been wonderfully preserved and conserved and is obviously lovingly cared for by the present head librarian and his staff. The quiet roads around the Library changed into busy thoroughfares long ago, and a bus route now uses the road I grew up in. The Library has become a listed building and is a thriving centre of the community. I hope the children's library is still moderately quiet! I remember it as an oasis of peace when I was a child, and loved the near silence that was then imposed by the head librarian.

Although I had been on my own in my old job, I was always busy and there had always been a lot of responsibility, interest and friendly telephone contact with the patients and pharmacists. I was now in my new 'job' and I was still alone, but now had no contacts, no busy life and no telephone. Why ever were new wives expected to give up work in the past when they married? It was crazy. However, new responsibilities and interest soon appeared.

Our YPF leader moved soon after my marriage and I was asked to take on the leadership. One didn't volunteer for a church position in those days; I wouldn't have dreamed of volunteering to become the leader, but I had been considered, and then approved by the deacons, one of whom then asked me if I would accept this responsibility. I have always preferred to be asked to do something rather than feel I was pushing myself forward, and have ever since found it difficult to volunteer but prefer to be asked.

We continued with our usual YPF activities and country rambles after I became the leader, (what an old-fashioned term in youth work this seems now) but I began to expand our activities a little. I wrote to our MP asking if he could escort our group of young people round the Palace of Westminster. He replied, telling us that he would be delighted to personally be our guide. So, on the appointed Saturday, we all set off for an afternoon tour of the Houses of Parliament, feeling very privileged to think we were to be escorted around by our local member of parliament, but on arrival we found, not our M.P., but an official uniformed guide awaiting us, who told us that our M.P. had been called away and he sent his apologies. We were disappointed at first, but the guide was excellent, and I am sure he told us more than our M.P. would have been able to do. He took us not only through the House of Commons and the House of Lords but we were privileged to be taken up into the Clock Tower and saw the huge bell of Big Ben at eye level. There were so many steps for quite a large group of people to climb up, but when we were assembled around the bells, the guide told us that the Big Ben bell had cracked as it was being installed in the middle of the 18th century; it was never repaired and has been cracked ever since. We saw – and heard - the bells in action as we waited for them to strike. It was unusual for the public to be allowed to visit this part of the Houses of Parliament, and I think it was a special extra for our YPF because the MP had let us down.

We retraced our steps down very carefully, and on reaching ground level were then taken even lower by going into the crypt, where there is a little chapel where MPs and their family members can be married. We finished our tour by visiting the vast and ancient Westminster Hall, where King George the VIth had lain in state after his death a couple of years earlier. We had had the full works, and were all quite excited as we went into the small, old-fashioned Lyons teashop afterwards (that used to be opposite Big Ben) and had tea together. What a lot of noise we must have made in that rather small teashop with our excited chatter. The block of little shops that had been on this site for years is now occupied with the new fortress-like Parliament buildings.

On another occasion we had a guided tour round Faraday House, which was then the London Telephone Exchange; we visited what used to be the main London Postal Sorting Office and on another occasion went up to Fleet Street and had a guided tour of the printing works and watched the printing of the Evening Standard. Both printing works and the Evening Standard disappeared years ago.

I arranged a tennis tournament with another youth fellowship one Saturday, and we had a good time battling it out on some local tennis courts that we had hired for the afternoon. Not many of our members played tennis, but there were enough of us to make up a team, and the rest came along to cheer us on – and to enjoy the tea afterwards that was supplied by our opponents. It was the first official contact we had had with another church. Other contacts came along in due course.

In time our occasional socials in the church hall, were replaced by a 'squash' in somebody's home. They were called squashes because as many people as could be squashed into someone's living room made for a successful occasion. They were held on a Saturday evening, usually at our home, and we opened the dividing glass doors between the two downstairs reception rooms in my father's house to make a larger area, which also enabled us to use his piano to accompany our singing. My dear father spent the Saturday evening after his return home from work, sitting alone in Maurice's and my upstairs living room, no doubt listening to all our chatter and singing down below. We could invite any friends; food and coffee were served, some games were played, some choruses were sung (it was still a pre-guitar age and someone was required to play the piano) and a short talk was given.

Nobody got drunk, or took drugs, nobody smoked, and nobody slipped off to a bedroom. Nobody blasphemed, swore, or used foul language, but we had all had a good evening. Did we actually think of 'enjoyment' or 'happiness'? I don't think so, but I think we were content and had enjoyed our evening. Why has life changed so much? Why is a moral, wholesome life so disparaged, belittled and despised or laughed at? Why has our language been so demeaned?

Our youth Fellowship even got around to producing its own magazine, with short articles provided by various members, accounts of outings or meetings we had taken. It was typed out each month on my old portable typewriter and then duplicated by Janet, who was the editor, and then each copy was stapled together, and circulated in the YPF and in the church. I still have some old copies, and although they seem very amateurish, formal and old-fashioned now, I marvel as I write this at what we achieved with modest talent, few facilities and limited opportunity.

The Queen's Coronation took place eleven months after our marriage. I can very clearly recall learning of her father, the late King George VIth's, sudden death in February the previous year. I was still at work, and in my boss's consulting room taking dictation of the morning's letters, when the phone rang. I answered it and a very solemn voice asked to speak to the doctor. I handed over the phone, and saw the change of expression on my boss's face. He seemed to blanch, sounded very shocked, and as soon as he put the receiver down he looked across at me and said, 'The King is dead'. Apparently it had come up on the ticker tape at the stock exchange, and Doctor's stockbroker had telephoned to tell him the sad news. My boss had been the informant of the two first deaths I had experienced. I wasn't among the crowds lining the streets watching his funeral procession, and may have been at work sitting at my typewriter.

But Maurice and I decided to go up to London to see the Coronation of Queen Elizabeth the second in 1953. We took a late train into London the night before so that we could get a position as near as possible to Westminster Abbey, and be able see the dukes and duchesses and other important guests arrive and have a good view of the grand military parade and the royal procession. We found a good spot, right opposite the north transept of the Abbey, and sat on the pavement for a while to stake our claim to the space. Lots of other people were doing the same and the pavement was soon crowded, but we had managed to get a spot in the front row. However, we soon stood up again as there was a lot going on and the pavement was cold and very hard. When the paperboys appeared in the early hours we bought a couple of newspapers and placed them on the paving stones, curled up on the pavement and had a snooze, but I don't think we really got to sleep; there was too much activity going on and we were too uncomfortable. It became very exciting when the newspaper boys began shouting out that Edmund Hillary and Tensing, his Nepalese Sherpa, had reached the top of Mount Everest. Together, they had conquered this mountain, and the news had arrived just a few hours before the Queen's Coronation. Everybody cheered. The weather had been dull and there were a few brief showers, but this cheered us all up and the atmosphere soon changed to one of expectancy as more people began to arrive at the north transept entrance to the Abbey.

We were wide-awake now, as we watched the various guests and dignitaries arriving in large cars throughout the early part of the morning. At last we heard the sound of the drums and trumpets in the distance and knew that the Royal Procession was on its way, with all the carriages seating kings and queens from many countries, other dignitaries and representatives from the Commonwealth countries whose names were mostly unknown to us. The weather was cold and grew more showery as the morning wore on, and I can recall the Queen of Tonga, a huge lady sitting on her own in, if I remember correctly, a rather small open carriage, braving the rain and the chill of England in June. The wonderful golden coach with the Queen inside appeared at last. We were able to see it all with a kerbside view as it passed by towards the main doors of the Abbey. It was all vividly memorable for many years, but the memories are now rather hazy.

I made my first friendship since my marriage soon after this when a young couple moved into a house on the opposite side of the road. After a little while I called on them, taking with me a bag of plums from our garden as a welcome gift. We soon made friends, and Pat became a source of help and wisdom after I had my first baby a couple of years later. Our husbands soon met, and a long-lasting friendship developed between the four of us. I remember a Saturday evening visit to London with Pat and David, when we walked down Regent Street to an Indian restaurant – unique, or at least very rare at that time – called Veeraswamy's, where we had a very hot curry meal (too hot for my taste, but it was an experience).

Two years after our marriage we had our first holiday abroad, which came about quite unexpectedly. I had seen a small advertisement at the bottom of the page in a magazine, giving details of a two-week holiday in Norway, costing £32. We thought it would be wonderful to have a holiday abroad before we settled down and had a family. Tourism was beginning to develop by 1954, but this was a private party, not advertised by one of the large companies that now run so many holidays. It was organised by one retired gentleman, who, I think, arranged these holidays more as a hobby than for profit as a business.

We decided to go for it, got our first passport, and early in June we were in our seats on the overnight coach from Victoria to Newcastle. My husband wore his only suit (his going away one) and I wore a hat, together with my best coat for the journey, and neither of us had much sleep. It seems incredible to recall how one dressed for travelling in those days; there really were no, what we would now call, informal clothes, but we preferred to wear, rather than to pack, our 'best' clothes. The following morning we met the rest of the party of twenty, and discovered we were the only married couple amongst the eight younger people in the group. The S.S. Venus took us across the North Sea to Stavanger where we stayed the night before we began our tour.

We travelled in a small coach to a landing stage, where we embarked in a small open-deck ferryboat and sailed through the grand Suldal Gateway on the Hardanger fjord. We found our coach awaiting us at the next landing stage and we passed through several small villages, sometimes exchanging our coach for a ferryboat. We viewed the magnificent Seljestad Gorge and visited a wonderful waterfall before an overnight stay. Our party travelled in similar transport for the next day or two before sailing through a smaller fjord to reach the village of Utne, where we were to spend the following week. The ferryboats carried sacks of mail and other goods as well as passengers to remote villages; sometimes a few goats accompanied us on deck; we met a group of school children on the boat one morning who were eager to talk to us, practicing their little bit of English. We met many of the local people, which made the holiday very interesting and added to our pleasure. The journey was an experience far removed from that of present day cruise-ships. From our small boats we were almost in the fjord and could view the magnificent scenery almost from water level, as well as enjoying conversations with the local people and learning a little of how they lived.

The family-run hotel at Utne was an old, unaltered building, which still had a very a traditional interior, with a typical Norwegian stove in the corner of the main room that provided central heating for the whole house. The proprietors of the hotel at Utne were very welcoming, and the waitresses were charming and looked so attractive wearing their traditional costume. The travel, the scenery and the food were all such new and interesting experiences. A magnificent smorgasbord was spread over the dining table for breakfast, including a large bowl of stewed rhubarb – which my husband loved. It all looked attractive, but I didn't care much for many of the various ways of eating herring, and wasn't overwhelmed with Norwegian cheese. I have no recollection of what our other meals were like. Tourism was not apparent in this remote place in Norway, and we felt we were simply guests. I wonder whether this traditional building still exists, or whether a large, impersonal modern hotel has replaced it.

The Norwegians we met were very friendly and very kindly disposed to British folk after their war experiences. During our week at Utne we visited Ulvik, now a large tourist resort but then undeveloped, and gazed in amazement at Fossli Falls and enjoyed the beautiful local scenery. Our love of mountain walking really began at Utne, where we clambered up to the snowline on the mountain behind our hotel one day, paddled in the icy water in the pools and streams made from the melting snow and threw snowballs at each other. This was on my birthday and we were playing in the snow in the middle of June! It was exhilarating after our day's hard walking. No one else in the party had ventured beyond the local tourist attractions.

The roads were sometimes almost unnavigable, just single tracks along a mountain edge, or beside gushing streams. The mountain snows were melting and the streams were full in June. Sometimes we peered out of the windows of our little coach to see the steep slope of an evergreen forest immediately below us as we clung firmly to our seats.

Several of us went on an unescorted trip to another village in this rural area one morning, travelling on a local bus, and it half-tipped over the edge of the narrow, muddy, single-track lane on our return journey to our hotel. We were teetering over the edge and we were asked to sit still in this vehicle until assistance arrived. We were told not to move while the driver tried to rustle up some help to get us out of our predicament, but to keep absolutely still in case we jolted the bus and caused it to tip over into the valley below. We were literally looking out of the windows at a deep ravine below us, with a forest of young pine trees partially obscuring our view. The delay seemed interminable, but help came at last in the form of a substitute bus. The two drivers somehow cranked our bus up a little and we were told to move very cautiously towards the exit, where we were helped out of the bus. When we arrived back at Utne we were pleased to find that our lunch had been kept for us. I hope they retrieved the bus before it tipped right over. It was quite a frightening experience.

On a return visit to Norway many years later we discovered that the old main road we had travelled on when we were driven to Bergen at the end of our holiday was now redundant. A little bit of it had been left, and had been made into a tourist attraction; it was now an unofficial, short-term, tourist-coach lay-by. A tunnel had recently been excavated through the mountain and two new safe carriageways built through it. Before our coach driver drove into the new tunnel he pulled into the lay-by, to show us the disused remnant of the old road, now a showpiece for tourists. Everyone trooped off the coach to gaze in wonder at the fragment of the old road ahead that was cordoned off. It still clung to the side of the mountain for a short distance before it fell away towards a yawning chasm below. We recalled our previous journey in 1954 when we had travelled to Bergen in the small, rather dilapidated, old Norwegian bus, as it clung to the edge of this self-same very narrow road. We held our breath, scarcely daring to look out of the window, as the bus swung round the bends, while the driver shouted to us over his shoulder that there had been many who had fallen into the valley below over the years and lost their lives.

We went back to our seats in our new comfortable coach with gratitude that we had not been among those who had died on that old, narrow dangerous road. We felt reassured as we drove on in safety through the newly opened, tunnelled highway into Bergen.

Our holiday in 1954 ended with a day in Bergen. We were sitting in a little coffee shop with Ellen, Philip and Ken, from our party, after we had visited the famous fish market. We were wondering what we should do with the free day, as our holiday money had run out and the weather was cold, wet and windy. A Norwegian gentleman was sitting at our table, and overheard – and understood - our conversation. He began chatting to us and asked us what we had seen in Bergen, and we told him. He immediately politely excused himself and went outside, spoke to a taxi driver, gave him some money and told the driver to take us to see the local sites. We were overwhelmed with this kindness and generosity, quickly finished our coffee, thanked the stranger and all piled into the car. We were driven off to Greig's home, which was open to the public; we had a tour round the house and were shown his composing hut in the grounds. We were then driven on to visit an historic Norwegian Stave church. The driver took us back to the dockside, ready for our journey home. We couldn't believe the stranger's kindness in the café, who paid for us to have this free tour before the S.S. Leda brought us back to England. We couldn't thank him again because he had left the café.

Ellen lived in Scotland and Philip lived in the south of England. They were both singles, but we could see that a friendship was developing between them on this holiday. We kept in touch with them and from our correspondence I grew aware that romance was developing. Their Norwegian holiday resulted very happily in their marriage and Ellen moved to Kent. I am still in contact with her but very sadly her husband died many years ago and she is now living back in Edinburgh.

This was our first holiday abroad, and our, as yet unborn, children were well in their teens before we had our second. But within a fortnight my husband was once again in Europe, this time in Switzerland. On his first day back at work after our holiday he learned that he had to go to Switzerland to undertake high altitude tests on an aircraft engine that was being developed at Hatfield. The engine was to be tested in the special cold chamber test facilities that were used by a Swiss aircraft company on an airfield near Lucerne. We felt very sad that after a very memorable holiday we were so soon parted.

Two weeks later my husband flew out to Lucerne. We wrote to each other, but we were not on the phone at home, so were unable speak to each other for the next eight weeks. I went back to Harley Street for two weeks in August to fill in while my successor had her holiday, but although the surroundings were familiar, it didn't seem the same; it was no longer my office and I noticed the absence of daylight much more than when I had worked there full-time. My ex-boss was on holiday too, so life was pretty quiet, with a locum seeing any patients who were in need.

At the end of his two months abroad, Maurice came home at the end of the summer and was given a few days leave, but he was soon very busy at work preparing for a second spell of work abroad. Soon he returned to Lucerne for another two months. It was sad that so soon after a wonderful, memorable holiday abroad, we were parted for two lengthy periods.

Chapter Ten

LIFE CHANGES

My husband returned to Switzerland at the end of September and not long afterwards I realised I was pregnant. No more jaunts abroad for me for a while! Apart from a letter telling my husband the news, I told no one that I was expecting a baby until after he had returned home in December, not even my father or my mother-in-law. Maybe she guessed, and my father may have been aware of my horrible morning sickness and knew what it indicated. I didn't go to the doctor until after Maurice came home. I had felt too embarrassed to make it known to anyone whilst my husband was abroad. I am sure I would have told my mother if she had been around, although I don't think that thought occured to me then.

Maurice and I were unable to have a single telephone conversation during the entire period he was away. What changes there have been in communication since then; not only in telephone usage, mobiles, emails etc., but also in the actual expectancy of having constant communication. We didn't have a telephone in our home until 1956, and even then the phone was not used for long conversations. When my, then unborn, son was at university eighteen years later, we kept in touch with him through weekly letters. The 'phone was only used in an emergency – such as when funds occasionally ran out at the end of term. (I do remember receiving a surprise telephone call from him late one afternoon asking me how to cook braised lambs' hearts! His landlady was on holiday and he was experimenting with some of his mum's – originally my mother-in-law's – recipes!)

My husband flew home from Lucerne a few days before Christmas and I went to meet him on a bus. I sat in the observation room of the, then, very modest London Airport, sipping tea in the café from a china cup, watching the planes land before his flight came in. It was all very peaceful and civilised, and is an almost impossible memory when I think of the hubbub at Heathrow today. We met, and came home on the top deck of a 140 bus, pleased to be together again, exchanging our news. Maurice had had wonderful experiences at the weekends in Switzerland, going up Mount Pilatus and the Rigi mountain with his Swiss and English colleagues, seeing the Christmas decorations in Lucerne and the mountains covered in snow, whilst being superbly looked after in the lovely old hotel in which de Havilland's (or its' Swiss counterpart) had arranged for him to stay. Great time – I just wish I had been there. We visited Lucerne together twenty years later.

We told the news of my pregnancy to our friends and relations soon after Christmas. I wrote to my cousin Daphne to tell her my news. She replied and greatly surprised me by telling me that she and her husband had just had a letter from his cousin, Dorothy, to inform them that she was also expecting a baby. Quite remarkably Dorothy's cousin, Leslie, was married to my cousin, Daphne! Even more remarkably we not only both lived in the same town, but we both lived in the same road! I began to look out for a lady with a big bump walking up Kenton Lane to the shops. I hadn't noticed any expectant mums in our area and I found it quite easy to approach this obviously pregnant lady (with a bump like mine) and ask if her name was Dorothy. Dorothy immediately knew who I must be, and we developed a friendship that lasted until she very sadly died some years later. It was a very strange coincidence that we had met because my cousin was married to her cousin, made even more unusual in that we discovered that we lived about thirty houses apart in the same road.

I began to make preparations for our first child who was due at the beginning of June. I was busy sewing babies' vyella nightdress on my Singer sewing machine and hand knitting woolly vests and little matinee jackets. We bought a smart black Harris pram and a modern carrycot, loads of terry nappies as well as muslin ones. Pat lent me a baby's bath. There were no local informal anti-natal classes then, just occasional check-ups at the hospital.

My baby should have been born in Edgware General Hospital. I began labour very early on a June morning before it was light. Maurice hurried to the 'phone box outside our local shops to telephone for an ambulance, and soon I set off with my little case, rather frightened as to what lay ahead. The noisy, bumpy vehicle roared along the empty roads until it stopped with a lurch when we reached the hospital entrance. The male ambulance attendant who was sitting next to the driver, got out, banged the door shut noisily, and I was left in almost complete darkness, with my ears pricked trying to understand what the loud conversation could be about that I could hear outside. I wondered what was wrong. When the attendant came back he told me that the maternity unit was full. He had to take me elsewhere. The ambulance door was banged shut once again, and off we drove in the half-light to I knew not where, as I sat in the back with my large bump, feeling like a sack of rejected mail.

I had no idea where I was when the ambulance driver eventually pulled up with a jerk. The attendant opened the doors at the back once again, and I was told I had arrived. But, where was I? I went inside this apparently very large house, said who I was to someone in the entrance hall, and asked where I was. A nurse told me I was in Bushey Maternity Hospital, but I had no idea exactly where Bushey was. It was very cold that June morning, not at all summery. I had got very cold on my early morning drive, and my reception seemed pretty cool too. I was taken to a small room, told to get undressed, get into bed, and await examination. After this I was left alone to proceed with my labour, and told to ring the bell when I needed help. I didn't know when I was considered to need help, and didn't want to appear to make a fuss as my labour pains grew stronger. I felt cold and shivery in bed with inadequate bedcovering, so I got out of bed, put on my thin summer dressing-gown, pulled the blanket round my shoulders and walked around the tiny room, tense with cold and apprehension, coping with my ever-increasing contractions. The room was so small there was really no space to walk about, so I got back into bed with my dressing gown still on, and pulled the small, thin blanket over me. Did I need help? Should I ring the bell? I didn't know when I was supposed to need help. I didn't want to bother them. I was reluctant then to ask for help, and realise that I have remained the same throughout my life.

 I could hear distant sounds that didn't help me to relax at all, but eventually a midwife remembered me, burst into my room and almost immediately shouted out, 'Quick! She's about to deliver'. Someone rushed along the corridor, and I was wheeled rapidly in my bed to the delivery room. I was told afterwards that they had been very busy – too busy, I think, to look after me. I had kept quiet, not made a fuss, and in their busyness I really think I had been forgotten. After all, they weren't expecting me. I had been put into the spare room!

Childbirth was not a well-supported experience in those days, certainly not for me, anyway. I had been left entirely alone and had had nobody with me throughout my labour – so much for midwives, I thought. There was no time for preparation or deep breathing, gas and air, pushing, or not pushing – the baby was really on the way! It was all a bit scary. My baby was born at around mid-day but after showing him to me he was immediately whisked away, while I was given some stitches before being wheeled into a large ward. I didn't see my newborn son again until he was brought to me at the evening feeding time.

When Maurice had telephoned Edgware General Hospital in his lunch hour to see how I was getting on, he was told I had been sent to another hospital in Bushey, which is near Watford. He had never heard of this maternity hospital, and didn't quite know where it was. I don't know exactly when, or how, he heard that he had a son. He had to wait until after his day's work was over before finding his way to the hospital on his motorbike – no Sat. Nav. in those days, and I don't think he even had a road map. He arrived at the end of the evening visiting hour having got lost on the way. He was dressed in his motorbike gear, carrying his crash helmet and smelling of petrol. A nurse had just put my baby into my arms, as it was the evening feeding time. It was the first time I had held him since he had been born earlier in the day. I don't know who I was most surprised to see, my husband or my new baby!

All the babies were looked after in the nursery by the nurses, and were brought to the mothers at regular feeding times during the day. New mothers were not allowed out of bed for the first week, and had to stay in hospital for a second week. No wonder the maternity ward was full at Edgware General Hospital, and the nurses at the extension were too rushed with other confinements to keep an eye on me - they already had a nursery full of new babies to care for and a large ward full of new mums too. We were still in the baby boom era. After a week in bed the new mothers were allowed to walk along the corridor and look at their babies in their cots through a glass wall. We peered through the glass at about fifteen or twenty new-born babes, neatly tucked into their little cots, wondering which baby was ours. You could barely see their faces, and we found it was quite difficult to decide who was your baby. They were, I hope, cared for during the night, and given a bottle if needed.

My baby had great difficulty in latching on to the idea of breast-feeding, and even after I was allowed to get up I continued to have difficulty in getting him to suckle. I think I should have been expressing milk, but nobody suggested it, and I had no idea that this was possible. I developed a high temperature during my second week, and had a persistent headache, felt uncomfortable, and couldn't be discharged. At last, one morning in my third week in hospital my temperature was normal and I was told I could go home immediately. My husband was contacted – but I don't know how - and he arrived later in the morning in a taxi to bring me home. I didn't feel too good after we had had some lunch, but Maurice had to get back to work in the afternoon.

New fathers were the only visitors allowed in the maternity hospital, so my father saw his first grandson when he returned home from work that evening. I wonder whether my mother might would have enjoyed holding her grandson. My father told me many years afterwards that he was 'worried stiff' when I had told him I was pregnant. When I asked him why, he had replied that he was 'worried stiff that you would go like your mother'. That is the only clue that I have that my mother's mental illness possibly began as post-natal depression, and that severe psychotic illness developed subsequently. Would this have become her 'life sentence' if it had been known how to treat post-natal depression in the 1930s? What a blessing that this condition is now understood and can be properly treated!

There was a lot to do after returning home, and a lot of men's clothing needed washing after my absence from home for more than a fortnight, but by the time Maurice came back from work that evening I was in severe pain in my breast, I didn't know how to manage with trying to feed my baby, let alone doing the washing or cooking a meal. I had had a difficult afternoon. A breast abscess seemed to be developing. Two men who were not at all domesticated, who knew little about new babies, breast abscesses, (neither did I!) or new mothers, were not the most comforting or helpful folk to be around me, and although they were concerned it was very difficult for them to understand or know what to do. How could I cope with looking after my menfolk, washing the baby's nappies, and bathing, dressing and feeding this new member of our family when in such pain?

When Maurice came home from work the next evening he realised that the doctor should be called in; kaolin poultices were prescribed to put on the abscess – very difficult for my husband to accomplish - but the infection grew nastier and nastier. We got through the weekend, and when the doctor returned on the Monday she prescribed penicillin, but I reacted badly to it and it was stopped. The huge variety of antibiotics that are now available had not been developed in the 1950s and the following day my new baby and I had to be admitted, this time actually to Edgware General Hospital, for immediate surgery. A general anaesthetic was necessary. I had never been in hospital before my confinement, and here I was in hospital for the second time in one month, and quite scared at what was to come. Although I had worked in the medical field for some years, surgery was a rather frightening word that had not been in the vocabulary I had used during my years in Harley Street and Weymouth Street. I had never worked amongst surgeons. I had no idea what removing a breast abscess would entail and, inwardly, I was scared stiff.

Nowadays, a breast abscess would not be allowed to develop without early treatment with antibiotics, and I think much more care would be taken with new mothers to ensure that such conditions did not occur, and I believe that my abscess was really due to neglect and inadequate care in the hospital.

The horrible abscess was removed and a drain put in to clear any residual infection, and I spent the next few days trying to change nappies, bathe and feed my baby one-handed – and one-armed. It was quite a difficult procedure when holding such a precious, tiny, bundle. My right arm was not very comfortable when nursing my baby while at the same time having to avoid hurting my tender bosom, or dislodge the rather bulky draining tube. Three other new mothers were similarly affected (all from the same maternity hospital) and we looked after our new infants, all of us totally inexperienced, so most probably a little incompetent, in a little room beside the sluice, just beyond the double doors of the ward. Our nerves were continually shattered by the noise of the constant banging of these double-doors night and day, as nurses rushed in and out of the busy surgical ward. We, the new mums, were ignored and left to fend for ourselves. It was like being in a prison cell, as we tried to care for our babies in such confined surroundings, with no room to move around, feeling awkward, disheartened and a bit freakish as we half breast-fed and half bottle-fed our babies. It was a nightmare.

A day later and the other two mums were discharged, but I think my drain was removed too soon and my breast didn't heal. The new 'treatment' then prescribed for me was to spend an hour each day, seated on a bit of flat roof at the top of Edgware General Hospital, bare-breasted in the midday sun at the height of the summer. A chair was placed on a patch of flat roof and a small screen was placed around it, and I sat with the sun shining on my bare bosom, watching the traffic roar along the Edgware Road far beneath me. The sun was supposed to encourage the wound to heal. I could see and trust I could not be seen, but I felt solitary and exposed. Nobody had as yet considered the dangers of exposure to the mid-day sun.

All this anxiety certainly removed some of the delight my husband and I should have had at this time. We were relieved when I was eventually allowed home, and we thought we would be able to settle down to enjoy our baby at last, but I found that this enjoyment was fraught with the weariness of coping with a very restless baby who cried a lot both night and day. I had broken nights, sometimes getting up several times a night to pick him up, feed him, change his nappy, give him a cuddle, and when he was a little older we would look out of the window at all the darkened houses of our neighbours and those on the opposite side of the road as I softly whispered to him as he nestled in my arms that. 'Auntie Pat was asleep, Mrs. Brown was asleep, Mrs. Holding was asleep, Mrs. Jones was fast asleep, Mrs. Siggers was asleep and ...all our neighbours were sound asleep'. Then I would lay him gently down in his cot, stroke his cheek and soothe him to sleep – for a little while, and then he was off again.

After the morning bath and feed it was customary to put one's baby in his pram outside the front door, where he would have a morning sleep, and Andrew had a good snooze in the open air while I got on with the housework and the washing. But he was soon awake and restless. When he was a little older he soon grew bored with his little baby toys, and I couldn't think how to amuse him. He was happier when being taken for a walk in his pram, and really contented when he was old enough to be sat up and strapped safely in his pram and look at the world around him. I must have walked miles during that period; he stopped crying as soon as he was 'on the move' – I think he has been busy and 'on the move' ever since.

Feeding was a somewhat complicated business, as Andrew was part breast-fed, and part Ostermilk-bottle-fed, as I could only provide a one-sided natural feed. I don't think the approved practice at that time of strict four-hour periods feeding times was appropriate for my lively son. He would have preferred more frequent snacks and also the present day busyness and stimulation, with his mum spending much of her of time playing with and cuddling her infant. That didn't happen in the 50s' before the days of washing machines and refrigerators and a weekly supermarket shop. Shopping for food was done every day. There was not much spare time to play with one's baby or encourage their mental development, although more good toys were becoming available in the shops.

Housework included the daily boiling of nappies in a large aluminium bucket on top of the stove. New babies wore Viyella nightdresses, and baby boys were dressed in 'romper suits' during the day when they were a little older. These were an absolute pain to iron before easy-iron cotton and man-

Sheila Brook

made fabrics appeared. This applied to shirts too; practically every item of clothing needed ironing in those days. No wonder many mums were unable to provide enough nourishment for their offspring; 'home-made' milk disappeared and the baby was put on the bottle. I think we were all worn out ourselves, and my milk supply soon diminished and Ostermilk took over.

When Andrew had given up having a night feed, my dear father gave up his little bedroom once again, so that his baby grandson could be put down to sleep in his carrycot in what we always called the 'little room' - the bedroom over the hall. My father was once more sleeping on the put-u-up in his dining room.

I seemed to take quite a while to recover after my first confinement. My fretful baby didn't help; my sleep was disturbed nearly every night as I paid several visits to his bedroom, standing on the cold lino trying to coax him back to sleep. We had these broken nights with our first son until shortly after his little brother arrived three years later. When Ian was three months old we transferred his carrycot into his brother's bedroom, and he was soon blissfully asleep each evening. Andrew was by now in a large cot, and he suddenly began to sleep through the night. I always felt that Andrew was, in his childish way, comforted when knowing there was someone else in the room with him – his three-month-old brother. Or maybe he woke and in a sub-conscious way realised that if he made a noise his little brother would wake and start to yell! So maybe he kept quiet and then dozed off to sleep again. Who knows? But quiet nights at last came to our household, and I was able to get a full night's sleep.

I had made no friends when I was in the maternity hospital, which was not in my local area; there were no health visitor calls once I came home, and no new-mother's support groups then. As long as the baby was gaining weight when taken to the clinic each week new mothers were expected to cope on their own and learn as they went along. I was very pleased to have Dorothy's friendship. Her son was born less than a month after mine and was a very contented baby. When we visited each other, my son was nearly always crying, but Martin was very placid, sitting up in his pram smiling benignly at everyone, or propped up in a corner of a chair, cooing contentedly, or fast asleep. What bliss – to have a baby who slept! The two babies became good friends as they grew up, and eventually started school together.

Pat was another very supportive friend who lived opposite our house. She had a family of daughters, and Andrew had many happy times when he was a little boy, playing with them while we chatted over a cup of coffee. She and her husband David became firm friends, as did Dorothy and her husband Ted. They all lived in Kenton Lane. Pat's mother visited her regularly, but I never thought that I missed out on this motherly support, and yet… did I? I have a faint recollection of feeling how lucky she was to have her mother visiting her, and I think I used to feel…something; was it a sense of something I had missed when I saw Pat's mother? I really don't know.

I bumped into an old classmate one day, also named Dorothy, as she was wheeling her baby in his pram around our local Woolworth's. We almost literally bumped into each other's prams, but although we had been in the same class at Chandos School we didn't know each other well until this casual meeting. We began to play tennis together in our local park, leaving our respective offspring safely strapped in their prams outside the courts. They should have become tennis champions with these opportunities of studying our play – or at least enthusiastic supporters, with this early introduction to the game as spectators, but they were obviously not impressed. After a few weeks our babies grew bored, wanted to be out of their prams to develop their own skills in their newfound crawling ability, and our tennis had to cease.

Nevertheless our friendship continued, and developed with afternoon cups of tea in each other's homes, as our children played, and later on when our husbands met, it grew into another friendship. Dorothy and Frank introduced us to the game of Contraband, when we had a hilarious time with them at Christmas before they moved away from the district. We kept in touch over the years, but sadly this friend Dorothy also died in her early sixties. She was a lovely, carefree lady, who had brought up four children and was always sunny, warm and reliable. How odd that both my friends named Dorothy died in their middle age. They were very different in character, but I missed them both, and they are not forgotten.

My mother-in-law lived nearby, and we used to have tea with each other on alternate weeks. She enjoyed holding her new grandson, watching him as he played with his toys, and reproving him when he was a little older saying, 'All right! I'll remember…' accompanied by a wagging finger when he did something naughty. She never did (remember)!

My father and my father-in-law got on well with each other; I think they were both rather lonely men, and it is good to think back and realise that they were quite good buddies. We sometimes sat together on warm summer Sunday evenings in the little arbour my father-in-law had made in his garden. It was covered in roses and honeysuckle and the scent on warm evenings was delectable. It must have been a comfort for my father to have another man to chat with, although I don't think he would have chatted about my mother to my in-laws. She, poor lady, was still an unspoken subject. One didn't talk about personal matters between families in those days. I didn't know much about my husband's family background either.

My mother had to wait a few more years before she was able to meet her grandsons. When her second grandson was about eighteen months old we did meet, and she held Ian on her knee. Many years had passed by, and I not seen her since before the war. There was no photo of her on display in my childhood home and I had no picture of her in my mind.

The year after our first son was born my father and my husband shared the cost of £200 for a second-hand pre-war Austin Cambridge. My husband drove it to Hatfield each day for one week, and my father drove it to his shop in Ealing the next. Maurice had to take a driving test, but my father was exempt, as he had driven since before tests were enforced. Maurice did all the maintenance on the car, bending over the engine in a white overall, or lying in the driveway on his back beneath the car giving it a service. On one occasion after a day's work he spent the entire night doing a de-coke (whatever that may mean!) on the engine, before we drove off to Essex to see his grandmother. I lay in bed throughout the night, hearing the metallic clash as spanners and other tools were dropped onto the concrete drive, wondering if he would ever come to bed, and worrying whether the car would be ready to drive in the morning, and almost wishing we had never bought it – but yes, it was ready, and we did visit his grandmother and she was able to meet her great-grandson. Thank goodness car engines are far too complicated for home servicing nowadays, but I think my husband enjoyed maintaining his own car, and his engineering background made the exercise a challenge – but even, possibly, to him, an enjoyable one.

I didn't take my driving test for another two years. I didn't have the opportunity to do much driving, as the car was in use throughout the week by my two menfolk. Local shops were near at hand and I did the daily shopping, filling the large basket fixed over the handlebars of the pram with fresh bread, vegetables and meat etc. It was loaded – or overloaded - when I added our groceries and potatoes once a week.

As yet we had no fridge, but how glad I was when we were able to afford a washing machine before our second son was born. Monday was washing day, when the machine was wheeled into place in front of the sink. It was about a metre square in size and the lid was hooked on to the back of the machine when in use to form a tray to hold the washing after it had been put through the wringer. The little hand wringer was lifted out of the tub before beginning the week's washing. A short hose was fixed to the hot tap and led into the tub. The white cottons, sheets etc. were washed first and the more delicate articles having the last, coolest, but dirtiest water. A lot less water was used than nowadays in the weekly wash. Nappies were soaked in a bucket of disinfectant outside the back door, then rinsed and boiled on the hob in fresh water and soap powder the following day. Washing was still hard work.

Our first holiday in our £200 pre-war car was to Torquay when our son was not quite firm on his feet. No seat belts or car seats for babies then; Andrew sat on my lap in the front seat of the car. As we drove through heavy rain over Dartmoor we discovered that the flooring leaked, and when we drove through large puddles I had to lift my feet off the floor of the car as the water seeped through. Andrew was a plump baby when he was just over a year old, but we managed to reach the top of Hay Tor on Dartmoor with the baby in the pushchair on one fine afternoon, and so continued our love of getting to the highest spots wherever possible on our holidays.

Chapter Eleven

ALL CHANGE!

We had been married for three years when our son was born, and were still living in the first floor rooms in my father's house when Andrew had his second birthday.. Our living room became more crowded at Christmas, when we found room for a decorated Christmas tree, a high chair, baby toys, and, for Andrew's first birthday, a toy Airedale dog on wheels to encourage his walking. A further year of carrying Andrew's toys and high chair up and down the stairs, as well as all the food and crockery whenever we ate a meal together or had visitors, made us feel that it was impossible to live like this on a long-term basis. Accommodation was still very difficult to find, and we couldn't afford to take on a mortgage and buy our own house yet. We also felt it would have been unkind to leave my father to cope on his own. I think we had just accepted the situation, and at the time didn't think we would ever have our own home. Grown up sons or daughters cared for their elderly relatives then, (as even my comparatively wealthy ex-boss did, with his very elderly aunt living in his home) and men were not expected to be able to look after themselves. We didn't dream of leaving my father to cope on his own.

I don't remember whose idea it was but eventually an acceptable solution was found, and it was decided that we would move our living room furniture into my father's downstairs rear reception room. He never used this room, which had always been known as the 'drawing room', and I have no memory of it being used when I was little. I think it was a 1930s version of the Victorian 'parlour', only used on special occasions – of which my father had experienced few. We agreed that my father's very old, leather-backed armchairs with the squashy velvet cushions and my mother's old Singer sewing machine should be disposed of, and his more up-to-date, just pre-war Berkeley armchairs and my mother's piano were moved into the front room. We managed to roll up our carpet, get it downstairs, unroll it in the rear reception room, and then carried all our furniture into our new living room. It all fitted in very well. I made a pair of heavy curtains to cover the glazed doors that divided the two reception rooms, which gave us both some privacy. My father was now able to sleep in the main bedroom once more, instead of on the put-u-up in his dining room. He had been unable to use his own bedroom for so many years. His living room in the front of the house was lovely and sunny, and looked much nicer with more modern furniture in it and there was still space for his dining-room table and chairs. The house space was better used; everyone had a proper bedroom and both Maurice and I, and my father, had a downstairs living room. The new accommodation was much better for all of us and made daily life much easier.

What a nightmare it had been before we moved downstairs! Every time we had visitors to tea all the food had been carried upstairs. I invited my ex-boss and his wife to dinner shortly after I was married, and I cringe as I think of the performance it must have seemed to them, as Maurice and I carried all the warmed dishes and the food upstairs for our meal. I hope everything was still hot as we ate roast beef and vegetables on the beautiful dinner service they had given us as a wedding present. It must have been quite an experience for them to be eating a meal in the first floor room of a modest semi-detached home, with dining room suite, two fireside chairs and a bookcase crowded into one room! We continued to live *en famille* for another six years, eating at ours' or my dad's dining table and listening to one or another's radios in the evening. As yet there was no television in either of our homes.

My husband, my father and I sometimes visited the aunt and uncle with whom I had lived at times when I was a child. My uncle was then a teacher in London. I was living with them during the summer of 1939 when he and my aunt were evacuated to Devon with his school immediately after the outbreak of the war. My father had to find a new home for me at very short notice as my mother had had a further severe nervous breakdown. I had missed these relatives during the six years of war, and think that my aunt must have been almost a substitute mother to me when I was very small. We visited them regularly after their return to their home in Beckenham after the war. It had always been an awkward journey, either by rail in earlier years or even by road after we had a car.

My aunt and uncle came to see us shortly before Andrew was born, and I had quite a shock when, over lunch, my uncle told me that as he had now retired they had decided to move to Bexhill-on-sea. The long trail from Kenton, north of London, to Beckenham, then in Kent (now both part of Greater London) then seemed no distance compared with a drive to Bexhill-on-sea so far away, and I felt rather bereft.

I didn't see my aunt and uncle for a couple of years after they moved, but when Andrew was about two, they kindly invited me   to have a week's holiday with them in their new home. They wanted to meet their new great-nephew too. These relatives were childless, but they had looked after a nephew whose mother was ill with tuberculosis for a long time before I was born; sadly both the mother, and a few years later, the nephew, Bernard, died. Some years after this they had cared for me several times during the 1930s. They would appear to have sacrificed having their own children in older to care for their relatives' offspring. It was a very kind gesture for this elderly (well, they were quite a bit younger than my present age – but they seemed 'elderly' to me then!) childless couple to have another youngster invading their home for a week.

Maurice drove us down on the Saturday, and stayed for the weekend. Bexhill did seem a long way away then. It was quite a complicated route in the 1950s, even after we had driven across London, before we reached Bexhill. (Motorways – even with their hold-ups - have made travelling so much simpler) Maurice left on the Sunday evening, and I discovered on the Monday morning that my uncle had hired a beach hut for my two-year-old and me, when after breakfast he drove us down to the seafront. Between us we carried the pushchair over the pebbles, together with all the other paraphernalia that goes with a toddler, helping Andrew over the hard, knobbly stones, and eventually reached our beach hut, which seemed a long way from the promenade. My uncle returned home for a peaceful morning with my aunt, thinking I was having a pleasant holiday, some relaxation, and was taking the sea air, and that Andrew was going to have fun at the seaside.

But we were marooned, stuck on a deserted late-September beach, surrounded by large pebbles that spread before us across a wide stretch of stony beach towards the distant sea, the sole occupants of a line of otherwise empty beach huts. A strong, chilly wind was blowing and the sunshine disappeared as grey clouds swept across the sky. What were we to do for the rest of the morning? Andrew couldn't make sand pies without any sand, nor could we go for a walk on these knobbly pebbles. I was stuck! It was no place for a fidgety toddler who couldn't stand this hard, uneven base for his little feet, who was supposed at some time in the morning to have a nap in his rather uncomfortable 1950s pushchair, which had nothing like the comfortable padded seating, good design, or the safety measures of today's baby carriages. I couldn't leave all our stuff in the beach hut and carry Andrew and the pushchair to the promenade to take him for a little stroll. We were both trapped in the confines of the beach hut.

It was low tide; I couldn't get Andrew to the water's edge over all those pebbles so he couldn't even paddle. Oh! for a sandy beach, where we could have made a sandcastle and he could have made sand-pies, or we could have walked across the sand to the sea and paddled together. Bexhill may be '-on-sea', but it is also '–on-pebbles' and the sea is a long way away at low tide. I grew cold as the morning dragged by. There was nobody to talk to in this end-of-season period as no other beach-hut was occupied.

It was a very long morning, and I was very relieved to see my uncle arrive to pick us up at lunchtime. He assumed we had had a pleasant morning, but I had just been looking at the horizon and my son had shown his displeasure as only two-year-olds can. My childless relatives did not appreciate that their kindness in paying for a beach hut was more like banishment – even a punishment - for Andrew and me. I couldn't disillusion them, but I would have been much happier walking along the promenade, or strolling round the shops, finding things to look at and talk about to Andrew. My uncle had been a teacher, but teaching maths to senior boys was entirely different from entertaining and occupying toddler boys! We had to get through the rest of the week, and the September weather remained blustery.

My aunt always rested on her bed in the afternoons, so Andrew and I played quietly for an hour after lunch while my uncle dozed, with the newspaper spread over his lap. After her rest my Auntie Ada made a flask of tea, and off we went in the car; 'Bert' took us for a 'little drive' – just as we had in Beckenham when I was a small child! Going out for a drive in the afternoon was still a pastime in those days, and I think post-war motoring was still a bit of a novelty.

We parked at the top of Galley Hill and gazed out at the sea while we all had a cup of tea. This was my relatives' regular outing, which they really enjoyed after their retirement to the coast. Auntie Ada still had her smart little hat on, and Uncle Bert still wore his leather gauntlet gloves for driving just as they had done when I was living with them before the war. Life didn't change much and my relatives' routine remained the same. I know that they enjoyed having Andrew in the home, even though we must have been quite an intrusion into their quiet lives. We were all very fond of these relatives, and my uncle was a particularly kind, quiet, gentle man. He tolerated his nephew sitting on his potty in the kitchen in the mornings, often forgetting Andrew's name and called him Bernard, the name of the other little boy my relatives had informally fostered. Considering their age, their personal childlessness, and the period in which they grew up, I think they were amazingly kind, adaptable and very caring.

Andrew developed a chest infection towards the end of our week's holiday, which developed into a whooping-cough-type cough after we had returned home. The blustery late-summer weather may have affected him. He had recently been immunised against whooping cough, so we presumed it could be a reaction to this, but he was extremely poorly. Whooping cough still occurred then and a single vaccination against this disease, which is now renamed pertussis, had only just been introduced in 1957. He was among the first recipients.

Soon after our return home my husband, my father, and later we learned, my uncle, and I all developed similar symptoms and we were all quite ill with high temperature, vomiting, 'flu-like symptoms and a wracking, whooping type of cough. I think my elderly uncle was very ill. During this period I realised I was pregnant again. I was very sick and ill with unabated sickness twenty-four hours a day, and at first we didn't know whether it was whooping cough or the early signs of pregnancy – I suspected the latter! The slightest movement produced severe vomiting; I couldn't keep any food down and I began to lose weight. I was eventually admitted to a London hospital, and at one stage the removal of the foetus was considered. I had never before heard the term 'abortion'; it was only legal in a life-threatening situation then. I am thankful that I didn't get to the position where I had to make that kind of decision. I was eventually discharged from hospital, but it was nearly Christmas before I felt really well again.

Chapter Twelve

BETTER NEXT TIME AROUND?

The rest of my pregnancy passed without incident; my baby was due in June, so we decided to have a brief holiday at Easter. After I had left work my husband and I had developed a warm friendship with one of my old boss's patients. Some years later they had moved to the island of Jersey and we had been invited to come and see them in their new home. We flew to St. Helier, our first flight for Andrew and me (and for our unborn baby!). Sadly, Mr. B. was terminally ill in hospital by the time our holiday arrived, and my husband went to the hospital to visit him, but on a couple of mornings his wife took us around some of the local beauty spots. She had a large, 1930s, Wolseley car which she assumed that Maurice would drive. Jersey roads were notoriously narrow, but he successfully chauffeured us around the island, with Mrs. B. calling out directions. One morning she led us down a very steep hill to a tiny harbour, with parking along the sea edge of the harbour wall, she assumed that Maurice could safely reverse her car into a parking space! He managed it; and, with his heart in his mouth – and our lives, her car and the deep sea - immediately behind him; it must have been a nightmare, and one that we both remembered. He had had no experience of parking in such dangerous conditions, and certainly not in someone else's car!

This couple had lived not far from our home in Kenton prior to their move to the Channel Islands, and after our marriage we had been invited to tea at their home. As we sat on the bus going to Northwood we had wondered what on earth we were going to be able to talk about with this elderly retired couple that we scarcely knew. On arrival at their home we had found them both most welcoming, Maurice and Mr. B. were soon chatting together about similar interests, and his wife and I got on well. Instead of coming home on the bus, Mr. B kindly drove us, with a cabbage, tomatoes and some fruit grown in their very large garden, in the boot of his car.

We learned that they had lost their only son during the war. He had started his degree course in Cambridge University just before the start of the war, but joined the Air Force when the war began, became a pilot and was killed in one of the big air battles. They were still grieving, but liked to talk to us about their son Martin and I think we became almost like their adopted family. Mrs. B. hand-knitted – in the traditional Jersey manner - a beautiful shawl as a gift when Andrew was born.

I was invited to their home in Northwood for a day when Andrew was still in his carrycot, and Mr. B. drove to my home to collect us. When we arrived at his home I found his wife pulling dead flowers off her pansy plants. She told me that dead-heading these plants would encourage them to continue flowering; I always think of Auntie Phyllis, as she had asked us to call her, when I deadhead pansies. It was the first gardening tip I had been given, and maybe she initiated my subsequent interest in gardening.

A year or two later they decided to spend their remaining years back in her homeland in Jersey, but Auntie Phyllis visited us on several occasions whenever she came to England after her husband died. It was on one of these visits that she said, 'I think it's time you called me Auntie Phyllis'. We felt very touched by this. I remained in contact with my adopted aunt until she died in Jersey many years ago. I never thought to ask her whether she was living in Jersey during the war. People living on the mainland had no idea for many years of the travails of the Channel Islanders during their German occupation.

Only first confinements were allowed in hospital during the baby boom in the fifties, and when I was referred to the maternity clinic at my local hospital I was told that my baby was to be born at home. I was quite pleased to learn this, as I had not had a pleasant experience in hospital with my first confinement. I was determined that this time round all would go well and the way I wanted: I would be comfortable in my own home; I intended to remain dressed, warm, and busy, until the last possible moment.

Once again I went into labour in the early hours of a June morning. My husband brought me my breakfast in bed and waited until my father had left for work before ringing the midwife. We didn't want him to be unduly anxious during his day at work by knowing that I was in labour. Andrew was taken across the road to be looked after by my friend Pat for the morning. Everything was going well until the midwife arrived at about 10.30 a.m. when I discovered that she was not the one I had seen from time to time during my pregnancy. It was Sister Speight's day off. It was the first thing to go wrong.

Her replacement examined me and told Maurice to ring our doctor to inform her that I was two fingers dilated when examined at 10.30 a.m. and that she thought I would 'get going' early in the afternoon. Both the midwife and my doctor were expected to be with me for the birth. The midwife left me to do her very busy double round and she said that she would return at about 2 o'clock. She left a list of contact telephone numbers by the phone in the hall in case of emergency (we were on the phone by 1958), and went off to do her two rounds of new mums. I was sorry Sister Speight wouldn't be with me during my confinement as I had had a little contact with her but had never seen her replacement before. After informing our doctor my husband felt he had a couple of free hours before he would be needed at home, and went off to deal with a little problem at the Edgware factory of de Havilland.

It was a warm and sunny day, unlike my first confinement. To take my mind off my 'inner' labour I did some light household jobs between contractions, and for a while I felt confident, and pleased to think that it would all be over before my father came home from work. My middle-aged spinster doctor arrived. 'You look fine,' she greeted me with a grin. 'That's a good idea,' she continued with a glance at the Hoover in the hall, 'Get your housework done while you can. You won't have much time to spare in the next few weeks'. I told her the midwife was returning at 2 o'clock. She was aware that I was alone in the house, and observed me through another, rather strong, contraction, then told me that she had to get away to a meeting in London, and left.

As soon as I had shut the front door I had a further very strong contraction, and wondered how I was going to last for two or three hours before the midwife returned. I was still leaning against the back of the front door when a few moments later there was a ring at the doorbell. 'Thank goodness', I thought, 'the midwife', but I found that my doctor was on the doorstep. Apparently, she had been sitting in her car, pondering on the strength of my contractions, wondering whether I would be all right to be left until the early afternoon, and had returned to see me through another contraction. I very soon obliged. She asked me again when the midwife was expected to return, and when I told her, she replied, with some hesitation. 'Oh... I should think you will be all right until then' and left to drive to London for her meeting. I thought my contractions were very frequent and awfully strong if I was not expected to 'get going' for another two or three hours, but I presumed that the professionals knew best.

Very soon afterwards I felt an urgent need to go to the toilet, but after I had waddled upstairs I discovered that my 'urge' was actually the baby's head. I had had some difficulty in getting upstairs but now I was afraid to try to go down the stairs again in case in doing so, in stepping down and unbalancing my body, I might damage my baby's head. I was trapped upstairs and didn't know what to do. I had completely forgotten that the phone was downstairs on the window ledge in the hall when I had walked upstairs. I waddled across the landing from the toilet to our bedroom, and yelled for help from the bedroom window, but no one heard me. I opened the window in the front bedroom and shouted from that, but nobody was walking along the street. I grew more frantic as the minutes passed and my contractions increased. I walked very gently to and fro across the landing, was scared to sit, but soon felt so exhausted that I thought I should try to get on to our bed. It was a difficult process, and for a while I was half on and half off the bed. When I was at last lying down, I found I couldn't sit up again. I was still dressed, and grew even more fearful that my underclothes could be stifling the baby, but I couldn't lift myself off the bed to do anything about it. The contractions seemed to have stopped for a while, but I – or rather the baby - seemed stuck half way. I was petrified!

It had developed into a blustery day. I had left the window open, and a sudden blast of wind banged the bedroom door shut. I felt even more trapped. I was beyond yelling for help when I heard the car engine in the drive and knew my husband had returned. I managed to scream at him to bring up some scissors – I needed them to cut my pants off! Having got my behind on the bed I couldn't manage to lift myself up to remove them. Not understanding why I needed scissors, Maurice picked up the kitchen scissors and rushed upstairs, and had to tear down again to get sharper scissors to cut through the material and get my underpants off! It was a nightmare; I don't remember anything from then on until after the baby was born.

As soon as he could leave me Maurice 'phoned the midwife, who was shocked and rather cross to hear that the baby had arrived, and said we should have phoned her at one of the numbers she had left on the hall window ledge; but I had been unable to get downstairs to the 'phone in the hall. She didn't understand the circumstances! She warned him to do nothing until she arrived. Within a few minutes there was a ring at the doorbell; it was the midwife, who rushed up the stairs. When she saw the kitchen scissors lying on the bed, she had a fright, thinking that we had tried to cut the cord with them! The baby was lying quietly on the bed, and I left her to finish things off. I don't really remember anything until I saw her holding up a fine baby boy for me to see. She weighed him in a net bag, before wrapping him up and placing him by my side in bed. She told my husband to inform my doctor that I needed some stitches, which she was unauthorised to give. We were relieved that neither baby nor mother appeared any the worse for the experience, and I was just thankful that our new baby son was whole and healthy.

At the time, and afterwards, I made light of my experience and made a joke about it, but - what a day I had had. What a scare! Later on I was not sure how much sound had come out when I was screaming for help. I think that when you are very frightened, fear perhaps stops the sound coming out. But either way there was nobody around at the time to hear me.

My doctor telephoned about an hour after the birth. She told Maurice that she had been rather concerned about the strong contractions I had been having earlier in the day, and was wondering how I was getting on. She appeared surprised to learn that the baby had already been born an hour previously, although I don't think we took note of the actual moment whilst in the throes of delivery and its' aftermath. Maurice told her I needed some stitches, and the doctor said she would be unable to do this until she returned from her conference in the evening. (This was in the days of single doctor GP practices.)

Where is the Key?

It was about 8 p.m. when the doctor arrived. My father was back at home from work, my three-year-old son was in bed, and our newborn baby was asleep in the carrycot at the side of my bed. The doctor opened her medical bag and exclaimed, 'Oh! I haven't got any local anaesthetic with me; well, never mind'. An exceedingly painful procedure followed, occurring several hours after the birth, when I was feeling very sore and tender. I wanted to yell when these stitches were inserted but I felt I couldn't allow Andrew and my dad to hear me, and held it in. I have since been told that there is a kind of natural local anaesthesia immediately after childbirth, but that a few hours later the area is particularly sensitive to pain.

That night I had a very severe headache, but thought that a night's sleep would make me feel better after the trauma of the day, but I had little sleep and retained the headache the next morning. I began to feel pain in my face a few days later, beneath my cheekbones and in my lower jaw. A 'home help' came in each morning for the first week. She was a real treasure, did everything that was necessary in the house, and cooked me a midday meal. Different ladies came in from the church each afternoon during that week and I think the purpose of this was to enable me to have a rest while someone looked after the baby and Andrew, but they sat and talked to me, and I think I had to talk too much, and the pain seemed to get even worse after any conversation.

Maurice took some holiday leave the following week so I was able to take it easy for another few days but every morning I woke with a headache, which developed into raw pain across my cheeks soon after I got up, and as the day wore on my temples began to hurt and feel very tender. I developed an intense throbbing pain at each side of my throat.

Our new baby looked beautiful as he slept peacefully beside our bed, but I couldn't get to sleep at night because of the pain. Ian was a very contented baby, quite different from his brother who was still unable to sleep through the night. Ian didn't cry much, soon settled after a night feed and seemed quite content in the day. He slept in his carrycot in our bedroom for the first few months, and when he no longer needed a feed during the night we put him to sleep in the same room as his brother. His carrycot was on a firm frame, and fitted in to the little bedroom very neatly. Our first son had noise, anxiety and confusion surrounding him after his birth, and our second son must in some way have been aware of the anxiety and panic that accompanied his entry into the world. Not a very peaceful beginning for either of them – nor a comfortable time for me.

Andrew was at last sleeping through the night in his full-size wooden cot, but often woke early in the morning and called out, 'Mummy… (short pause)… salty biscuit, salty biscuit, mummy,' in a loud pleading voice. He wasn't calling me a salty biscuit, but he was proclaiming his longing for a Ritz cracker biscuit! I would find him standing up in his cot, clutching the wooden side as he swung to and fro in rhythm with his singsong cry, waiting for his 'fix' of salt! Ritz cracker biscuits had just come on the market, and Andrew adored them. We knew nothing of the risks of too much salt in those days, and packets of otherwise unflavoured crisps always contained a little screw of dark blue paper containing salt. My son's early developed longing for a savoury biscuit has remained with him to this day! Ian seemed to sleep through these early morning demands.

Did the circumstances of the nightmare of my confinement have any relevance to the subsequent constant pain I have endured? Over many years the doctors didn't appear to understand the nature or the intensity of my facial neuralgia, try to think through to what caused it, or knew what to do to relieve it, and as the years passed by I felt 'written off'. Nobody seemed able to give any answer, or made any connection between my confinement and the start of the many years of pain I subsequently experienced. Maybe there isn't a connection, but the trauma surrounding the birth of my second son was ignored, dismissed as irrelevant, and was even laughed at by one of the various male specialists I saw over the years.

Did the site of my pain – in my temples, cheeks, jaws and throat – have any connection with the screaming and straining and holding back that I had done while yelling for help while in labour?

I now know that I have a number of food intolerances, and the fact that I (and later my older son) was allergic to penicillin may have been a clue that there were other possible intolerances too, that lay unsuspected for years. Nobody knew much about food allergies at that time, and only a little about air-borne allergens. I now believe that food intolerances seem to develop in some people after trauma, or a period of extreme stress, but I had no general awareness of allergy – but had often wondered why Andrew seemed to suddenly develop a cold when he was a baby and a toddler after I had cut the lawn; at that time one didn't even know about hay fever. His cold symptoms usually disappeared as suddenly as they had developed.

Nobody seemed to try to pinpoint a cause, which I think might have led to more understanding of my pain – and thus, perhaps, to appropriate treatment. Can sudden shocks or traumatic experiences trigger illnesses or unexplained conditions or multiple allergies? Doctors didn't seem to think 'outside the box' of their training. I was prescribed various medications, whose names I have long forgotten. I don't think they did much to relieve the pain, but made me feel a bit woozy and perhaps disconnected from it. It's so long ago now, I don't remember; but I can remember the all day, every day, presence of the facial neuralgia that I had for many years.

In the meantime, life went on. My home help had enthused to me about the benefits of a refrigerator so a few months after Ian was born we had saved enough to buy one. We now had a car, a washing machine, a telephone and a fridge. The modern age was approaching us, but oh! for a mobile phone when I had been in labour – or a downstairs loo that would have precluded the need for me to go out of reach of the telephone. It was quite difficult to look after my family and keep cheery, to cope with a new baby and a toddler and lead a normal family life with constant neuralgic pain in my face. Nevertheless, ordinary life had to continue, and we enjoyed our children's development.

Our friends Dorothy and Ted also had their second baby at about the same time that Ian was born. They had arranged a self-catering holiday later on that summer at Holland-on-sea, near Clacton in Essex, and they invited us to spend the weekend with them. Between us there were two small babies in carrycots, two three-year-old boys and four adults in a small rented house. We arrived late on the Friday evening at the end of our friends' first week, and the next morning, when the sandwiches had been made after breakfast, and the thermos flasks filled, we set off to see the sea. The adults were well laden with food, drinks, towels, and spare nappies for the babies, and the small boys carried their buckets and spades, as we walked to the beach. The weather was fine and we enjoyed the day on the sand, paddling and making sand castles with the children. There were no knobbly pebbles on this holiday! The two babies slept peacefully in their carrycots on the beach most of the time, unaware that they were spending their first holiday at the seaside. I wonder whether they had a sense of their changed surroundings. There is a tangible difference in the atmosphere near the sea. I always find the sound of the waves splashing in and then the rush of receding water, the sound of distant voices and the sense of great space with so much sky visible, gives me a sense of exhilaration. I always feel a thrill when I am by the sea, be it rough or smooth. Perhaps babies feel the same combination of peace and excitement and are soothed.

Maurice and I shared our bed with Andrew over the weekend, and our peace was suddenly – and frequently – disturbed during the night. Andrew soon went off to sleep after a day in the fresh air, but when we carefully crept in to bed on either side of him later in the evening, it soon became a different matter. The excitement began in earnest as he thrashed about in the bed, suddenly flinging his arms out, bang, right across, first, my face, and then his father's; then came a sudden heave as he turned over, taking the bedclothes with him. Ian slept peacefully in his carrycot in the corner, but in our area of the room it was as if a mighty storm was raging. The peace and relative tranquillity of a day with two lads and two babies certainly changed for Andrew with the setting of the sun. The weekend soon passed, but its' memory remains with me.

My in-laws retired to Holland-on-sea the following year.

The little church we attended had the opening ceremony of its' new building later that year. The old wooden hall (which we often referred to as 'the hut' had been rented by the church on Sundays and for evening meetings since before the war) had been pulled down. Mr. Dalton, our landlord, and the headmaster of the small, private prep. school, had retired, and Kenton College had closed. It probably did not meet with the requirements of the 1944 Education Act as this became implemented after the War. The large house, the wooden school hall (our church 'hut') and quite a substantial area of surrounding land were up for sale. The church members had had a building fund since before the war and had saved enough money to purchase part of the site, and our own permanent church had now been built.

The Opening Service of the new brick-built church was a very important event on a Saturday afternoon in the autumn, and Maurice walked to the church early in the afternoon to help in some official capacity. I drove the car there a little later on, with toddler Andrew at my side and baby Ian lying in his carrycot on the back seat. The modern carrycot gave mothers so much more mobility in those days as baby and carrycot could be laid in the back of the car – providing one had a car, of course.

I parked the car, and Andrew ran off to be with his father. The service was to be relayed to me in the new kitchen, which was also intended to serve as a crèche. Ian and I were the sole occupants of this new facility as I was the only young mum in the church. Within minutes of the opening service I found the volume of the relayed sound was too loud in the small room. I could not stand the loud voices of the various speakers leading the service, and began to feel a bit claustrophobic and soon felt a little faint. As soon as the organ played the introduction for the first hymn I couldn't bear to stay in the room any longer. I couldn't stand the noise felt I would collapse but managed to stagger out of the kitchen with Ian in the carrycot. The volume of the new P.A. had been set up far too high, and I think the sound was possibly made worse by the harshness of the kitchen environment – tiled walls, tiled floor, metal saucepans and cutlery, cups and saucers all set out for the tea that followed the service. I managed to get to the car, sat there for a while, too limp and shaky and drained of energy to do anything, and almost in a faint and then I think I drove all over the district before I eventually got myself home and collapsed on the bed with Ian in his carrycot beside me. When Maurice got home he couldn't understand what had happened to me.

I saw my doctor the following week, and I think she thought it was a bit of a joke that the usually cheerful, unemotional Sheila should have got herself into such a state, but I could not understand what had happened, and it was no joke to me. I was soon back to normal, but couldn't stand any loud noise, and I soon found that if the organ in our new building was sometimes played a little too loud, or certain organ stops were used, it almost felt like a physical attack on me. Certain frequencies made me feel very limp and weak and if the amplification was a set little too high I just collapsed in a heap on the floor. I flinched if our minister stressed any words by raising his voice. My first experience of a public address system appears to have affected me permanently.

I began to feel weak when standing for any length of time – when waiting for a bus, in a queue at the shops, or singing a hymn in church. I can recall friendly shop assistants (in the days before the supermarket check-out appeared) commenting and showing concern about how ill I looked. I used to rest my body on the pram as I walked to the shops. I could hardly walk back home again, wheeling my baby in the pram, with the shopping balanced in the pram basket, and Andrew by my side. Life was a daily struggle with pain and exhaustion. I had no appetite and lost weight. I am now even more sensitive to loud noise of any kind but weight loss isn't a problem!

I was referred back to the hospital I had been in during the early days of my pregnancy, and the consultant suggested that I was ill because I wanted to back out of social life, and was using pain as a barrier and excuse. This caused a lot of unproductive heart-searching and upset, only adding to the difficulties of coping with daily life, and seemed to produce more problems than solutions. I had given up my church commitments when I had my first baby, and had always enjoyed being involved and active. I would have enjoyed a social life, but there were no mother and toddler groups then, I had no relatives nearby to visit, my husband and I didn't go out in the evening, as babysitting circles didn't exist. Where was I to find a social life anyway, I wondered? In any case, I wasn't able to stand the noise! I saw my friends regularly, but not every day. Where was I to get the energy to go out in the evenings? Fathers were not left 'holding the baby' in those days and, in any case, my husband was often at work in the evening.

Maurice's parents moved away to the coast the following year. We visited them from time to time, driving to Holland-on-sea (where we had spent a weekend with our friends Ted and Dorothy) on a Friday evening, with Ian prepared for the night, placed on the back seat in his yellow sleeping bag, and Andrew sitting on my lap on the front seat – there were still no child safety regulations then, and no seat belts were required.

Maurice and I spent the night on the put-u-up in my in-laws dining room, but I can't remember how beds were made up for Andrew and his brother. After chatting over the weekend I was often urged to have a rest on mum's bed before we drove home on Sunday afternoon, but I couldn't lose consciousness in a short nap because of the dominance of the pain, and sadly it didn't help. When the children were a little older and the motorways appeared, we were able to visit them on a Saturday and return the same evening.

I had been very fit throughout all my childhood, and as an adult, until I had children. Many years later I was to learn that my mother had her first experience of depression after the birth, then death, of epileptic and/or brain-damaged Peggy, and her serious mental illness would appear to have started after my birth, although of this I am not certain – because she was never mentioned. Talking made my pain worse, my jaws ached and my teeth felt like burning metal in my mouth. I found it impossible to cope with the rather hard acoustics of our new church building, or the volume of the organ as it was sometimes played. A change was needed.

For a while I stayed at home on Sundays until the lady who lived at the bottom of our garden invited me to the Young Wives' group at her Baptist church. I began to attend their fortnightly evening meetings, and was gradually drawn in to the larger church fellowship, and eventually my husband and I left our smaller childhood church. The Baptist church building was much larger, with a very lofty ceiling, and the PA was used in moderation. I can't remember any problem with the organ volume while we were there and the late Revd. Barry Morgan had a soft voice. There were also other young families in the church and I was not the only young mum.

After a while I was asked to become secretary of the Young Wives' group. The lady who lived at the bottom of our garden was the leader, but we never addressed each other by our Christian names in those days. She was always Mrs. Rayner. Nowadays people who scarcely know me address me as Sheila. In time I fear that surnames will tend to disappear.

The following year the leader of the primary department in the Sunday school moved away. I was asked to take her place. I had a group of about forty children to interest, enthuse and keep in order on a Sunday morning, and six young teachers to encourage. But the noise was not overwhelming. Nobody could now say that I was trying to withdraw from social contact. I enjoyed both of these activities very much, but came home from Sunday school in agony, my jaws ached so much that I dreaded having to speak at all. I went to bed after I had got the Sunday lunch, hoping that an hour or two's rest might help, but once again sleep escaped me, as without mental or physical activity to distract me, I was more aware of the pain.

On Tuesday evenings I usually returned home from Young Wives' with my face and throat searing and throbbing with raw, sore pain. The pains always grew worse as the day lengthened. I was again unable to sleep, and tossed and turned in bed, with restless legs and burning feet adding to all the other problems. I often had to get up in the middle of the night to bathe my feet, dangling them in a bath of cold water, with a cold flannel pressed against my cheeks.

As I write this I find it difficult to believe that I could have coped with all I did; yet in spite of it all life went on as usual. Dorothy and I had set up our own mini-playgroup on Tuesday mornings. Martin spent one Tuesday morning with Andrew at our house, and the following week I took Andrew down the road for a morning with Martin. Dorothy and I both tried to give the boys some pre-school experiences with water and sand, and painting, but we knew little about pre-school education.

Andrew played with Pat's daughters, sometimes in our home and on other days across the road in theirs. In those days it was quite safe for the children to play along the very wide pavement on that side of the road, and the youngsters had a lot of fun, and many imaginative games were played out there. We often went to the park and all the usual childhood activities and outings occurred, although these were all far simpler than children enjoy nowadays. Our meals were all home-cooked from fresh food, purchased daily at our local shops; cakes were all home-baked and desserts always made.

My father retired during this period. He was given a retirement present of a television from his employer, which was a delight to him for many years. Andrew had enjoyed Listen with Mother on the radio with me, but now both the boys could watch Andy Pandy, the Flowerpot Men, Popeye and all the other children's programmes in granddad's living room. In time Maurice and I found we were spending more of our evenings in my father's living room too, watching programmes on his TV. That retirement gift gave my lonely father hours of pleasure until his death twenty years later.

Family holidays in Norfolk with both the boys didn't provide us with any mountains, but I think they were 'high spots' in the children's young lives. We rented a cottage on the cliff top at a little-known place called Ostende, near the village of Walcott, with Bacton not far away. We were able to walk from the door of the little sun lounge of our bungalow, across a field and down some old, wooden steps that lead directly on to an unspoilt golden beach. The children were able to sail their boats, paddle and splash around in the shallow pools in safety, search for sea creatures and unusual shells. At low tide the sea was a wide expanse of indigo blue in the distance, and we paddled in the shallows when the gentle waves lapped the sand as the tide went out. Sometimes a storm blew up and white rollers came crashing in and the following morning we walked along the beach looking, unsuccessfully, for treasures amongst the driftwood.

I always think that bathing in the sea is a wonderful experience, and I made the most of it on holiday. My husband was less enthusiastic, and remained on the beach making elaborate sandcastles with children. As the tide came in it swirled around the old water-worn timber groynes, before the waves broke with a splintering crash on the sand. When the tide went out it left long, calm, cool pools of water along the beach between the groynes where the boys could sail their boats, and we could wade through them taking a knee-high walk in the sea! No ugly sea defences had then been built across the beach to stop the sea from encroaching upon the land and dragging the cliffs into the water.

A mobile shop drove around the unmade-up road where the semi-circle of bungalows was built on the cliffs facing the sea. We listened out for its distant bell announcing its imminent arrival around midday, and often rushed out in the middle of our lunch to buy any food we might need in the next day or two. The bungalow was not equipped with a refrigerator in those long ago years. We queued up to buy fresh fish, and freshly cooked prawns and crabs from a local fisherman who had a little wooden stall in the village.

In the afternoons we went off in the car and explored the local farms, watching the pigs snuffling in their sties, the chickens wandering about the farmyard, the ducks in the pond. No factory-farming methods were used then, and the farm buildings were old and weathered; nothing had changed for years. We stood watching while the wheat and the oats were harvested in August in the old traditional way, with no combine harvester in sight. Farmhands were busy gathering bundles of hay and propping them up in stooks, and once we watched in the early evening while a traditional haystack was being built. My husband made a beautiful photographic record of this traditional harvesting, which totally changed in the course of the next few years.

Our drive back to our little bungalow was sometimes held up by a herd of cows that commandeered the road, and we sat patiently waiting while a young lad with a dog slowly moved them on. We took a lot of 'goodies' with us that I had baked before we left, and two weeks later we stopped on the way home and filled the empty cake tins with blackberries. We holidayed at the end of August for three years running, in the same place, in the same accommodation. I suppose this was the only time we were in our own family abode in those early years of our marriage. I'm sure those memories are still remembered by my sons. We enjoyed our holidays despite my constant pain, which I tried to conceal from others and ignored as far as was possible myself. I don't know how I did it!

A huge oil installation has now totally transformed Bacton, but there were no unsightly oilrigs sticking up out of the sea on the horizon when we spent our holidays on the cliff top at nearby Ostende. This was possibly an ancient name meaning East End – on the cliff's edge somewhere along England's east coast? How far out in the sea may the ancient settlement be now, I wonder?

Factory farming had not yet appeared to alter the life of farming folk either. Despite the subsequent construction of what appeared to be immensely strong sea defences all along that part of the Norfolk coastline, the cliffs are still being eroded, and one or two of the semi-circle of bungalows at our holiday village has slipped into the North Sea. There is no longer direct access to a beach that has been ruined by the section of these very necessary, but very ugly, sea defences. The erosion is bound to continue, and it is possible that the neat little semicircle of bungalows will eventually disappear, as the inevitable march of the sea takes place.

Chapter Thirteen

WE MEET AGAIN

During the latter part of the 1950s I began to sense that my mother's mental condition might be improving. My father was visiting her more frequently and he seemed less tense and withdrawn when he returned home. I felt able to ask him how she was without dreading the answer I had always been given – 'She's about the same, dear'. On his return from recent hospital visits his response to my question was now something on the lines of, 'Not too bad today, dear', or 'She seemed a little better', or 'She was quite chatty today'. I didn't really know what a 'little better' meant. How had she been previously? Nevertheless, all these replies from my father were more positive than those I had been used to hearing nearly all my life. I kept all these thoughts to myself for some time until I plucked up my courage to speak of her. My father just couldn't bring himself to talk to me about my mother, and I think that had somehow prevented me from mentioning her in conversation. She didn't really exist as a person in my mind.

It was years later before I became aware that the antipsychotic drugs that had been developed after the war were then beginning to be used on patients who were mentally ill, and my mother appeared to be benefiting from chlorpromazine, or Largactil, as it is more generally known. At the time the general public had not heard of the term 'antipsychotic drugs'.

I had not seen my mother since I was eight years old and I began to feel I would like to know something about her. I had never heard her tell me stories of her childhood, or of the work she had done before she married. I knew nothing about her. What did she look like now? I couldn't even remember what she looked like when, as a child, I had last seen her. I had not said 'good-bye' to her then; she had just disappeared from my life. What was the hospital like? I knew nothing concerning her life or surroundings, but found it was very difficult to start a conversation with my father. I, too, found it difficult to speak about my mother, but I became more curious, and wanted at least to see where she lived.

In the summer of 1959 I asked my father if I could accompany him on one of his Sunday afternoon visits to Shenley. He seemed a little doubtful at first, but agreed when I said it would give me somewhere different to take Ian for an afternoon's walk in his pushchair. So I drove with him on his next visit to the hospital, with Ian sitting on my lap in the front seat and the pushchair in the boot. My father dropped us off at the bottom of the hill leading to the hospital entrance, and then drove on into what was unknown territory to me - the hospital campus. While he was talking with my mother, I walked up and down the hill that ran alongside the boundary of the hospital site, pushing Ian in front of me, wondering all the time what the inside of the hospital was like, what did my mother look like, how was my father's visit going. Did he talk to her of their grandchildren? Did he speak to her of me? Did she even know I was married? I had no idea, but I somehow doubt that he told her I was walking around outside the hospital.

After several similar visits, my curiosity and my desire to meet my mother became more intense, and I asked my father if I could go with him into the hospital on his next visit. He appeared very thoughtful, a little apprehensive perhaps, and then said he would speak to the ward sister about it. Would it be practical, beneficial, or might it upset my mother? Apparently the medical authorities considered that we could meet, so a few weeks later I accompanied my father, together with my baby son on a sunny summer, Sunday afternoon and made my first visit. It had been decided by the staff that I was not to go into the ward, but that we should meet in the grounds, so my father left me sitting with Ian on my lap on a seat under a large tree in the very extensive gardens while he went inside and, I hoped, would bring my mother out to meet me. I waited while he went into the large two-storey, brick-built building. A few minutes later I watched as he and my mother walked across the lawns to where I was waiting. I saw a lady with snow-white hair approach, arm-in-arm with my father. She was quite stout, not very tall, and there was nothing about her that I was able to recognise as the mother I last saw when I was eight. We greeted each other with a kiss, and I said, 'Hello, Mumma' (my childhood name for her) and then we all sat down. She was very reserved in her greeting, didn't use my name but was quite amiable. We found things to talk about. I handed her grandson to her and she sat him on her lap, and was quite natural with him. She had not seen or held a baby for many years, probably not since I was Ian's age. Her leg was shaking uncontrollably at times, and she seemed generally a little ill at ease – which is not surprising. The meeting must have been very difficult for her, but it was tricky for all of us really. But I was so pleased that it had gone well, so after this initial meeting I accompanied my father each time he visited my mother and we met in a similar way for several months but, although she always seemed pleased to see us, she appeared to be unable to accept that I was her daughter. Neither could she remember any of the little incidents I spoke of that included her when I was a child. She could not understand or accept that I was her daughter. Conversely, I couldn't regard her as my mother. She was an unknown elderly lady, but I knew that she was my mother. That was the difference.

With the approach of the colder weather we began to meet in the ward on our Sunday afternoon visits, and for the first time I saw the large lounge where a number of elderly ladies were sitting around in upright upholstered chairs. They were doing nothing, not chatting to each other, appeared rather isolated, and seemed well sedated – but it was a Sunday afternoon and they may have been having a little snooze after their midday meal. The room looked bright and clean and there were a number of pot plants dotted around, but there appeared to be nothing to do, no newspapers or magazines, nothing to occupy their minds or attract their attention. I went into the lounge to greet my mother, but at first found it quite difficult to make out which lady *was* my mother, as they all appeared to have white hair. When I spotted her I went over, and she seemed pleased to see me. I think I remember that she said, 'Hello dear'. I escorted her to where my father was waiting in the visitors' area.

We sat chatting for an hour just outside the ward lounge area, which was well screened from the resident patients with a group of large foliage plants. There was rarely more than one other patient with a visitor on a Sunday afternoon, but we were often the only family. It was very thoughtful to screen off a little area for visitors so that it would be less upsetting for patients who may have had nobody to come and see them. It also gave a little more privacy for those who were visiting relatives. I fear that many of the patients were quite alone in the world and may have been abandoned by their relatives.

Soon all the family visited my mother on a Sunday afternoon. She met my husband, and her other grandson Andrew and she was friendly towards us all, and very gentle with Ian. Sister Brown usually joined our little family group for a few minutes, to check that all was going well. She joined in our conversation, and often tried to persuade my mother to acknowledge that I was her daughter, and that she had a son-in-law and two fine young grandsons. But my mother vehemently refused to acknowledge that the two little boys were her grandchildren, or that she was my mother. She said that she 'had no idea where I came from'. She called the boys by name, and was friendly, unemotional, but interested. She joined in the conversation about everyday events, the children, our friends, etc., and I felt that Sister Brown's coercion was not worth pursuing, as the more she tried to force my mother to acknowledge our relationship, the more adamantly my mother refused to accept it. It seemed to me to be better not to try and make her admit to a relationship that she had obviously forgotten. It was sad but true. There is a hymn that we sometimes sang in church, which I always found very hard to articulate: 'Can a mother's tender care, cease towards the child she bare?' I knew in my heart that yes, it could; it had ceased.

Some time later she was moved from the large Ward 4A into a villa. The villa was on the ground floor of another building, which was the only difference I noticed between the two and I don't know the reason for the move, but it had a very pleasant lounge and I think there were fewer patients. I think patients who were requiring less supervision may have lived in the villas, but that is only an assumption. My mother seemed to quietly settle in, but I began to think how nice it would be if she could come home for a Sunday, eat her Sunday dinner with us all, and later on in the day drink her tea out of a nice china teacup, and have a piece of home-made cake before returning to hospital.

I suggested to my father that she might be allowed to come home one Sunday, and he seemed rather hesitant, but agreed to talk it over with the new sister in charge of her villa. After some consideration it was agreed that my mother could come home for a day. The visit went very well, and my mother behaved as if she had never been away, was quite calm and, literally, 'at home'. She spent several Sundays with us throughout the following year with complete equanimity. She seemed quite relaxed with my family, chatting naturally to Maurice and the children, calling them by name. They called her 'Grandma' and she accepted this term, and we almost seemed a normal three-generation family – except that my mother didn't believe that I was her daughter or to believe that Andrew and Ian were her grandchildren. I don't think she addressed me by my name, but always called me 'dear'.

Maurice and I found it very easy to call her 'Mumma', which was the name I used when I was a child so there was a possibility that hearing it might help her to recognise and remember that I was her daughter. I had kept both my early childhood names for my parents, and still called my father 'Dadda'. I don't know why I didn't change it to the more usual 'dad' when I was young, but he was always my dear dadda. I don't think I met other children's fathers to even hear the word 'dad' and so continued with what I was accustomed to. Perhaps it was good that when everything else had changed for him, 'dadda' was the one thing that remained the same. In everything but name and memory, my mother behaved as if she had accepted that she was my mother and the children's grandmother. She was interested in our activities, the boys' development, our car etc., but no affectionate and could not relate to anything I mentioned about the past.

I became very fond of this elderly, white-haired lady, even though she was unable to make any connection with the few memories I tried to remind her of my early childhood. This made it almost impossible for me to think of her as my mother, who was vitally connected to my past,. It appeared that anything connected with me had been blotted out of her memory. When I related some incidents I remembered from long ago, it seemed so strange that she didn't appear to know what I was talking about. She never spoke of anything from the past that had any connection with me. She couldn't remember taking me to school on my first day, or going to the library, going to the seaside in the car, when I learned to swim, or the tricycle my parents gave me, or anything about me. She couldn't understand that the lady whom I called 'Auntie Ada' must b closely related to us both, although she would talk about her sister Ada. Her memory about everyone else seemed quite good, but there was no memory at all about anything connected with me. I was unable to make any real links between us. I tried to jog her memory, but she could not connect with, or admit to, our relationship.

Any emotional connection had been severed in my case because she had never been talked about in my presence for twenty years. I could not connect with her physically, because she had changed and now looked like an elderly lady, or emotionally, through shared memories, but in time I grew very fond of her. My mother's memory of me had possibly been wiped from her mind through ECT therapy. Was my birth the cause of her illness? Post-natal depression was not recognised until fairly recently, and I am sure that many women spent their lives in mental institutions in the past because post-natal depression had not yet been understood. They could not be treated and some were left in secure institutions for the rest of their lives.

I had not thought about my mother for so many years, and it was so sad that having met once again, the connection between mother and child could not be made. I was able to recall more incidents about my childhood when I was writing my book 'Child of the Thirties' a few years ago, than I remembered about her when she was still alive, and which maybe we could have shared way back in the 1960's. What a pity! It might have jogged her memory and helped us to build a real relationship. We got on well together, but I really didn't know what a mother was, and she believed her daughter had been taken away from her. By different means both of us had our relationship wiped from our consciousness

Her Sunday visits were occurring more frequently and she spent Christmas Day at home with us in the following year and we had a very happy time together. A few days later we all went to a matinee performance of what I think was the first production of 'Holiday on Ice' at the old Wembley Stadium. It was the first big show our children had seen, and the first time my mother had been to a public performance of any kind for many years. It was spectacular! It must have been quite a shock for my mother to see such a huge stadium, to be among so many people and watch such a spectacle, but she appeared to take it all in her stride and was quite calm. It seemed to me that we were just a normal family on an outing with my husband, my parents, our children and their grandparents. What a lovely memory.

My parents had enjoyed going to the music hall in the past and seen some of the light operas in the nineteen-twenties, and went to the early Henry Wood concerts in the Queen's Hall; they had experienced the development of the movies from the old silent films, and it must have been a real treat for my parents to enjoy the spectacular ice show together.

I don't know what my children had thought of this sudden appearance of a second grandmother a year or two earlier, when they were both under five years old. I don't think I ever explained to them the reason why they had never seen her before. They understood she lived in a hospital, and Andrew was old enough to know that granddad had driven off in the car on some Sunday afternoons to visit her. I now realise that I behaved in a similar way to how my father dealt with me when my mother became ill and disappeared from my life. I think that Andrew would have been more puzzled that Ian, who was not even a toddler when he first saw his grandmother. I must have assumed that my sons simply absorbed the information – I guess in a similar way to how I may have absorbed the circumstances that occurred during my own childhood. How differently a similar situation would be dealt with today.

We kissed on meeting and also when she returned to hospital, but I don't remember now whether she used my name. (One of her little individualities was that she never used contractions: for example, she would have said 'I *do not* know where you come from'; or 'I *do not* understand why you say this'.) I don't know whether this was a way of speech when she was young, or whether it was said for emphasis – I really *do not* know! Neither do I know whether she really accepted that Andrew and Ian were her grandchildren when she sent them birthday cards each year, signing them 'From Grandma', or whether she had possibly been persuaded by nursing staff to sign her cards to them in this way. She once stated that she 'had had two daughters, but they took them both away and I do not know what they have done with them'.

This in a sense was true: Peggy had died when she was eighteen months old. My father spoke only once to me of her, and that was in response to my question. Bad things weren't talked about in those days. Peggy would have been my sister if she had lived. I have since read that there is a 10% risk of epilepsy if a child has a parent who suffers from schizophrenia. I wonder whether there were signs of schizophrenia in my mother's earlier years. My father once told me that she was never the same after she was very ill with 'flu in the 1918 influenza pandemic. My mother later told me that the sister I never knew was also blind and deaf and couldn't walk, but I have no idea whether these details were, in fact, true. She had sadly lost Peggy, but I was still around, and she couldn't remember me.

My neuralgic pain continued, and I was referred once again to the same London teaching hospital as previously, where music therapy was now suggested. The battle to discover relief for persistent neuralgic pain is still ongoing, as the strong pain relieving drugs are not very effective for this type of pain and the side effects can make life intolerable in other ways. I think this was but an early attempt to help the sufferer by distracting the mind with absorbing activities. I had already realised that distraction appeared to be the best kind of relief for my on-going pain; if my mind or my body were actively engaged, it helped me to be less aware of pain, thus diminishing my awareness of it.

I was asked to attend at a new unit where I was encouraged to extemporise at the piano, but, sadly, this had no beneficial effect on my pain. I was hopeless at extemporisation, and didn't like the discordant sounds I produced, but it did make me interested in playing the piano again. I decided to try and improve the basic piano teaching I had received as a child. I gave up the therapy with its requirement of a regular journey to

London and started having lessons with a piano teacher who lived nearby. I enjoyed this far more; it did help to distract my attention from my facial neuralgia while I was playing, although practising at the piano gave me pain in my shoulders! I tried to fit in some practice on my father's old piano each day. I knew my mother had played the piano before she became ill; indeed, one of my few memories of her in my childhood was of her sitting on the piano stool while playing the piano All her old music was in the piano stool, but when I sat down to do my practice I didn't make any connection between my mother and the stool on which I sat, or those old sheets of music inside. (Why hadn't I thought to ask my mother to play the piano when she visited us all those years ago? It would have been interesting to see if she could have sat down with some of her old music in front of her, and play. I think this is one of the things – like typing, or swimming, or even pain – that once learned, gets imprinted on the brain, and is never forgotten. She might not have played well, but I think it quite likely that she would have remembered where her fingers should go.)

I was now having lessons with a far better qualified teacher than my much-loved childhood one. Miss Iveson was a professional, and I had my weekly piano lesson sitting at her grand piano. I encountered music theory for the first time, and – yes – I enjoyed it. I was well aware of the many gaps and drawbacks in my own education during the war, and perhaps education is more appreciated as an adult. I worked hard for Miss Iveson, but I soon found that the childhood tremor I had had in my left hand was much more noticeable when I was playing the lower reaches of the piano, or doing scales or arpeggios, when my hand wobbled terribly. It didn't trouble me so much when doing my practice at home, but was more apparent when I played in front of my teacher.

However, I persevered, and passed one or two examinations at the Royal School of Music. My examinations were on a Saturday afternoon and when they occurred the family drove up to London together. My husband parked outside the imposing Royal School of Music building in Marylebone Road; yes in those days you could park your car in London, and it was free. He and the boys waited in the car while I went in for my exam. I remember my left hand wobbled a bit when I was asked to play some scales and arpeggios in such august surroundings. Of course it was partly because I was nervous, and playing on an entirely different piano, but my performance was made worse by the persistent tremor, which I believe is called 'intention tremor'. It comes on when the affected hand has to act independently – cut a cake, hold a cup of tea, write, or play the piano. After my examination we all went for a walk in Regents Park before driving home. I passed two examinations, taken at different periods, with a reasonable, but not outstanding mark.

Andrew also began to show a lot of interest in the piano, and I asked Miss Iveson's advice as to when would be the best time for him to begin lessons. She felt that as he was a bright youngster it would be a good idea for him to start before he went to school, so that learning the basics of musical notation would not clash with early reading, so Andrew began to have piano lessons too. He did very well, and I took him up by train to London just before Christmas to the Guildhall School of Music and he took his first preliminary grade examination before he was six. We were able to see the Christmas lights in Regent Street afterwards, and to have a walk round Hamleys toy shop, looking at the toys and the wonderful train layout. Andrew was impressed, and I fear that his subsequent Christmas present of a Hornby train set was rather boring after the incredible display he had seen in this famous toy shop. He couldn't do much with a small train set, a tunnel and a station! We both did our practice – at different times of the day - on the old piano in my father's living room. I can't remember it ever being tuned, and one or two of the notes made no sound at all when played.

Chapter Fourteen

TIME FOR SCHOOL

Nursery schools and recognised pre-school education had scarcely been thought of in the 1950s, but one or two very small, unregulated, so-called 'nursery schools' had opened in the district towards the end of that decade. I found one within walking distance from home that was conducted by a lady in the kitchen and rear living room of her small semi-detached home. It gave Andrew contact with a group of children of his own age and a couple of terms' introduction to school life. It is almost incredible to recall that in this small fee-paying 'school' a uniform was insisted upon, and I was required to buy my not-yet five-year-old son a blazer and a cap and, I think, a tie before he could attend this little nursery school five mornings a week. I don't think it had much else to commend it.

I rushed along the road each morning pushing Ian sitting up in the pram, and Andrew dressed in his little maroon blazer and cap hurrying along beside me. It was about a mile's walk before a 9.30 a.m start, and I left him at the front door to start his first day in school. There was no friendly gentle start; he was just accepted at the door and I had a brisk walk home again, wondering how he was getting on, followed by not very much time to do some housework before I had to strap Ian into the pram once more and hurriedly retrace my route to collect his brother at 11.30 a.m. I had walked about three miles by mid-day, and done some washing or a little housework in between. We now had a fridge, so shopping every day was not essential, and a washing machine, which made life a lot easier. These modern appliances were much appreciated years ago, although refrigerators had minute freezer compartments and washing machines bore no comparison with today's fully automatic appliances that do everything on the press of a button.

Andrew's morning had been spent doing simple jigsaw puzzles, learning some singing games and nursery rhymes. He learned his alphabet and basic numbers, played with other children and listened to a story, but it was not very inspiring, and I don't think the cost was really worth the effort, but it broke the ice for school, and Andrew was happy to leave nursery school behind him and start mainstream school when the time came.

He started in Priestmead Infant School after the Easter holiday in 1960, the term before he reached his fifth birthday. He went to the same primary school that I had attended in the 1930s. The two schools {the Bricks and the Huts) had now been combined into one JMI School; rivalry between the two had ceased, although the old, black-painted, wooden huts in which I had spent my early school days were still in use. The school uniform colours were grey and red, so Andrew wore a grey shirt, grey and red striped tie, knee-length grey worsted trousers, and grey, wool, knee-length socks. These infant school boys were expected to wear a grey school cap with the Priestmead school badge on the front, and another badge was also sewn on the pocket of the grey blazer. He looked great, and was proud of his uniform, which was identical to that worn by the boys when I was a pupil at Priestmead School.

We lived near to the school, and it was not long before he was able to meet up with two friends who lived nearby, and 'the three musketeers', Martin, Mitch and Andrew, went along the road together, unaccompanied by their mums. The school-crossing man was at the Belisha crossing and saw the children safely over the main road to the school. Independence was encouraged in those days, and children's safety was assumed. There was not much traffic, parents were not overly worried about speeding cars or child safety, and knew their children were O.K. It was a different world.

Andrew settled into mainstream school very easily, was a sturdy little boy, who had his little group of friends, and adored his teacher. There was a parents' open evening at the end of his first year, when we were able to look at his drawings and read through his news book. Then we met his teacher, who said that Andrew was doing very well. She related one amusing little incident to us, telling us that the children had written up their news one Monday morning, and when she read Andrew's she found that he had apparently been to Holland for the weekend. She thought this was something a bit special that she could discuss with the class, and told the children that 'someone has some very special news'. She then asked Andrew if he would tell the rest of the class what he had done over the weekend. (We had in fact been visiting my in-laws, who now lived at Holland-on-sea, in Essex.)

We were told that he was called to the front of the class, and proudly said, "I went to see my grandma and grandpa on Saturday and Sunday".

"Oh, Andrew, how exciting for you. Where do they live?" the teacher asked, prompting him to say the special word.

"At Holland," Andrew told them.

"Is your grandma or your granddad Dutch?"

"No," said Andrew not understanding what she really meant.

"Did you go by boat?" the teacher prompted him.

Andrew looked even more puzzled. "No," he said, "We went in my daddy's car". He must have thought his teacher had had an 'off' moment.

Apparently it took quite a bit of the lesson time to unravel the fact that the Holland Andrew had visited was called Holland-on-sea and was near the seaside resort of Clacton on the east coast of England and not across the English Channel!

Years later, when recalling this incident, Andrew told us that he was so pleased to have this bit of real news to record because he never knew what to write in his 'News' book on Monday mornings! He was probably right. We were usually doing jobs around the house and garden on Saturdays, and Andrew's Sunday consisted of going to afternoon Sunday school. We certainly didn't go out every Saturday, and didn't have many excursions on a Sunday in those days. I guess many children had the same problem with writing up their weekend 'news'. Sunday was a quiet day spent at home for most people, doing odd jobs, gardening, going to Sunday school, and for many, going to church. Dads were decorating, (I don't think it was called D.I.Y. in those days, although I think most people did, in fact, do their own decorating.) There were no local restaurants or cafés or coffee shops in our suburban area and certainly none open on Sundays; pubs didn't do Sunday roasts, and children were not allowed in public houses. Roast lamb, or pork of beef was the usual Sunday dinner, cooked at home; Sunday tea consisted of bread and butter, jam, maybe fish paste sandwiches or home-grown lettuce and home-made cake.

Andrew's first year had passed quickly and he was pleased to find he would have the same teacher for his second year in the infant school. He liked this teacher very much, but she had sometimes been unwell during his first year, with frequent periods of absence from the classroom because of a persistent cough. Our son sometimes came home from school and asked his grandfather for some of his 'Hacks' (throat sweets that my father sucked) to give to his teacher - 'Mrs. --- has a *terrible* cough, Granddad; can I take her some of your Hacks?'

I had been very concerned when I met her at the school end of year open evening at the end of his first year. I thought she looked very unwell and wan; but teachers are usually exhausted at the end of term. I commented to my husband as we walked home that I thought this lady was very ill, and was either suffering from cancer, or had TB. I have reflected on this comment many times; it seems very strange, as at that time I had scarcely heard of TB, and cancer was another of those unspoken diseases, but at that time I only knew one person who had cancer who was in our Young Wives' Fellowship. Why ever did I express this thought? There was not much treatment available then, but I am also sure that there were not so many cancer cases either.

His teacher was off sick several times during the autumn term in his second year, and had been away from the school during the last hectic few days of term before Christmas. However she came back on the last afternoon for the class Christmas party. Apparently she still had a terrible cough as she played party games with the children.

Andrew had also been unwell during the second half of the autumn term, with high temperatures, night sweats and a bad cough. He had one or two periods off school, with visits from our doctor, who had considered he was suffering from attacks of tonsillitis. I was worried, and the seemingly irrational thought, 'TB', again passed through my mind when I went up to his bedroom in the evenings and felt his sweaty forehead and his damp chest. I had never met anyone with TB, and had had no cause to fear it, but somewhere I must have heard of the term 'night sweats' being connected with tuberculosis. I had a secret unspoken fear that my son was really ill.

Towards the end of the following Christmas holiday all the parents of children in Andrew's class received a letter from the Local Education Authority saying that 'a case of tuberculosis has been found in the school, and that tests were being arranged for all the children in this class'. We were informed that the children should attend school as usual, and there was nothing to worry about, it was just a procedure that had to be followed. Mrs. --- had not returned to the classroom after the Christmas holidays and the parents were left to draw their own conclusions as to where the case of TB had come from.

With the usual bureaucratic delay, the tests the children were supposed to have taken a long time to materialise, but eventually all the class were tested for TB at the local chest clinic in Harrow. The weather had been very cold during this long waiting period, and was still bitterly cold as the anxious parents awaited for the results afterwards. The delay added to the general anxiety. I felt I already knew what the result of Andrew's test would be, could feel it in the pit of my stomach, and sure enough, it was positive. Yet it was still a great shock when we were officially informed in 1962 that our six-year-old son was suffering from tuberculosis. It still gives me the horrors as I write about it now.

A subsequent x-ray indicated that Andrew had a TB-infected gland in the chest wall. I wonder why Andrew, but not his close friends, was affected. Years later I was having treatment from a homoeopathic doctor, who reminded me of the theory of Hahnemann, the founder of homoeopathy - that we inherit what he called 'miasms', which are pre-dispositions to certain types, or groups of diseases. If you have a certain 'miasm' and come into contact with, say, tuberculosis, you would be more likely to fall victim to it than someone with a different 'miasm', who may, perhaps, be more likely to develop cancer or arthritis or some other common illness. I wonder whether Hahnemann's miasm theory would today be defined as a genetic disposition. I think it could be another way of expressing genetic involvement with particular diseases, and connected with the present unwrapping of our DNA. This could be why Andrew became a victim and not his equally sturdy, healthy friends Martin, Mitch and Roy who were in the same class.

About nineteen boys and girls out of a class of thirty had reacted positively to the TB test, and several were admitted to a specialist chest hospital immediately; the rest were told that they would be prescribed special medication to treat their condition. The LEA informed all the parents that it was quite safe for the affected children to continue to attend school, as they were not infectious, and they could go out in the playground as usual (in bitterly cold, late winter weather) for games lessons and at playtime. Some of the class kept away from the affected children at playtime, avoiding playing with them in the playground. Their parents had warned their offspring not to play with 'the TB children'. I can quite understand their concern; how were they to be sure that their children's classmates were not infectious? Do we always have confidence in official health pronouncements?

There was a further long, anxious delay before the affected children were at last given the prescribed drug, Isoniazad, early in March. Andrew began taking his medication of one packet of Pasinah, the trade name of the drug Isoniazad. It was quite a large packet a powder that had to be mixed with water then swallowed. It had a horrible taste.

There had been a delay of almost three months since the initial letter of information had been received just after Christmas, after the unnamed, initial case of TB had been diagnosed with active infective tuberculosis, (meaning that she was infectious). Andrew's teacher should have been thoroughly investigated much earlier because of her persistent cough.

I had the greatest difficulty in getting my young son to swallow his medication. Any powder is difficult to swallow, even when mixed with liquid. It had a very bitter taste that was overlaid with an artificial, strong orange flavour, and we had real scenes each evening trying to get Andrew to swallow his daily dose without choking. He soon developed side effects to the drug, with distended tummy and he felt very unwell and nauseous. His tummy was soon so swollen that he couldn't fix the belt of his school trousers. Antibiotics, which we take for granted now, were still in their early days, and drug treatment for tuberculosis was also comparatively new. Andrew had no cavities in the lung, was not infectious, and when he was first diagnosed the only evidence of tuberculosis was in a gland in the chest, but three months had passed since we had learned of the initial case of TB immediately after Christmas. The saying, 'Time is of the essence' comes to my mind.

The weather was exceptionally cold and very windy in March that year, too blustery for children who were coping with an invasive bacillus, plus the side effects of powerful drugs, to be out of doors at playtimes, but it was considered quite safe for them to spend their break times in the playground. Before long Andrew developed another chest infection, had pain whenever he coughed, ran a high temperature, and soon complained of a sharp pain in his side, and had to be kept home from school again. This time it was certainly not tonsillitis.

Another home visit was required from the doctor, who sounded his chest and diagnosed pleurisy. Perhaps our son would not have developed this additional illness if the authorities had acted more speedily, or had allowed these children to stay in the classroom in playtimes during the cold weather? Penicillin was prescribed (the first time he had been given this antibiotic) but Andrew reacted badly, and large wheals developed on his arms, and the drug had to be stopped. The doctor visited once more while the pleurisy raged on untreated, and the tuberculosis spread from the gland into the lung. He became very ill, needed urgent hospital care and the doctor telephoned for an ambulance. This crisis occurred while my husband was at work on the 20th March, his birthday. It was all such a sudden shock. Our sturdy, stocky young son was now weak, feverish, and very ill with a life-threatening illness.

The ambulance arrived and there was a sudden burst of activity as the attendants shot upstairs to Andrew, then lifted him from his bed down the stairs into the ambulance, while I followed, carrying a bag with all his essentials - clothing, pyjamas, a few 'Famous Five' books (his favourites at that time) and one or two small toys. I assumed there would be plenty of toys and books in the children's ward. My father had recently retired, and followed closely behind the ambulance in the car, with Ian beside him, to bring me home. He didn't know the route and had to keep the ambulance in sight, and it must have been a traumatic day for him too. He had had more than enough bad experiences in his life.

It all seemed like a nightmare; I was so worried as I sat beside Andrew who was strapped into the narrow bed in the ambulance. He must have been frightened by this experience too, but he remained very calm. I think he felt too ill, or else he was very stoical – I think it was a bit of both! My husband was at work without the car to enable him to get home quickly. Communication and travel were not easy in those days.

We arrived at the entrance to the children's ward of a specialist chest hospital, and remained inside the ambulance while the driver went to the ward entrance. We could hear some conversation being exchanged and wondered why there was such a delay, when there had been such a panic earlier. Eventually the driver returned, flung open one door and asked me if my son had had chicken pox. The ward sister had informed him that chicken pox was rife on the ward and they could not admit Andrew if he had not had the disease. He hadn't, so he was refused admittance. Why couldn't this information have been given before we had had the ghastly drive in the ambulance? The door was banged shut and we were driven straight back home, with my father driving behind us in the car feeling rather confused, not knowing what had happened. Neither of us could understand why we had had this ridiculous journey with a very sick child. (Can it really be possible that I have twice been refused admittance to hospital; on two occasions the ambulance doors had been banged shut while I remained inside? It seems incredible, but it's true!)

Our GP had been informed that Andrew was not admitted to the hospital, and he arrived soon after our return home. He examined Andrew's chest again, and told us we had to bring his bed downstairs where it would be easier to care for him; he had to have total bed rest and was not permitted to get out of bed or go up and down the stairs. I think he had received these instructions from the hospital. The following day the chest specialist arrived, bringing with him a portable x-ray machine. He examined Andrew, took some pictures, and recommended that Andrew's horrible Pasinah powder be changed to a more acceptable peppermint-flavoured liquid medicine that was easier to swallow. It was essential that he took the whole dose. He seemed to understand why Andrew had been unable to swallow his powdery medicine. The liquid medicine was much easier to take, but he still had the discomfort and nauseous side effects together with loss of appetite. His tummy was still distended and now he couldn't do up the button to hold up his pyjamas. A couple of days' later Andrew's skin, pyjamas as well as the bed sheets began to reek of peppermint. The smell was over-powering it permeated everything. When I went shopping for our food I smelt strong peppermint as soon as I opened the front door on my return.

When the consultant left, carrying his rather primitive portable x-ray apparatus, I offered to carry his medical bag to his car. As I opened the car door for and placed his bag on the back seat I was immediately assailed by the smell of stale cigarettes. The car reeked of tobacco. I think he must have had a cigarette just before he visited Andrew. The doctor had obviously not yet learned of the dangers of smoking in relation to chest diseases – or else, despite the knowledge, he was unable to give up the habit. My memories of that period include two very strong memories of smell – peppermint and tobacco!

Andrew was considered to be so ill after a week at home that a bed had to be found for him in hospital, and we returned once again by ambulance. We drove in procession, with my father following behind the ambulance in the car – he could see our vehicle, but Andrew and I couldn't see anything. It is an unpleasant experience to be driven without being able to see where you are going. It was rather like being transported in a prison van.

Chapter Fifteen

A TIME OF TROUBLE

When we arrived at the hospital I was stunned to discover that my six-year-old son still couldn't be admitted into the children's ward. A small room had been made ready for him in an adult men's ward. The tiny room had no window, just four bare walls; it was like a prison cell, and similar to the room I had nursed him in as a baby a few years earlier in Edgware General Hospital. We stayed with him for a while but as we were driving home I noticed the newspaper stand outside our local train station had the latest news headline, 'Another child admitted to Hospital' blazoned in thick black ink across the news board. I was horrified; that was my child making the headlines! The episode was a brief item in the news, with several paragraphs on different days in several of the daily papers. I had telephone calls from the press later that day asking for information, but I didn't feel I could cope with it. Today there would be a huge outcry and a public enquiry, but then it had a certain amount of publicity that soon died down, and the incident was quickly hushed up.

Visiting time was an hour and a half every afternoon, so my husband, who was at work during the day, could only visit Andrew at weekends. Our concern for Andrew was immense, my father and I visited him the following day his greeting as we entered his little room was, 'Granddad, granddad, you must stop smoking', and then in a strong monotone, he added, *'If you smoke, you will get congestion of the lungs, and die'*. We learned that this message was broadcast periodically to the men in the adjoining ward, to warn them of the dangers of a crafty puff under the bedclothes. The warning was transmitted to the ward several times a day, but because Andrew's tiny room was part of the adult male ward he also heard the message. Andrew was scared that his beloved granddad would suddenly die. He repeated the message to us exactly as he had heard it. He sounded like a robot – a Dalek - as he slowly and clearly repeated the warning word for word. Since his admission the previous day he must have spent hours in anguish after repeatedly hearing this message, fearing that his granddad was going to die. We consoled him, reassuring him that granddad was not going to die. My father had been a light smoker for most of his life, but he told Andrew he wouldn't smoke again. He never smoked another cigarette, and lived until he was nearly eighty-eight. I wonder how many years Andrew's message may have added to my father's life.

About a week later we were told it was now safe for Andrew to be moved to the children's ward. I believe some of the male patients (probably smokers!)

came in to talk to him from time to time, but apart from that and our daily visits, he had really been in solitary confinement with no view of the outside world at all. He had coped so well, and we felt that now the epidemic of chicken pox was over, things would immediately improve. We were so relieved, imagining that he would have the companionship of other children, and that life would be much more fun. How wrong we were! Although we had been assured that our son's TB was not infectious, we found that Andrew was now isolated in one of a long row of glass-walled cubicles, still on complete bed-rest and wearing his pyjamas night and day. His lung had been artificially collapsed at some time without our knowledge or consent, presumably to allow it to rest and recover, but my husband and I were not informed that this was going to be done, nor had the procedure, or the need for it, been explained to us. Maybe the TB had infected the lung during the long delay before treatment had begun? We never saw a doctor, and rarely observed a nurse in the corridor that ran alongside the back of the row of single occupant, glass-walled cubicles. The young patients were facing away from this corridor, so saw no activity at all, but faced a blank wall at the foot of their beds.

Andrew could see the boy in the cubicle on one side of him through the glass walls, but the bed on the other side was empty. He was unable to chat or play or have any contact with any other patients in this cubicled ward. Visiting was only allowed for a set period in the afternoon. Occasionally we found that the children's' beds had been wheeled outside their cubicles, to breathe the rather chilly spring air, and they were snuggled down beneath their blankets, ranged along an open veranda like a lot of parcels. Modern drugs to treat tuberculosis were relatively new, but this hospital combined them with the old regime of bed rest, fresh air and isolation. Perhaps the doctors thought the drugs were too new to be entirely relied upon to cure the disease. Andrew was in this ward over Easter, and enjoyed his Easter eggs in solitude once the Sunday afternoon visiting period was over. I can picture him now with various boxed Easter eggs adorning his locker, but without any company once we had left him. He tells me that he can still remember one particular dark chocolate egg that he had received.

The regime was very harsh in the children's ward, the food intolerable, the care and attention inadequate, and several worrying incidents occurred. Our son was scared stiff of the sister, who tried to force him to eat unpalatable food, and to make him swallow what his stomach couldn't tolerate, so he secreted food he couldn't eat in the drawer of his locker before she came into his cubicle to check that his plate was empty. He said he was frightened to leave any food on the plate. When I visited in the afternoon he sometimes anxiously asked me to 'hide this in your bag, mummy, and take it home'. I often returned home with a couple of cold, unappetising-looking, barely-cooked roast potatoes or a chunk of tough meat wrapped up in a paper serviette in my handbag. The food seemed quite unsuitable for a very sick little boy who was also suffering from the side effects of his medication, which still made him nauseous and gave him considerable abdominal discomfort. His previously chubby body was beginning to look rather thin.

On another day I found his locker drawer was alive with ants crawling all over the place, on the floor, the pillow and elsewhere. I expect the 'free grub' supplied by Andrew's endeavours to avoid issues with the sister had attracted them! However, someone should have noticed the infestation of ants before I did. We were frightened to complain as we felt we did not know what the consequences might be with regard to the treatment of our son. It was a very difficult situation.

When we arrived one afternoon we found him sitting up in bed, looking very anxious, with very red cheeks, damp pyjamas and a wet chest. He told us that he had been taken to the bathroom and told to get in the bath, then the nurse suddenly left the room and he was left sitting in a large, high-sided, old-fashioned bath of hot (or possibly, warm) water. He told us that he sat there for a while, and then thought that perhaps he was supposed (or had been told, or not understood) to bathe himself, but there was no soap or sponge or flannel. Nobody came back, and he just laid in the bath as the water cooled down. The nurse didn't return, so he decided that perhaps he should get himself out. He had clambered out of the deep-sided bath, dried himself – insufficiently – and walked along the corridor back to his cubicle in his pyjamas. He had just climbed into his bed when we arrived.

He told us he was worried that he was going to get into trouble for climbing out of the bath on his own. He certainly hadn't dried himself properly. I think the nurse must have had an urgent call, but had then forgotten all about him. Further unacceptable incidents occurred, and almost daily our son begged me to 'please ask sister to speak kindly to me'. Life was made very unpleasant and frightening for our sick son and probably other youngsters supposedly in the sister's care. There were not many visitors during the week. The ward must have been understaffed, but kindness doesn't cost much.

I often spent part of the visiting period with the little boy in the next cubicle. He never had a visitor, seemed neglected, appeared to have no toys of his own, and none had been provided by the hospital staff; he just sat up in his bed looking around. We waved to him from time to time through the glass partition, but I soon felt compelled to spend a few minutes with him. I left Andrew for a little while and went into this boy's cubicle, and tried to amuse him. He seemed unable to tell me his name, and he was rather incoherent when he spoke. I think today it would be said that he had severe learning difficulties. I took in a few toys for him and some simple children's books but found he couldn't read at all, so I read to him for a little while from some of Andrew's Noddy books. He loved listening to stories. Every time a picture of Mr. Plod appeared on a page I was reading, he jabbed his finger on it, and shouted gleefully, "Copper, copper". He seemed to know about policemen! I would wave to Andrew while I was with this young lad, then return to my son and waved to the Mr. Plod fan. I never learned his real name.

For a day or two there was an empty cubicle on the other side of Andrew, but it was soon occupied when another Priestmead School boy was admitted.

I don't know whether we were more anxious about Andrew's recovery or concerned about the conditions he was in. I think it was probably the latter, and that we had more confidence in the modern drug treatment. It was a terrible period in our lives. With hindsight I realise that we should have made an immediate complaint, but in those days the public was rather in awe of authority, and people were much less likely to complain. There was the fear that the patient would suffer in some way as an immediate result of a complaint.

We heard that a child on the open ward had broken her arm, but we didn't know the circumstances. We knew there was a large open ward somewhere, as we could sometimes hear the sound of children's voices, and I think that the nurses and the sister spent more time there and the few children in isolation were forgotten. The hospital served a large area and I think many parents, like my husband, were only able to see their children at weekends, but poor young 'Master Plod' appeared to have nobody who visited him.

We were allowed to take Ian round to the outside of the building to Andrew's cubicle, where the two boys were able to wave to each other through the floor-length windows, but he couldn't enter the building. Our son sustained his ordeal in that hospital with a great deal of courage, telling me not to worry about him as he had his 'pretend brothers' with him, and that 'Jesus was looking after me'. He read voraciously, devouring all the books I could bring him with much quiet pleasure and his reading ability must have increased dramatically while he was in hospital. Some of the parents in his class asked for donations of toys or books for the 'TB children' who were in hospital, and one book, 'The Red Balloon' became another of Andrew's favourites.

We were distraught for several weeks until my husband found out that there was a small specialist chest hospital in Hertfordshire that was also much nearer to his place of work. He visited the hospital, explained our situation and conveyed our worries about our son. He felt there was a much kinder, more informal atmosphere in the children's ward in this hospital. He managed to arrange a transfer for our son, and the hospital was able to accept him immediately.

Where is the Key?

Andrew was overjoyed at the prospect of getting away from his glass-walled prison. We informed the hospital of our intention. Maurice got time off work and we were told to collect Andrew at 9.30 a.m. for this transfer. On arrival we found Andrew, sitting all alone on the draining board in the sluice. He was fully dressed with his outdoor coat on, looking very anxious. He told us he had been sitting there ever since his breakfast, which had been a long time ago. He had apparently seen no one since being placed on the draining board. We then had to wait for a while before the sister arrived with his discharge notes. I don't think she wanted this patient transfer to be noticed, and kept him hidden in the sluice until we arrived. She made some comment to Andrew as he left to the effect that she hoped he found his next hospital satisfactory. It immediately put doubt, and a bit of fear into his mind, but perhaps she meant well. We were relieved to get away.

We drove together in our own car to the new hospital, and didn't have the trauma of a long bumpy ride in the ambulance, shut off from the outside world. Why, I wondered, was an ambulance essential when he first went in to hospital, but considered unnecessary when he was being transferred from an isolation ward to another hospital? I think it was probably because this hospital transfer was initiated by us, the parents. It was lovely for Andrew to be able to enjoy the sunshine and see the countryside and I think we all felt a weight lift from us, and the journey almost felt like a family outing.

The ward in the new hospital was very quiet and a little gloomy when we arrived shortly before midday, with curtains drawn at the windows and around each bay. The children were lying on their beds having a morning's rest before their lunch. As Andrew was taken to a bed in a four-bedded bay, we heard the sound of plates and cutlery being laid on a table in the middle of the wide, open ward of six bays. Suddenly the curtains were drawn back and sunshine filled the ward, and the children got off their beds and chatted together as they sat down to their midday meal. It was a total reversal of our previous experience.

A nurse suggested that we stayed with Andrew while he had his lunch and that he might prefer to eat it quietly in his bed while he got used to his new surroundings. He could then meet the other children more informally after their meal. How thoughtful! So soon after our arrival at Clare Hall Hospital we could see that both the attitude to the young patients and also aspects of personal welfare were totally different – and the food was palatable. Andrew ate all his dinner.

I was told that Andrew could see his brother, and when his granddad, Ian and I visited the following afternoon I was momentarily shocked to see Andrew up and dressed and playing outside on a seesaw with the other children. Ian was invited to join them. As I watched I noticed how thin Andrew had become. His sturdy young legs now looked like matchsticks. We had only seen him in bed wearing pyjamas for some weeks. After their play the youngsters came indoors and sat down to have their tea. Ian was invited to join them as they all sat in small chairs around a large table. It was someone's birthday and there was an iced cake with candles. What a contrast! Andrew was given the same medication, but total bed rest was not practiced. The young patients sat companionably around the table for their well cooked, tasty, and easy to eat meals, instead of eating poorly cooked, unsuitable food from a bed-tray while sitting solitarily in their beds. It was a great comfort to see our son up and about and playing with the other children. They went outside for periods of recreation every day, with a variety of play equipment in a garden that had a seesaw and a few swings.

We soon discovered that pyjamas were for night-time only. I am sure that wearing normal daytime clothes must have been a great boost to Andrew's recovery. The children were dressed during the day, and there was a relaxed, friendly, caring atmosphere. Ian was allowed in the ward whenever we visited, and Andrew also saw more of his father, who was able to call in at the hospital on his way home from work in the evening. The mother of another boy in Andrew's bay told us that her son had previously been in the children's ward of the hospital I have described, and she had also been very concerned. He then came home for a while but had to return to hospital, and she refused to allow him to return there. She declared that the sister in that ward didn't like little boys. Maybe that was the problem.

There were a few lessons in the little ward school in the mornings before the short period of bed rest before lunch. I have no idea what Andrew learned in his morning lessons. How one teacher could teach anything to a group of children of different ages, from different schools, in varying stages of recovery and different levels of treatment for a short period each morning is beyond me. I was just relieved to know that Andrew was very well cared for. One didn't interfere with educational matters in those days, and parents were not encouraged to have anything to do with their children's education. But Andrew's reading had progressed so well during his time in bed, he was now having new experiences, meeting new people and he was a bright lad. One didn't worry so much about education then, and we just wanted him to get well. TB takes quite a long time to cure.

The mother of another boy in the children's ward was also being treated for TB in the women's ward. She came down to see her son every day and was sometimes allowed to take him for a little walk outside the hospital perimeter; Andrew was invited to join them. It was in all more like a holiday. Our relief was immeasurable.

We found that the completely different treatment approach and the totally different atmosphere in Clare Hall Hospital meant all our fears were completely allayed. Andrew quite enjoyed the rest of his time in hospital and made a good recovery in the care of the late Dr. Hounslow, but hospital closed many years ago. Andrew's ward was an ex-army hut, part another group of black painted, wooden huts, similar in appearance to my sons' and my own Primary School and also our church.

I believe the teacher recovered from her advanced tuberculosis, but she didn't teach at the school again. She was such a nice lady, and I understand that prior to her diagnosis she had made several visits to her doctor, complaining of her persistent cough, but it was only taken seriously by her young pupil, who came home to his granddad, saying, 'Mrs. – has a *terrible* cough, granddad, can I take her some of your Hacks?' Her doctor had made no investigations and she had quite a long period in the classroom while she was ill and infectious - long enough to spread the dangerous bacteria to more than half her class.

We contacted the father of the other boy who changed hospitals telling him that we were considering making an official complaint and asking if he would back this up with his own experience. He assured us of his and his wife's strong support, that they had been so worried about their son's treatment in the isolation ward that his wife had been on the verge of a nervous breakdown. We wrote to our local MP with details of our experience. He was very concerned and met us almost immediately. We told him about the other couple. He requested a meeting with the hospital authority, which we attended with him, and two of the consultants. (We had seen neither of these doctors while Andrew was in the hospital; the only doctor we saw during that entire period was the doctor who came to our home, the one with the nicotine-filled car!)

The chairlady opened the meeting by decrying any possibility of anything wrong in 'her' hospital. To our amazement the other parents didn't attend but had sent a letter declaring their satisfaction with the treatment, and stated that it was only because the father found it difficult to visit his son that they had considered moving him to a nearer hospital. They had 'chickened out' of a meeting that concerned all the other children in that ward, because they didn't want the personal aggravation. Our case had no confirmation or support, and the meeting ended abruptly.

During all this difficult period I continued to live with incessant facial neuralgia, along with the anxiety and complexities of serious illness and poor hospital care. I was never able to forget the pain, but had to try to ignore it.

As I write this in 2010 I appreciate how life has changed for the better with regard to the treatment of TB, as well as attitudes to childcare in hospital. In the early 1960s it was unusual to hear of this disease, certainly not in my part of the country, although in the hospital where Andrew was first a patient, there was a big male TB ward, and, presumably, a large women's ward, and there were many boys and girls in the large children's ward, although we didn't see them. I think that understaffing and overcrowding, and a ward sister who was probably overworked, and may have been better suited to an adult ward, caused the bad experience we had. But if this was so, it should have been admitted at the meeting, and an apology given for the reasons for the unsuitable treatment. An admission and an apology make all the difference in all manner of disputes. With the advent of effective drugs the hospital in Hertfordshire had adapted the care and treatment of TB to a much more modern approach.

The scourge of tuberculosis has largely been removed from this country, and I understand that TB testing and BCG inoculation has now been stopped in schools. Reduction in smoking and improved drugs are the main reasons of this change for the better. Andrew was at the beginning of a modern approach. There was still some trust in old methods by some specialists, and some doubt about the new. Andrew was given Isoniazad but there is now a selection of much more reliable, approved drugs. There is still a need to provide treatment for the disease in its early stages to ensure success. Tuberculosis is still a scourge in undeveloped countries, but now occurs mainly in deprived areas in Great Britain. I would certainly not consider the suburban area in which I grew up to be a deprived area, and Priestmead School pupils would have been considered mainly middle class, although I don't think anyone had much money. TB has not been eradicated; there has been an increase in incidence in recent years.

For some weeks before he was discharged from hospital we feared that we would be unable to have our usual summer holiday, but we were told that it would be 'just what the doctor ordered' and that a few weeks at home to settle down again, followed by a holiday would be ideal preparation for Andrew's return to school in the autumn. We were able to stay on a farm in a remote village on the edge of Exmoor. We were so grateful for Andrew's good recovery and we all had a really lovely holiday on 'Somerset farm' as the boys called it. We visited Porlock Weir, Dunster, walked up on to Exmoor and Dunkery Beacon, drove down Countisbury Hill, which I had cycled down on my bike years before. We drove up Porlock Hill and found a beautiful narrow lane that led us down to the tiny church at Oare, made famous in Lorna Doone. We managed to get to Wellington and visited the lady I had been evacuated with for a few months during the war, and took her out for the day. We watched the tide come in to the little harbour at Watchet, and I thought of the poem, 'The Ancient Mariner' by Samuel Taylor Coleridge that I had studied, and learned a lot of by heart while at school, which he had been inspired to write when living nearby. Some years ago my husband and I were staying in the area once again and tried, unsuccessfully, to find the old farmhouse in the hamlet of Bicknoller where we had stayed. Nothing seemed familiar.

Andrew soon settled into his first year of Junior School, caught up with his old friends, and seemed none the worse for his unpleasant experience, but had to be monitored annually for the next ten years.

Where is the Key?

It was now time for Ian to have a term or two at nursery school before he started his mainstream education. I enrolled him in another of the early, unregulated nursery schools, run in private homes by probably unqualified teachers. He was a shy, retiring little boy who went to his first morning at nursery school without any protest, but he kept repeating to me as he pedalled home on his tricycle, 'I've been to school, mummy', and a few minutes later, 'I've been to school'. 'Yes dear', I replied each time he made this comment. I thought it was a sign of his approval, and that he had enjoyed his first morning and was looking forward to the next. I didn't realise the significance of what he had said until the following day, when he again told me quite firmly, as I began to get him ready to go to nursery school, 'But mummy, I've been to school'. He appeared to consider that his education had been completed in one morning – he had gone along with this idea of education, and had *been* to school. He'd been there, done that, got the T-shirt!

It was with great difficulty that I kept his tricycle heading in the right direction the following morning, as I gently – or firmly - edged it in the general direction of his destination, while he kept twisting the handlebars, turning them strenuously towards home, with the firm statement, 'I've been to school'. I suggested that we looked out for yellow front doors (yellow was a popular colour at that time for painting front doors) as I tried to keep his attention, and his feet, pedalling towards his little school. We had protestations for several days, until he accepted that there was no option, and that school was permanent for the foreseeable future.

Chapter Sixteen

THE MOVE

My mother spent Christmas Day with us again in 1962. Very heavy snow fell during the day and my father had a difficult time driving my mother back to her ward on Christmas evening. No one was about when they reached the Shenley campus (although that word would not have been used in those days to describe the hospital buildings and the surrounding grounds). My father found that the little roads in the grounds of Shenley had been obliterated by snow; and these hidden, snow-covered lanes made it difficult for him to find where he should park the car. In the end he apparently just left it, and he and my mother trudged through the snow across the lawns until they reached the little side entrance door to my mother's villa. They found the door was locked. The staff had forgotten that Lily Brook had been out for the day. My father later told us that he had great difficulty in getting an answer to his repeated ringing of the doorbell. Were they all asleep, I wonder? Someone eventually appeared just before my father decided he would have to bring my mother back home for the night. He was relieved when a light appeared and, at last, the door opened. My mother went up the stairs to her bed in the dormitory, but my dad had to find his way back to his car in the snow, cold and alone, before driving home in the 'white-out'. On his return home he told us that he had to shout and bang hard on the door as well as ring the bell for quite a while before anyone realised a patient was waiting outside in the freezing cold. The snow was much deeper in Hertfordshire than in Middlesex. Shenley is 400ft above sea level and is situated on the ridge of the largest plateau in Hertfordshire; the weather had been much more severe there than in Kenton.

I am not aware that any other patient in my mother's villa ever had a day out. Whenever we visited we found we were among the very few, if any, visitors in the ward. I am sure that most of the ladies, like my mother, had been there for years, but that many had been abandoned by relatives, who had possibly moved far away from their former home in Harrow, Wembley, Ruislip, Willesden or any of the other suburbs of north London that made up the hospital's catchment area.

Their former home could have been bombed in the war, and their relatives – possibly their children - could have been among the fatalities. Maybe someone's husband had been killed when on active service. Some men might have been unable to bear the stigma attached to them by their wife's illness, and had just walked away and made new lives, others had possibly found other partners and had remarried (bigamously) and the poor mentally ill wife was forgotten. Others may have formed another partnership for the sake of the children who were left without their mother.

To be abandoned by your relatives, receiving no visits, no attention or consideration from your family is an intolerable situation for anyone to be in. But it was possibly the hard truth for some of the patients in long-term care in Shenley hospital. I knew of nobody's personal history. I am just feeling my way, trying to see reasons, and understand all sides of some of the tragic possibilities brought about by severe mental illness at that time. I wonder how many of these ladies had initially suffered from unrecognised post-natal depression in the 1920s and early '30s. How many of them had lost contact with their children because of the illness, as my own mother had, and thus forgotten their existence?

I now realise how fragile my childhood had been, and that if my father had received no suitable answer to his advertisement for a housekeeper when my mother was admitted to a mental hospital in 1939, I may have been put into care. There was nobody who could have looked after me, and my father had to keep his job. There was little social care provided in those days. I realise how constant had been my father's care and contact with his very ill wife. It is unlikely he ever had any commendation for this. I wish I had considered this when he was alive; I have only begun to understand the difficulties my parents had as I wrote this book. When nothing is said, no thoughts are brought alive.

Andrew had missed one-and-a-half terms of Primary School, but soon settled in fairly well with a new teacher in the junior school in the autumn term. He began to tell us that some of the children at school were avoiding him and were not playing with him and with the other TB victims, even though most of them were now recovered. We heard that the children, who had not needed to be admitted to hospital, but had had a positive reaction to their TB test earlier in the year and been well enough to remain at home while taking their medication, were also being ostracised by some children in the playground. Parents, understandly I suppose, were worried that their children might catch TB from them, but none of the children affected had been infectious. None of them had infected sputum, or cavities in the lung. The situation rather unsettled us, and may have helped to germinate the seed of thoughts of moving.

We had lived in my father's house for the first eleven years of our marriage, and my father had now retired and was around the house all day. Andrew and I both did our piano practice on his piano in his living room, which meant quite an intrusion on his privacy, and our children's activities were spreading over the house. Granddad's television (his retirement gift) was a great attraction for the boys, and I know he enjoyed their company. My husband I often joined my father around his TV in the evenings too.

I had cared for him and looked after the house since I was fourteen, but I began to feel restricted by my father's presence all day, especially when my friends Pat, or Dorothy came in for coffee or a cup of tea. I didn't know where to take them; I felt I was excluding him if we sat in the kitchen, or in our living room, with only glass-panelled doors between my father and us. It felt a bit odd if we went in to join my father. Did he want us there, chatting away while he was reading the morning paper? Our kitchen is where we often ended up, but it still had an old-fashioned Ideal solid-fuel boiler, which did make it nice and cosy on a winter's morning, but was rather ugly. We now had modern, strongly patterned (ghastly!) plastic curtains at the windows, but old-fashioned lino on the floor, and two old-fashioned kitchen chairs. Red Formica had replaced the old enamel-top of the kitchen table. It was still largely a pre-war kitchen; the curtains the replacement tabletop together with modern wallpaper on the walls were the only concession to modernity. Looking back I can see that the colours and the patterns were hideous and the colours too bright, but that was the fashion in the fifties and early sixties.

We began to think that we would like to live in our own house in another area, although I didn't like to feel I was abandoning my father as he grew older. We had been saving hard for quite some time and suggested to him that we bought our own house and that he could come and live with us. He could then have the privacy of his own bedroom and sitting room while we would be able to spread ourselves a little more in our own home. I would continue to housekeep and cook for us all and we would share each other's company, but not live in each other's pockets.

He then dropped a 'bombshell' and told us that he had been considering whether my mother might be well enough to live at home again. Although her behaviour sometimes appeared to be a little unfriendly towards my father, she always enjoyed the Sundays she spent back in her old home. But she had been away from home and housekeeping for twenty-four years, and was now nearing seventy. Would she be able to cope? Was it safe for her to return home? The possibility of my mother returning home again had not entered my thoughts.

As she had improved so much with the modern drugs I believe that my father felt it was his duty to have her home, feeling that people might think he was allowing her to remain in hospital because he didn't want her back. I believe he thought that his sister-in-law, my Auntie Ada, who had looked after me in pre-war years when my mother had a nervous breakdown, might consider that Lily, her younger sister, should no longer be shut away. My father discussed it with the sister in charge of my mother's villa, and after consideration the hospital authorities said she was free to leave the hospital if she so wished, and she could return to her own home at any time, although I don't think my father was altogether confident about this decision, but felt he was doing his duty by his wife.

After her death many years later I asked to see her consultant who told me that my mother's medical notes indicated that neither were they confident that things would work out well, but that as she was no longer sectioned, my mother was free to go home if she so wished. That was the only time I spoke to a doctor in Shenley. I never heard, or over-heard in my childhood, my father speak of her seeing a doctor, nor of him having a consultation with a doctor about his wife.

My mother appeared to pass much of her time in hospital in recent years in writing long lists of names and figures, which she called her 'business' considering it to be private and important. She kept these lists in her handbag, guarding them closely. She had some old-fashioned phrases that I think were a hangover from her own upbringing before the First World War, phrases that seemed rather old-fashioned, but were somehow attractive. She was interested in our lives and in her (unacknowledged) grandsons; she was rational and showed no aggression either on a home visit or when we saw her in Shenley. But it seems amazing that she was allowed to return home without any preparatory, short periods living at home, to see how she would manage.

Before my mother could come home my husband and I had to find somewhere else to live. It was time for us to start looking for our first house.

There was still a lot of snow around in January 1963, when early on a Saturday morning Maurice and I, together with our sons, began our first house-hunting expedition. At that time houses were cheaper in the area around Hatfield and St. Albans than in Kenton or Harrow. We felt that it would be sensible to move nearer to my husband's work. We also felt that it might be a good idea to move away from Kenton because of the slight discrimination perceived at school by the ex-TB patients. We had both grown up in the Harrow district and we were perhaps keen to strike out on new ground. It would be nice to live nearer to the countryside. The snow was very deep as we trudged around building sites and looked at half built houses that were far too expensive, but very tempting. It was bitterly cold, although the scenery was really beautiful as we drove through the outskirts of St. Albans, with low snow-covered hills, stark white against the sky, with silhouettes of big old trees, fields thick with untouched snow, marked out clearly by the winter-black of the hedges. There was certainly a lot more snow in Hertfordshire than in Middlesex. It was surprising to notice the difference in the weather eighteen miles further north.

The Saturday morning house-hunting visits passed so quickly, and we hadn't seen anything that either appealed to that or us was within our budget. Time was flying by and the daffodils were blooming when Maurice visited a house on his way home from work one Friday evening. He came home quite excited. This is the one, he was sure. He had been much taken with the house, told the owners that he would like to bring his family to see it the following afternoon. They had kindly invited us to have a cup of tea with them after viewing, so once again we set off to St. Albans the following afternoon. The house was very attractive, rather small, but it had a lot of useful inclusions in the price. The hall and landing had fitted carpet in a lovely rich shade of blue that was included in the sale. We had no fitted carpets at Kenton so this was a big attraction for me. The tiny kitchen was fully fitted but there was really only space for one person to work in it. We would certainly be unable to have breakfast in the kitchen, as had been our practice. There was a very pretty garden in which the children played as we looked around indoors. It was a smaller house than the one I had lived in for most of my life.

We were sitting talking to the owners while having tea and homemade cakes when Andrew asked for the toilet. He went upstairs, and after a while I realised that he had been absent for a long time. I looked around and couldn't see him anywhere downstairs or in the garden, and as I went up the stairs I heard a quiet voice call, 'Mummy, I can't open the door'. I pushed the toilet door, and it didn't budge. My son had bolted the toilet door, but it was a bit stiff and he hadn't fathomed out how to unbolt it, so he sat on the toilet seat, quietly and politely calling for help and waiting patiently for a response. I think he had bolted himself in through childish curiosity rather than the necessity for privacy. He had only seen toilets whose door was locked with a key.

This toilet had a bolt, easy to slide in, but difficult to undo if you don't know how it works! Where was the key? This time there was no key. He had been too shy to shout out in these unfamiliar surroundings, and had been patiently waiting until one of his parents noticed his absence. He was much relieved to regain his freedom after instructions had been called out to him and he had successfully unbolted the door.

We decided to buy this house. I still remember the bowl of beautiful daffodils that the owner had picked from the garden and put on the landing windowsill, which I had noticed as soon as we entered the house. They appeared very welcoming as the sun shone on to them through the large window. They contrasted so well with the blue carpet. It just shows you what little things can influence an inexperienced house-buyer!

We moved to our own house at the end of May. As all our belongings were being stacked away in the removal van, we went around saying goodbye to our neighbours, and then kissed my father goodbye, before we drove off to start our new lives. We were not going far away, only thirty minutes drive by car, and after a day or two we would be back in Kenton to return the car to my father for his fortnight's ownership.

I didn't appreciate then how emotional our move to St. Albans may have been for my father – we didn't have emotional moments in our family. I am sure that people generally were not as open with their emotions, or aware of them, as they are today. I think tough times make one unaware of, or else bottle up, feelings. My parents' generation and my own had lived through shortages, war and deprivations, and there had also been plenty of additional difficulties in my family. I now realise that my father may have been feeling very apprehensive about my mother's return, and rather sad at losing the lively presence of his grandchildren in the home. I should have realised that he may also have grieved that his only daughter and companion of thirty-two years was leaving home. He was alone in the house for the first time since the last few months of 1939 when my mother had gone into Shenley hospital, and I was being cared for elsewhere. I was leaving the house I had lived in since I was a child of four. It must have seemed very empty to my father that first night, half empty of furniture, and without his family or the sound of his grandchildren playing. But it was very exciting for us as we arranged our furniture in our new home. It was a nice little house in an attractive tree-lined road with a local primary school nearby.

So in the early summer of 1963 my father began an entirely new phase in his retirement. He had a busy time rearranging some of his furniture to fill the gaps the removal of our furniture had made and purchasing some replacements. A few days later he brought my mother back to the home in which she had only lived for four years before becoming a long-term patient in a psychiatric hospital in 1939. She came back to what we all hoped would be her home for the rest of her life. It was quite an eventful time for all of us; first house ownership for Maurice and me, new schools for the boys and a real home again for my mother.

For the first time in eleven years of marriage Maurice and I were on our own with just our children. We had our first mortgage on a very pleasant, semi-detached house, built in the mid-1920s in what was then the country town, or rather city, of St. Albans. Our mortgage was £20.9s. a month, which sounds a trifle now, but was quite a good proportion of our income then. I had to walk a little further to do my shopping in the local parade of shops, where there was a small grocer's shop that delivered a weekly order. There was a fresh fish shop, two butchers, a chemist's, two small greengrocers, a barber and hairdresser's shop, a paper shop and post office, together with several other little shops, but their businesses declined some years later when a large supermarket was built close by. The post office combined with newsagents and a tiny greengrocer's are the only survivors although other, alternative, shops have thankfully filled the spaces.

A van came round the local streets on Saturdays selling vegetables and some other goods at the door. We found a good bakery a little further away – opposite the city cemetery, and we tended to call it the 'cemetery baker's, where lovely bread was baked on the premises, which was far removed from the 'pappy' bread available today. I knew that the city of St. Albans was built on a hill; but I soon discovered that nearly everywhere was a little hilly. My walk home from the shops carrying the shopping baskets pulled on each side of my neck as I walked up a long incline, which fired up my persistent facial neuralgia. I never seemed able to forget it or be unaware of it. I was not used to walking uphill, as Kenton itself was flat, although edged with hills – Harrow-on-the-hill, Belmont Hill, Clamp Hill, and Stanmore Hill.

We found that a large market was held in the main street of the city centre twice a week. This was something completely new in our experience, but we really thought we were in a rural country town when we took the boys to the cattle market that was still held every Saturday morning. We watched the cows being led in by the farmers, and we heard the dealers' rapid prattle, as it sounds to the uninitiated, hopefully followed by a good sale. But cattle farming was becoming rare in Hertfordshire, and soon the cattle market ceased. To mark the original use of the site a new road was built some years later near the old cattle market and called Drover's Way. It led to the new multi-storey car park. The twice-weekly general market is still thriving, as it has for hundreds of years.

St. Albans was a quiet Cathedral market town when we first moved, but during the 1960s everything began to change with the electrification of the railway into London and the building of the motorways. House prices rocketed as the City became commuter land A ring road was built in the early sixties, which almost encircled the town, passing through new housing estates, on the edge of others, and through well-established residential streets of pre-war houses, whose quiet gardens were to be filled with the endless sound of traffic in the coming years. The area gradually became much busier for the residents around this new ring road as the traffic that had been tempted away from driving through the city centre now drove along their street. Eventually the sense of living in a country town vanished. The ring road now has traffic passing through continually, whilst other transport is often held up as it drags through the city centre. St. Albans is too near to the Ml, the M25 and the A1M, none of which had been constructed in 1963.

New uniforms were required with a change in school, and the boys looked very smart in their new dark brown blazers and caps with the Fleetville School badge on the front of the cap and on the blazer pocket. Short grey worsted trousers were still worn right through primary school years and also the first year in secondary school in those days. Boys remained 'boys' for much longer before they became 'lads,' and girls were also 'girls' until they left school, and not 'ladettes,' into make-up or fashion.

Their new school was an old building with high windows, and not at all like their previous school. I think Andrew missed his old friends, as he had left behind a little group of real 'buddies' in Martin, Roy and Mitch, but I think the new area had excited his curiosity and he soon settled. Ian was in the middle of his first term at school before our move from Kenton and hadn't really had time to settle there so I thought he had accepted that school was obligatory for the foreseeable future. For a while I walked with the two boys to school each morning and met them in the afternoon.

After I had registered my two boys in the respective departments of their new school, I came home and decided it was time to do some washing. We had brought with us our very reliable twin-tub Hoover washing machine, a much-improved successor of the single-tub earlier model. It tucked neatly under a removable worktop adjacent to the kitchen sink in our new home. I fixed the short hose onto the hot tap and dipped the other end into the tub, then turned the tap on to fill the tub while I went into the garden to fix the washing line. I pulled the kitchen door shut behind me, and heard a little click. My heart lurched as I realised that the kitchen door had a Yale lock, and I had shut, and locked, the door. I was shut outside my new home, stuck in the garden, unable to get into the house, with the tap running hot water into my washing machine! For a moment I panicked. I knew nobody; I had not met either of my neighbours; what could I do? I suddenly felt so useless. Here I was, shut out of the house I had only lived in for a few days. There was only one thing I could do – and I must do it quickly, the hot water was still filling (or, I feared, would shortly be over-filling) my washing machine. I would have to break a window.

French doors with small windowpanes led from our lounge to the garden. I found a jagged piece of flint in a nearby flowerbed, knelt down in front of the doors and smashed the stone into one of the bottom windows. I quickly pulled away the larger pieces of glass and then picked off the tiny shards that were still attached all around the frame. I carefully eased my head through the hole, then my arms, and turned my body a little to edge my shoulders through the tiny window frame, placed my hands on the carpet and slowly pulled and wriggled and squeezed my body sideways through the small rectangle of space I had made. I rushed to the kitchen, and found the tub almost up to the brim with hot water, but, amazingly, I had reached it just in time. Where was the key? It was, of course, safely on the inside of the lock. I had lived with a mortise lock in our kitchen door at Kenton all my life and had never thought of a kitchen door with a Yale lock. I felt awful; to have smashed a window of my own house, and broken into my new home after living there for just a few days was almost unbelievable, but I had done it, and I didn't have a flooded kitchen. Looking at the small aperture afterwards I could hardly believe that I could have got through it. I didn't pull that door shut from the outside again. When Maurice came home from work that evening, I told him my tale, showed him the evidence, and when he measured the size of the window that he had to replace, he found that it was 9inchesx12in. I wish I could squeeze my body through a hole that size now!

A few days later I was busy washing up the breakfast dishes after taking the boys to school when I heard loud bangs on the kitchen door. I was a little worried as to who was outside the door making such a racket, but when I opened it, I was most surprised to see my younger son standing on the step. 'I don't like school,' he said. He had walked out; nobody had noticed this not-quite-five-year-old new boy slip out of the classroom – or the playground, I never knew which – and take himself home, crossing the new ring road on the way. I persuaded him that school would improve when he grew used to it, told him that children liked being in the Infants' School, he would be bored all day at home and eventually, reluctantly, we walked back to school.

I went into the classroom and told the teacher that one of her pupils had left the class, but she was overly busy with a crowd of small children around her. She didn't seem very disturbed that this could have happened, and I had a feeling that she didn't even know who he was, or was aware that anyone had gone missing. There were no classroom assistants in those days. I think there would be quite a hue and cry if this happened nowadays. Ian was certainly confirming his opinion that 'I have been to school' after his first day at nursery school. He'd been, he'd done it before. He had already got the T- shirt - except that it was a new school uniform.

The school summer holidays soon arrived and Andrew began exploring the area on his Raleigh Explorer bicycle, which he had ridden on the pavement in Kenton. It was not long before he came home rather distressed because a policeman had stopped him and told him he could not ride on the pavement. (Yes, a policeman on a beat, walking around the local streets! I don't think I have ever seen one in my road. Andrew was very unlucky.) We had bought the bicycle for his seventh birthday the previous year and had understood that it was a 'pavement' cycle. It was certainly too small, and he was too young, to ride on the roads. It was a great disappointment, and rather spoilt his first summer in his new surroundings. One seems to see people of all ages on all sorts and sizes of bikes riding on footpaths or pavements nowadays.

The boys missed granddad's television, and it was quite some time before we owned one, and then it was an old, hefty TV, with a very small screen, which had been passed on to us by an aunt of my husband's. We had quite a tight budget, and were buying a piano on hire purchase as well as our mortgage. I think the piano was the only thing we ever bought on the hire purchase, apart from our gas stove. We didn't have credit; we saved until we could afford whatever it was we wanted. In time we bought a record player, then an early, cumbersome, tape recorder; items that are both obsolete now.

The boys were soon sensible enough to walk to school together in the mornings, and I met Ian coming out of his infant school in the afternoon. Parents didn't feel the necessity of escorting their junior school-age offspring each morning then, or consider they were at risk by walking home unaccompanied. Independence was encouraged.

Chapter Seventeen

HOME AGAIN!

My mother appeared to be settling happily into her old home, and managed amazingly well domestically, cleaning the house, doing the shopping and cooking the meals. She was very calm whenever we saw her, didn't seem excited or overjoyed at being home, but just took it all in her stride. It was just as if she had never been away, and she was doing the day-to-day things she always did, but it must have been very difficult for my parents to begin to live together in the same home after such a long period of separation.

My parents had some shopping expeditions for items needed in the house, which was a new experience for my mother, and for my father, too, as he had not updated anything since before the war. Fashions had changed a lot since then, and new styles of furnishings and household equipment had appeared. They bought a fridge, some new cushions, some china and saucepans, but I don't remember a washing machine taking the place of the one that went into our furniture van; a laundry was found instead. I think my mother enjoyed the shopping expeditions, but my father had always hated shopping. He used to say that he spent five-and-a-half days of every week in a shop and he didn't want to see any more, but he certainly took my mother shopping to Sopers, the local independent department store in Harrow, now a branch of Debenhams. I was very pleased to see all their new acquisitions, especially as nothing had been replaced in our home since we had moved into the house in 1935. It must have been an enjoyable experience for them both.

During that summer my parents were able to have a few drives together in the car as in times past, and they spent a weekend with my mother's sister and brother-in-law at Bexhill. My mother had not seen her sister Ada for many years, but she recognised her and acknowledged their relationship. They also visited my in-laws in Clacton. At first everything seemed to be going well. My mother was fine with the boys, was pleased to see them, and chatted naturally. She always greeted Maurice and me warmly. We were all fond of her, but I had been for so long without her since my early childhood, that I never felt there was a mother-and-daughter relationship. There couldn't be.

One knew nothing about mother/child bonding in those days, and many parents were a little remote with their children; this could have been a legacy of the Victorian era for many in the first half of the twentieth century. As I was growing up it was still thought that children were to be 'seen and not heard'. Praise or commendation was infrequently given; children were not encouraged to think too much of themselves, they might become 'swollen-headed'. I don't think the era of being natural, loving or showing appreciation was a characteristic of many families in my parents' or in my own generation. People tended to have 'a stiff upper lip' and children were 'kept in their place' and were expected to help in the home.

My family and I saw my parents every two weeks, when we exchanged ownership of the car. They drove over to our home, and we had a meal together before Maurice drove them back to Kenton, and then returned home to St. Albans again for our fortnight's turn with the car. Two weeks later we drove over to Kenton and saw my parents for a few hours and my dad drove us back home before returning home for his two weeks of driving. The following year we were able to afford our own car, and this strange and awkward arrangement ceased.

My mother had prepared a very nice tea for us one Saturday, even making some lovely light cakes without the use of scales and she was the perfect hostess. She had never had scales, and didn't see the need for them. She had always guessed the weight of flour, sugar etc., and had not forgotten how to make cakes after so long.

Sometimes I visited my parents for lunch. They had a little snooze after the meal was over while I sat reading the paper. I began to notice that my mother sometimes glanced across to look at my father in a strange, unfriendly way when he seemed to be asleep. Sadly, she occasionally began to behave a little oddly, and often looked suspiciously towards my father when we saw them together. I stayed overnight with my parents on one occasion when, on going to upstairs at bedtime, I found that the toilet roll had been totally unwound and sheets of toilet paper were strewn everywhere. I think my mother had become frustrated or angry over some way in which my father had tried to assist her in getting me a bedtime drink of Ovaltine. She had disappeared upstairs and presumably blown out her anger on the toilet roll. It made me realise that all was not right, and that my father was obviously under considerable strain – and as I realised later, possibly fear. I was anxious about his well-being and safety, and rather concerned about my mother's unpredictable behaviour. I could see that my father was very tense.

I wondered and worried over which of my parents would break down first, and wrote to Shenley Hospital to this effect, but no one responded to my appeal for help, or even replied to my letter. There had been no back up or support for my parents; nobody checked up on how they were managing, advised my father in any way, or visited to make sure that my mother was taking her medication. I realise that she must have seen her GP to get a further prescription for her drugs as I don't think repeat prescriptions were given then. She may, of course, have appeared quite all right in his surgery, but someone, somewhere, should have followed her up more carefully, or visited my parents in the home to assess how things were going.

I was preparing to visit my parents one morning during the children's autumn half-term holiday, and was waiting for my father to arrive in the car to drive the boys and me back to Kenton for the day, when the telephone rang. It was my father, telling me in very strained tones that he was phoning from his next-door-neighbour's house because my mother had attacked him with a knife at the breakfast table, and he had been forced to flee and had taken refuge in the house next door. I began to understand what might have happened at her previous breakdowns. I realised what my father may have been through so often in the past. I began to appreciate too, the possible reason why I was suddenly uprooted and moved to a 'safe house' when I was young.

I left home immediately with the children and travelled by bus, train and another bus, to my parents' house. The journey seemed endless by public transport. At last I was back in Kenton; I rushed along the road with the boys in tow, took them directly to a kind neighbour, and hurriedly explained to her what had occurred before going to my old home.

I found that my father had been able to return to the house; he had a plaster over a cut on his face and looked very shocked, but thankfully was not seriously injured. My mother had aimed a knife at his face, but fortunately had missed his eye and hit the side of his nose, and the knife was not very sharp. However it was an attack, and must have been frightening. My father was very slightly built, and my mother was much sturdier. My father had rushed to the house next door, and had telephoned the doctor and the hospital from the neighbour's house. I presume that the doctor had visited and attended to my father's cut face, and had told him that my mother would have to return to Shenley. My father never spoke about the incident.

My mother was in another room when my father returned to the house, and she remained there for a while after my arrival. She joined us later and greeted me as if nothing untoward had occurred., but she was eerily silent. It seemed so sad that, after spending four months at home, my mother had snapped, I feel sure, through lack of support, or advice to my father, with nobody checking that she was keeping well mentally as well as coping well domestically.

The atmosphere was so tense as the three of us sat there in silence, not knowing what to say to each other as we waited for the GP and mental health officers to arrive. I don't know what provoked her to attack my father, but suspect that she had not been taking her medication regularly. I think she thought she was doing so well in the home that she no longer needed medicine. I am sure my father would have kept a watchful eye on her, but I know he would have had to be careful, as she might have resented what she saw as his interference, and perhaps this is what actually happened, and the resentment turned to aggression and violence. I am sure that this is what my poor father had feared might happen. I know I feared that something, or someone, would snap, but I really had no idea of what might occur or who would turn out to be the victim. I was so relieved that he had not been badly injured. One hears of violent attacks nowadays, but many of these incidents didn't occur so frequently years ago as so many people with severe mental health issues remained in secure wards of large psychiatric hospitals. If you keep taking the medicine, things are usually O.K., but it is easy for those who now feel well to leave off their medication, when life can then soon go disastrously wrong.

I made a pot of tea, and we sat drinking cups of tea as we waited for the doctor and mental health officers to come and assess, persuade, or insist, on my mother's return to hospital. My father and I felt strained and very tense, while my mother seemed quite calm, and there was almost total silence in the room as we waited for the three professionals to arrive. I didn't know what to say, and neither of my parents wanted to talk about what had happened. It was all very strange.

At last the medics arrived; my mother remained completely calm and rational as they tried gently to persuade her that it would be better if she returned to hospital. She repeatedly and firmly said that she did her housework, minded her own business, and was certainly not going to return to 'that establishment'. My father sat quietly. I feared for him, and began to guess at what he may have gone through when I was a child, when perhaps she was taken out of her home by force. We seemed to be getting nowhere. What could I do? After a while I quietly left the room, found her coat and hat, her handbag and gloves, and returned with them to the living room. I brought the coat towards where my mother was sitting, held it out to her and said, 'Come on Mumma, just pop your coat on'. She stood up straight away and without questioning she allowed me to help her into her coat; she then asked for her hat, and put that on. There was no need for any persuasion at all as she picked up her handbag, and then asked, 'Where are my gloves?' The GP murmured to me, 'Good psychology, Sheila!' as we stood in the hall. The mental health officers asked my mother to go with them in their car, and she, quite imperiously (good for her) said, 'I will go in my husband's car; I'm certainly not going with you'. After a little discussion it was agreed that it was probably safe for my mother to travel back to Shenley in my father's car; I sat in the back seat, and the two mental health officers drove behind. It was a nerve-wracking drive. I sat, leaning forward, at the ready to do – I know not what – if there was any trouble, as my father drove rather nervously back to Shenley Hospital. My goodness, how anxious he must have been. I really don't know what I would have been able to do, or how those in the car behind could have helped if there had been a problem. I often wondered what would have happened if I had not had the idea to get my mother's coat and hat. I just felt that these polite attempts at persuasion were only making her more determined to stay put.

I found it hard to accept that there had been no support, follow-up, or reply to my letter or advice from social, psychiatric or medical services for either of my parents. Follow-up of discharged psychiatric patients did not appear to occur in the 1960s.

After my mother was safely returned to hospital care we drove back to Kenton, and I collected my two young sons from the neighbour, who must have wondered how much longer she had to care for my children. How had the day passed for them? They must have been quite bewildered, as they didn't know Mrs. Holding at all well. She had lived a few doors away from us since I was a child, and she knew my mother before the war. Everything, however, was okay when I called to relieve her of her charges and explained all that had occurred. She had been very kind.

I am ashamed to admit my children were not in the forefront of my mind during that day. In the stress of the emergency I really hadn't given the children – or the kind neighbour – much thought. Mrs. Holding had kindly taken them in when I knocked on her door. She may already have been aware that there was trouble along the road. I was never told exactly what had occurred that morning to spark off the attack, but I think she knew what had happened and so understood the situation. I can remember being taken out for a walk with her when I was a small child, and I think this may have been when a previous crisis had occurred with my mother.

My father's awful day was not yet over, as he had to drive the children and me home and then go back to his empty house. What must he have been feeling? He had been so loyal to my mother for so many years, and suffered so much, but I think there might have been a little sense of relief combined with his sorrow. He knew it would have been a precarious outlook for their future happiness. He had tried. He still remained loyal. My father never spoke to me of the incident, and I was never made aware of all that had occurred early that morning. It was all part of my upbringing – and possibly my father's upbringing too, as he grew up as an only child with his widowed mother – that we didn't discuss problems or personal matters. How different our behaviour might have been nowadays!

People didn't show their feelings much in those days; certainly not the people I knew. Emotion was something that I think was not recognised, let alone expressed, then; weeping in public was unknown and people kept their anxieties to themselves.

My mother never saw her home again. She was placed in a different, more closely watched ward and for a while and she obviously resented being there and was hostile to my father when we visited. The ward was not familiar, or so easy going, as in her previous surroundings in villa 4A. If there had been an appropriate and immediate response to my letter to the hospital about my mother's lack of professional supervision, things might have been quite different for my parents, but maybe in the long term it was better for them both that my mother returned to hospital.

They would both have been considered to be getting on in years at that period and may have found living together even more difficult as they grew older. Nowadays you are not considered to be 'old' until you are in your eighties and I have not quite reached that big 'O'. My mother had said she minded her own business and cared for the home, but her outward calm may have hidden an inward uncertainty. As time passed I think she accepted that she felt more secure back in hospital, and she never asked if she could return home, or even asked to visit her home again. The months she had spent back in her own home were never mentioned after this sad episode.

Chapter Eighteen

SETTLING IN

It had been another very anxious period in our lives, occurring less than six months after we had moved into our new home. My father was now looking after himself and living alone. It had been a very difficult time for him, and we saw him regularly, sharing the car, and he soon began to visit my mother every few weeks once again. At first she appeared to be very aggrieved at being back in Shenley and would have nothing to do with my father. She probably blamed him for putting her back in hospital – but she could equally have blamed me, as I had got her to put her outdoor clothes on. My mother was very subdued for quite some time, probably aided by increased medication until she had settled and showed no signs of aggressive behaviour.

My father sold our family home a year later. Although I had lived in that house with both my parents for only four years before the war, it was nevertheless the house I grew up in and had continued to live in after my marriage. It had been my home for twenty-eight years, and it held many memories for me.

My father bought a bungalow in St. Albans, where he lived contentedly for the next nineteen years, and grew to love his bungalow and garden. When I telephoned him during the week he always appeared cheerful although his voice often sounded gruff, and he would tell me that he hadn't spoken to anyone since he had last talked to me. His voice had not had enough exercise, as he knew nobody in the area and rarely saw his neighbours, but he always spent the day with us on Sunday. As I greeted him on his arrival at lunchtime, I asked him how he was, his usual reply was, 'I'm all right dear. Never mind about me. What's more to the point is, "How are you?"' with great emphasis on the YOU. His concern for me must have often been on his mind when at home alone, together with his thoughts of my mother living back in Shenley. He had been such a loyal and devoted husband and father for many decades. He had no other companionship apart from our family to cheer him, and was very fond of his grandchildren and interested in all their activities and progress. We had at last been able to afford our own car, and we invited my father to join us on our annual holidays once again, but I can now scarcely imagine how we managed to get three adults and two growing children into our second-hand Ford Prefect, along with all our luggage and food for a self-catering holiday.

Whilst in my new home I often heard the sound of the aircraft engines being tested during the daytime six miles away at the deHavilland test beds. Maurice was part of the testing team developing the Gnome engine that was installed into the Sea King helicopters in the 1960s, and was in service for the following forty years. My husband's careful skill over the quality control of the instrumentation must have helped to contribute to its' safety record and he was always proud when news of a Sea King helicopter rescue was on the news, and used to say, 'I had a part in that'. It has been a good, and safe, engine, a British product to be proud of. The demand for overtime work had lessened.

In the 1960s the distant drone from de Havilland's engine test beds at Hatfield was constant at certain periods, but the sound was well muted six miles away and it didn't affect me at all, but I was still very sensitive to any loud noise close by, an aircraft overhead, certain organ frequencies, loud music or resonant, penetrating voices, ambulance or police sirens. I really missed our old Baptist church at Kenton and we found it difficult to settle in a church in St. Albans. Maurice occasionally had to get me out of the church building before I collapsed during the service - like a dropped overcoat - if loud sound occurred, be it verbal or instrumental. One such occasion occurred soon after we had moved. The preacher at the morning service had a very loud, booming voice, and I can still remember the opening words as he introduced his sermon by quoting the text, 'Ho! everyone that thirsteth, come ye to the waters,' using the old Authorised version of the Bible, in a very penetrating voice. This caused me to cringe and then collapse at the very start of his sermon. One couple in the congregation took care of our two sons and even took them home to share Sunday lunch with their family. John said kindly to Maurice, 'Just look after Sheila. We'll take care of the boys'. He and his wife Madge took Andrew and Ian home to share Sunday lunch with their two children, who then played together until Maurice arrived to take our boys home. I remember they told us that John had played hide-and-seek with them in the house and garden, and I think they thought that they had had a good day out, and were unaware of the reason behind it. This kindness had relieved my husband of any anxiety over them and gave me a few hours of quietness in order to recover. That kindness is still remembered – as is that loud, almost explosive, 'HO!'

A few years' later the church we were attending had recently had a new organ installed. The last hymn was announced and the organist played the introduction with great enthusiasm, exploring the organ's capabilities. He played even more exuberantly as the last verse began, and the congregation sang with great fervour, while I began to wilt. Maurice urged me to get out while I could, but I hung on to the back of the pew in front of me and whispered that I would be all right. I hoped I could hang on until the end of the service. I didn't want to appear to be walking out before it was over. As the benediction was given, my husband began to help me make a discreet exit, but the organist suddenly produced a great blast at the start of his final voluntary, just I reached the end of the pew. I collapsed in the aisle from the overpowering sound and was spread over the floor obstructing the clergy as they processed up the aisle. At the first very loud chord I had completely lost it. The next thing I knew was that I was laid out on the hymnbook table at the back of the church! Here was another church we could no longer attend.

A year or so later there was an occasion when parents were invited to an evening disco at my younger son's weekend Cub Camp, but I soon had to leave the scout hut because I could not stand the noise of the musicians playing the latest pop music; the amplification was so loud I had to make a quick exit. I stood outside for a while, but I still felt weak and limp. I attempted to return to the event, but the noise had increased even more as the evening had worn on, and I had to leave immediately and be brought home.

My mother seemed happier when she was eventually moved into another villa, number 12A, where about twenty ladies lived on the ground floor of two-storey accommodation. I presume there was a similar villa on the floor above, although I don't remember ever seeing anyone going up or down the internal staircase. We visited my mother regularly and she was always affable, greeting Maurice, her grandsons and me, warmly. She was usually seated in a comfortable chair in what could have been a large hotel lounge. There were still very few, if any, other visitors present in the large lounge of, mainly, elderly ladies. There was a piano in the room, together with a few potted plants, but there was a noticeable absence of books, newspapers, magazines, crossword puzzle books, knitting, or anything that would indicate that the patients had any hobbies or activities. Their medication probably made them disinterested, but at least my mother had settled in contentedly. I had little knowledge of what activities might have been going on during the day, although I remember my mother telling me once that in the mornings they all sat at a table and filled little plastic bags with small items; I think my mother said they were screws.

On one occasion I met a young couple who were visiting, I assume, their grandmother. The young lady had a baby in her arms, and as we chatted a little, she asked if my mother would like to hold her baby. My mother said she would, and the lady kindly handed over her baby, who sat for a while on my mother's knee, as she held him and jogged him lightly up on down. It was a very thoughtful gesture on the part of this unknown visitor.

I was surprised to see one or two of the elderly ladies were smoking. Some long while afterwards I noticed that if a patient seemed a bit edgy, she would ask the Sister for a cigarette and one would be produced from the Sister's pocket and handed to the patient. This only happened very occasionally, but it made me appreciate how a cigarette can calm the nerves, but please understand that I am not recommending smoking!

Where is the Key?

The patients slept in a large dormitory, and there were also one or two small rooms off the main passage. My mother was asked at one time if she would like to have her own bedroom. She accepted one of these little rooms, and had far more privacy and the chance of an undisturbed night, and I thought she would enjoy having her own little haven, but after a few weeks she said that she preferred to be in the dormitory. I guess she felt a little insecure in a room on her own after so many years of communal living – and sleeping. The small room could have felt claustrophobic. It was similar in size to the little room Andrew had been isolated in only a few years previously, and also a bit like the room I had occupied when suffering from the breast abscess. Our family seemed to specialise in 'little rooms'.

I sometimes accompanied my father on his Wednesday afternoon visit. He continued to see my mother regularly throughout his life until about a couple of months before he died, keeping a life-time constancy, together with concern and regard for her. She was still a little off-hand in her attitude towards him, however. Sister sometimes led us to a little side room – one of the unused small bedrooms - that gave us privacy, but it may also have been her intention to avoid other patients feeling neglected if they had no family to visit them. I didn't feel totally at ease in this little room when sitting there on my own with my parents. My mother was never interested in anything my father said; I noticed that she often looked very strangely at him, and I was sometimes a little concerned that there might be another physical assault.

I wasn't aware of it then, but I understand that this disregard of loved ones can be one of the many and varied symptoms of schizophrenia: I have been told that sufferers sometimes turn against their nearest and dearest. The symptoms of my mother's illness have never been explained to me; nobody ever talked to me about her terrible life-long illness. She was obviously now considered to be a resident patient for the rest of her life.

However, the new official mental health policy only a few years later was to try and empty the psychiatric hospitals of all long-term patients as soon as possible, and only the violent or those whose medication was being established were welcomed for more than a very brief period.

Changes were occurring in Shenley Hospital long before my father died in 1982. Attempts were being made to transfer patients to smaller house-centred groups, and when we visited my mother she sometimes told us that she had been taken to Harrow to have meetings with a few other people. We didn't understand at the time what this was about, and my father was not informed of the purpose of these trips to Harrow, but it gradually became clear to us that my mother was being considered, or approved, or persuaded to change from residential care in Shenley to a smaller, perhaps self-sustaining group in Harrow. After my mother had spoken to us several times about these group meetings, she told us in no uncertain terms that she 'wasn't having any of it'.

These meetings may have been arranged with some other patients who were originally from the Harrow area, hoping that they would gel into a group who could live in a small, hopefully supervised, community. But we were not officially informed about this until much later, when my father received a letter asking him to make an appointment to discuss changes to his wife's care with a hospital manager. He was asked to agree to my mother's transfer to a small unit in Harrow, and he had to be very insistent that he did not want his wife to have to make another attempt at living outside the hospital community. Moreover, Shenley was quite close to his present home, which enabled him to visit her frequently. He said he was too old to drive *to* Harrow, an area he had moved *from* in order to be nearer to his wife and family, and he considered it to be a nonsensical proposition at her age. My mother was also adamant that she didn't want to move, and I believe that my parents' insistence prevented another change of residence becoming a reality for her. I don't think change would have been appropriate for my mother in view of her age, and after such a long period of institutional life. I think that she had cottoned on to what was afoot pretty early on. It was now too late for her to cope with living 'in the world'.

With the changes in attitude with regard to the mentally ill (or those with mental-health issues, to be politically correct) changes began to occur in the villas. A few years' later, after my father had died, I sometimes arrived at the hospital to find that my mother was having a cookery session, and I was directed to another building, where I found my mother and a few other patients had been cooking a meal together under supervision, and had just finished their lunch. This was something entirely new and gave some purpose to life, but I didn't feel that my mother enjoyed the experience, as she told me that she 'couldn't figure out what they were up to'. I think she felt that this was another attempt to prepare her for the outside world, and she seemed to be so insecure when out of her villa and her everyday routine. She seemed to be aware that some attempt at change was afoot and was tuned-in to it, and was suspicious.

The cookery sessions seemed a good idea to me, and made a change of scenery and a bit of activity for the patients, and an attempt at socialising, but they may have been intended as another preparation for moving out of the security of the hospital She was nearing her eightieth birthday, and I fear that she was now too old for change and shunned any personal responsibility for her daily life.

I sometimes arrived in her villa and found nobody there at all. I had to look around for quite a while before I saw a member of staff who told me that my mother was in the therapy room. I found this to be another single story, temporary-looking building, obviously built long after the original hospital was built. When I opened the door I saw a number of elderly people sitting in a circle, each holding a child-sized plastic hockey stick. They were playing a soft ball game, trying to hit it between the legs of someone else in the group to get a 'goal' if it reached the outside of the circle. I thought it was fun and very good for these elderly people, and would happily have joined in, but I could see that my mother was not really taking part. There was a lot of laughter and hilarity, but when their game came to an end and I escorted my mother back to her villa, she told me she thought it was all very silly. I don't think she thought it was ladylike to be playing games like that; maybe she just thought it was childish. I think she had stopped doing her 'business' as she called it, with the long lists she used to write and keep securely in her handbag. She had also got past carrying a handbag around with her.

On another occasion I found her in the reminiscence room. This was another a separate building from the villas, where a room had been thoughtfully furnished with a lot of old 1930s furniture, pictures, and other items including an old Singer sewing machine. This brought back memories for me from my childhood, and I talked to my mother about my memory of her sitting at her sewing machine when I was little. She seemed to recall the machine, as she declared that the one we were looking at was not quite the same as hers, which she was convinced only had drawers to one side. My recollection was that it had drawers on both sides, but I wouldn't be surprised if my mother's memory was the correct one; she would have used it far more than I had. But she couldn't make any connection with my early childhood memory of her sitting at the sewing machine making pelmets soon after we moved to our new home in Kenton in 1935. We took our time in looking at all the objects in the room, and I tried to interest my mother, but without much success. I thought the room was a very good idea, and was well presented.

Another attempt to bring these elderly ladies into the more modern era was to give them a perm. I went to see my mother one afternoon, and found her sitting in her chair looking rather startled. I think the startled expression arose from the frizzy hair-do she had been given. Her very fine, short, white hair had been permed and she looked a different person. It really didn't suit her, but she was given several permanent waves at regular intervals for some time, until either the hairdresser left, or the staff realised that this wildly wavy hair didn't suit my mother – or, hopefully, she felt able to say, 'I don't want any more perms, thank you'. Her hair was too fine to take a permanent wave. She looked a lot more like the person I had become fond of when her hair returned to its short, straight, rather boyish look, and her white hair had its former natural sheen. Another effort by the staff was to varnish the patients' nails. It was very nice for them to have this personal attention, but somehow, these elderly ladies didn't look right with bright red nail varnish on their nails, when they had nowhere to go. Perhaps they had chosen this colour, but a soft pink would have suited them better. I believe these new activities were part of the implementation of modern psychiatric practice, attempts to have closer, personal contact with the patients, with new approaches of treatment.

The general public knew so little, almost nothing, about the great spectrum of mental illness in those days, and the relatives of those suffering from some form of mental ill heath knew little more. Any indication or mention of mental illness (or 'nervous breakdown' as it was euphemistically called) was not discussed, but was swept under the carpet, sometimes made fun of, or whispered about. Vague expressions such as 'she's under the weather', he's got a 'health problem', or she's 'a bit low', were – and, perhaps, still are? – used. Sufferers from depression are still sometimes told to 'pull yourself together'.

Shortly after Ian was born I can remember being told about a young mother who was behaving strangely and couldn't look after her new baby; she had to go into hospital as she had 'depression'. I thought it very strange, and couldn't understand how this could happen just after she had had a baby. This was in 1958 or 9, when nobody had heard of post-natal depression. It didn't occur to me at that time that the mother I had forgotten might have initially suffered from a similar, misunderstood, and misdiagnosed, condition. It was a totally unspoken subject in society as well as within the family.

Someone suffering with 'bad nerves' was generally thought to be having imaginary symptoms, which were 'all in the mind'. Some still don't believe or understand that our nervous systems are actual, physical, though almost invisible, parts of our body. Recently the broad subject of mental ill health has been very much in the news: there have been programmes on TV and the radio, articles have appeared in the newspaper, and well-known people are beginning to pluck up their courage and talk of their own or their loved one's mental illness. Not so in my father's generation, or for most of my own life. He kept it all to himself and shared his troubles with no one – not even me. I grew up hiding my mother's mental illness from everyone. I didn't understand it; it didn't even have a name that explained to me what was wrong. 'Mania' was an old-fashioned term that I had heard my father use, and I think that term was used to cover almost the entire spectrum of mental diseases in those days. Nobody would have known the terms 'bi-polar' or 'post-natal' depression; they are comparatively new definitions. Just being able to say the name of one's illness gives a little confidence to the sufferer. I hope my mother's story will help to bring more openness, more understanding and more compassion.

Chapter Nineteen

A LITTLE DRAMA

When we had recovered from the shock of my mother's return to hospital so soon after our move, we realised it was time to find a new GP, who might be able to help relieve the wretched facial neuralgia was with me constantly. Our new doctor decided to refer me to the London hospital at which he had trained. I travelled up to London on a steam train to the old Kings Cross station, and then had a couple of changes on the as-yet unmodernised Underground train before reaching the hospital. I waited in a very old-fashioned outpatients' department before I was called in to see the consultant, who took my history and prescribed a drug whose name I never knew. In those days patients were not told the name of their medication. Perhaps it was thought that the mystery of ignorance would add to the effectiveness of the tablets, and that it was appropriate to keep the patient unaware of the name of their medication. I came home and after the first two or three of the little tablets I began to feel rather peculiar.

We were going on holiday to Cornwall a few days later and I was feeling very woozy as I packed our cases. We had a lengthy drive with a long hold-up at Honiton, (no by-pass then) before reaching our guesthouse in a quiet little village not far from Bude. It had formerly been a large country home with expansive grounds that still retained a tennis court, and croquet was set out on the lawn. I began to feel very unwell as the days passed, but we got out and about and visited some of the beautiful spots on the North Cornish coast. I have only a few very hazy memories of this holiday but can vividly recall a couple of little incidents that occurred.

Our spacious family bedroom contained two additional single beds for the children and two large sash windows that we kept wide open during the hot August nights. The boys were sound asleep when we came up to bed one evening and we had no sooner settled down for the night ourselves when suddenly we heard, and then felt, the loud fluttering of wings and a strange whistling sound as a swarm of small black winged creatures flew in through the wide-open window. As they swooped over our bed and around the room we realised we were watching the flight of a bevy of bats; the loud swishing noise woke the children, and they both shot up in their beds, a little frightened at first by what they heard. We soon got used to the late evening light as the family tried to catch sight of the small winged creatures whirring swiftly around, then just as suddenly the boys ducked under the bedclothes as the bats whizzed low over their heads. They quickly popped up again as we all watched while our visitors swung around to have another low flight around the room. We peered at the tiny bodies in flight, heard their high-pitched noise, felt the flap of many wings and could feel the air move with the force of them as they did one further rapid flit around the room before they streamed out of the window. For a moment we could see their black forms etched against the not fully darkened night sky. It was quite an experience; a little bit frightening until we realised what we were observing, but one that we could recall years later. I wonder whether the bats made a habit of scaring the occupants of this large bedroom with two wide sash windows to fly in and then out of on warm nights, and whether they had regular flight around the room.

I was feeling very dopey and having rather strange sensations as if someone was pressing hard inside the back of my head, but I continued taking my medication hoping I would get over these horrid side effects. The large old country house in which we were staying stood in its own grounds, with comfy old garden chairs for guests to sit on, and we decided to spend one afternoon quietly lazing about in the garden; it was a very hot, humid day and I wasn't feel at all well. The children were happily playing with another small boy, roaming around this old garden and making up their own games as we sat chatting to some other visitors and having a nap. It was in the Dalek era, and the peace of the afternoon was suddenly broken when these three young lads began marching around shouting, 'I am a Dalek' slowly and deliberately. They were having a good time, but hopefully not annoying anyone too much. The little incident has stayed in my memory.

By the end of the holiday I was almost in a state of collapse and we had a very difficult drive home as I kept flopping out of my passenger seat towards the car door. This was in the days before car seat belts had been thought of. Once we were safely home I continued taking the prescribed tablets three times a day and soon I began having frightening hallucinations with horrific dreams in which I was squirming with fear about something that I could not put into words. I can still remember this time quite clearly after so many years. The dreams were horrible.

I was not well enough to travel alone for my next appointment at the hospital, so my husband had to take time off from work to drive me up to London. At times I was semi-conscious in the car, nearly falling out of my seat. Maurice had an anxious drive trying to prop me up while still maintaining a grip on the steering wheel and keeping an eye on the road. When we arrived at the hospital I had to be taken to the outpatient department in a wheel chair. The doctor saw me almost immediately, and arranged for me to have what I learned later was a liver-function test. I was wheeled to the path. lab., and was hardly aware that I had the test or that I was then admitted to a ward, and couldn't go home. My husband drove home without me, and the children found that mum had not returned with him.

The ward sister insisted that I continued taking the awful drug I had been prescribed, and although I think the pain was less, I felt sure the thrice-daily tablets were the cause of my present condition. I felt more alive in the early hours of each morning, and I tried and get to the bathroom before the appearance of the drug trolley, but often a nurse would call out my name very loudly, telling me to 'Come out of there and have your medication'. I think she thought I was trying to hide from her in order to avoid taking the wretched tablet, but the truth was that I felt more able to cope with the simple task of washing myself before I had taken my medicine. Shortly after I had taken the tablet the terrible squeezing sensation in my brain recurred, and I soon fell into a deep sleep. The next thing I knew it was lunchtime, and a nurse was shouting my name, shaking me, trying to wake me up and pull me out of bed. I had to be assisted along to the ward meal table, where I slumped in a chair and did not have the strength to pick up my knife and fork. The afternoon drug round soon occurred, with the staff nurse insisting I must have a second tablet, which I swallowed with much reluctance and soon fell asleep again until the evening meal.

I had no visitors during the week, as my husband could not get up to London after work in time for the visiting period. I didn't see the consultant again either, and presume that I was asleep when the medical team came round. All I was told by the ward sister was that I had a urine infection and must drink a lot of water. I don't remember ever having to produce a urine specimen. I felt I was dying, and by the concerned looks and comments of, in particular, one old East End lady, she seemed to think I was too. She came over from her bed on the other side of the ward to peer at me each evening after visiting time and told me, 'You look awful yellow, ducky'. She then looked at me sorrowfully for a little while before walking back to her own bed. The lady in the bed beside me died the following day, and the curtains were drawn around her bed for a long time before her body was removed and I felt my East End visitor thought I would be the next one to go.

Late one night as I was drifting unsteadily towards the toilet I overheard a very young doctor talking to another doctor and saying something about drug jaundice. I pricked up my ears, as I heard the other doctor reply that this was nonsense, but I heard the first murmur quietly about '...she's looking rather yellow'. I couldn't be sure that they were talking about me, but although at that time I had not heard the term 'drug jaundice' I felt sure that I was the subject of their conversation. I could see that my skin had taken on a yellow tinge. I began to think that the little tablets must be the cause of my present condition – the yellow skin and the continual state of semi- consciousness - but nobody appeared at all concerned. I felt I was being treated as if I was mentally ill, brainless, or a criminal.

The following week I was told that the urine infection had cleared, and that I could go home. I didn't recall having a urine test done to confirm either that I had a urine infection the previous week, or a second one to indicate that it had been successfully treated. My only 'treatment' for this so-called urine infection was being told to drink plenty of water! Would I be kept in hospital for over two weeks with a urine infection? I had not noticed or complained of cystitis symptoms. I was told I could go home as soon as my husband came to collect me, but that I must continue taking the tablets. I felt like a package put in the disposal bin. I still felt desperately ill, but nobody would believe me, and I felt sure that they thought I was making it all up.

Maurice was so shocked when he saw me, as apparently I looked so ill and was a sickly shade of yellow. We drove home in silence. I was still in a stupor, in a worse state than I had been before my hospital appointment. I was pleased to see my family but I have no idea how my husband had managed or who had looked after the children while I was away. I think I was too 'knocked out' to even care at the time. Once home, I tried to cope, but I went around in a daze and often fell asleep.

One afternoon I fell into a deep sleep soon after I had taken my midday tablet, and I was not at the school gate to meet my younger son at 3.30p.m. I was 'flat out' on the settee. A constant loud banging interrupted some dream I was having and it eventually broke into my consciousness that the sound in my dream was actually coming from nearby. I woke up, sat up, and staggered into the kitchen; it was a banging on my own kitchen door and not from some action in my weird dream. I quickly opened it, and I found Ian on the doorstep – once again – this time he was puzzled as to why his mum had not been at the school gate to meet him. He had walked home from infant school, hopefully with classmates, and had crossed the ring road, once again, to get home.

On another afternoon I must presume that I had turned the gas on in the oven, but was too woozy after taking my medication at lunchtime to light it. I lay on the settee to have a little rest before meeting Ian after school. A little later I 'came to' and went to the kitchen to put a casserole in the oven for dinner. As I opened the door of the oven, and bent down to light the gas, there was a sudden explosion as the gas I had forgotten to light ignited. My hair, my eyebrows, eyelashes, and the hair on the back of my hands and arms suddenly sizzled. There was a horrible smell of burning hair and I seized a nearby towel and smothered my face and arms in it.

Then I dealt with my singed hair and when the immediate crisis had died down, I looked in the mirror, and was shocked to see where the front and sides of my hair had been burned; I saw the remains of my singed eyebrows were all crinkled. I had been so intent on my hands and my arms, which I could see, that I think I forgot about my hair and my face in the immediate panic. My eyebrows and the backs of my hands and arms were sore where the singed hair had slightly burned the skin. I gently rubbed the singed hair off my head and eyebrows before I opened the kitchen door and all the windows to disperse the awful smell of burnt hair, and immediately got on with the preparation of our evening meal. I didn't tell my youngsters what had happened, and hoped that they wouldn't notice the smell, or observe the state of my hair and eyebrows. A really serious accident was soon averted. The horrible smell of burnt hair still filled the house for some time, but it could have been so much worse. I just didn't know what I was doing, but I had almost been forced into becoming a drug 'junkie,' with the doctors as the pushers!

A day or two after this incident the telephone rang late in the evening. I was surprised to hear the voice of my GP. "Are you still taking the tablets the hospital prescribed?" he enquired.

"I am, Dr. Truncheon. They make me feel so ill; they are draining the life out of me. I don't know what I'm doing. I feel as if they are killing me," I replied.

"They're doing just that," he responded crisply. "Stop them immediately. I have just had a phone call from the registrar, urging me to contact you as quickly as possible. Apparently, the ward never received the result of your liver function test, which was sent to the outpatients' department and has been sitting there for the past three weeks. You should never have been discharged before the test results had been read. The results should also have been sent to the ward you were in. They couldn't understand how you were discharged from the ward. The outpatients' staff have just checked up to see why you had not returned to the clinic today, saw the test result sitting with your notes, and remembered that you had been admitted as an emergency in-patient. The test result was sent to outpatients' because that was where it had been requested. It has been sitting there for a month. As soon as they discovered what had happened I received an urgent phone call this evening telling me to get in touch with you immediately. You're quite right. These tablets were killing you – the liver function test result indicated that you are highly allergic to this drug". (I guess – or at least I hope – that nowadays the computer would have picked up this mistake earlier.)

"I knew that all along," I replied. "I kept telling the sister on the ward that the medication was affecting me badly. I told her I felt I was dying, and really feared that I was, and still feel that it is killing me. No-one would listen; no-one took me seriously".

My GP was quite angry over this incident; I think he felt that his old teaching hospital had let him down as well as mistreating me. It would appear that the ward sister really had no idea of why I was in her ward. My doctor wouldn't let me return there. (With hindsight this may not have been a good idea. They might have been more concerned to treat me aright if I had returned there.) I am sure I didn't have a urine test, but neither was I aware that I had had a liver function test until my doctor telephoned me. I didn't know that I had been given a further outpatient appointment. I think I was too ill to notice what was happening.) I was never told what the drug was, but guess it was one of the tri-cyclic group of drugs like amitriptyline, as I have since been told I am allergic to the tri-cyclic group or drugs and should avoid them. These drugs are often very effective in pain control; what a pity I couldn't tolerate them.

It took me quite a while to get over the effects of the jaundice. If I could have tolerated the drug, maybe I would not have suffered the subsequent years of pain. Sadly, this has been the problem with so many drugs that I have been prescribed over the years. The side effects have been more than my body could cope with; they added to the problem of the pain and made it impossible to continue taking them. But nothing had such a dramatic adverse effect as this particular drug.

Normal daily life went on once I had got the unnamed drug out of my system but I felt as if I was carrying my shopping bags from strings attached to the sides of my neck as I struggled home from the local shops. In the sixties our refrigerator only had a tiny freezer compartment, large enough to contain some ice cubes, a packet of fish fingers, half a pound of frozen peas and not much else. I still walked to the local shops two or three times a week for our food. My neck throbbed and felt swollen at each side, as if it would burst; the arteries felt hard and very painful, my face ached, my jaws throbbed, my temples hurt, and it was painful to speak. We take our present-day fully automated washing machines, large freezers and capacious fridges for granted and sometimes forget how comparatively swiftly they developed from the modest pieces of kitchen equipment of the 50s (but still almost a luxury in the 1960s) to become an accepted and expected household accessory in less than a generation.

I still collapsed from time to time, sometimes if there was a loud noise, but often for no apparent reason, but later on I realised it was often due to wearing tight clothing (a round-necked jumper for example). Many years later I realised that I also reacted badly to some frequently eaten items of food that caused a flare up of additional pain.

My two sons and I had been playing a board game after tea by the fireside one winter's afternoon when I suddenly grew weak and very limp before collapsing in the chair; I couldn't speak or move, although I was aware of where I was. Had we eaten kippers for tea, I wonder? I have no idea! The boys ran to a neighbour, who telephoned my doctor. I don't remember this, but apparently he carried me upstairs to my bed, with what he told me later was called a 'dead man's lift' – which is apparently a fireman's expression. When I came round I had terrific constriction in my throat and felt as if I was being throttled, and my temples and cheeks were extremely painful. My doctor gave me an injection, which knocked me out completely, and I slept all night and most of the following day. He returned the day after that to check up on me. I felt much better, but he told me to take it easy and rest for a further day or two. In the course of conversation we were led to understand that his wife suffered in some similar way to me. Apparently, although the wife of a doctor, nothing could be found to ease her painful condition and we learned a little of his concern for her, which perhaps led to his concern and care over me. He gave up his practice and moved away a year or two later, I think to make life easier for his wife, but I often wonder whether she ever found the key to bring her freedom from pain.

He thought I needed some neurological investigation and had already referred me to a specialist hospital. It was not long before my husband accompanied me to the outpatients' department of another hospital. We waited for some while in a large, rather imposing, waiting area where I was told I would be seeing a professor. Eventually my name was called. A nurse escorted me to the professor's equally imposing consulting room, and he examined me, touching the areas of pain very lightly, (but this didn't cause additional pain) after which I was asked to return to the waiting area. When the morning clinic was over a nurse came in and told me "Prof. — would like to 'use' you in the lecture theatre. Would you agree to his examining you again? He would then ask you a few questions in front of some students".

I agreed, my hopes rising, as I thought that he must have had some idea as to what was wrong with me.

"Come with me then," the nurse continued kindly. "I'll tell you what to do." I left Maurice sitting, waiting patiently; he had a long wait, and was so patient.

I followed the nurse to another part of the hospital, and I was taken into a very small room. It was rather like a fitting room at a department store. There I had to get sufficiently undressed for examination and don the usual ill-fitting gown –although it was only my head and my neck that were of interest! I waited and waited in the silence of this cubicle and eventually a door was suddenly flung open, and I jumped out of my skin as a nurse came in and ushered me briskly on to a kind of stage. I had no idea that I had to appear, as it were, out front, on stage, in front of a real audience. I didn't feel suitably prepared or dressed for my stage debut! The professor repeated my symptoms to the students. While he spoke, I glanced around me, and saw that there were tiers of benches rising up in front of the stage where I was sitting in my hospital gown. I could see rows of, I think, all male, students seated upon the benches. I was overwhelmed for a few seconds, as I had not been prepared for this degree of publicity, but I soon forgot the audience of medical students when the professor began his examination of my throat and face, interspersed with a number of asides and comments directed to the students. I couldn't understand what he was saying as he spoke rapidly over his shoulder in the general direction of the auditorium. He suddenly began asking me a few questions, to which only brief 'Yes' or 'No' answers were required. My 'performance' was soon over, but I didn't hear any applause from my audience as the nurse escorted me back to my 'dressing room'.

I returned to my long-suffering husband and told him what had occurred. We both felt that, although I couldn't sense it from the preceding mini-lecture, the professor must have found something amiss that he was going to teach these medical students about. I dared to hope that we were at last getting to the bottom of whatever was the matter with me. Maybe he had found the key to unlock my problem and would be able to set me free from pain. It must be something quite obscure, we thought, but just to be able to give it a name would be a little comfort.

Before we left I was told I would be admitted to the hospital very shortly to have some special tests, and as we drove home we really felt I was going to be helped at last. A few weeks later I found myself once again in a hospital ward. This time I was aware of all that was going on around me. The nurses wore stiff white uniforms and starched nurses' caps on their heads. The beds with their crisp white sheets tightly tucked in at the sides and the tops turned neatly down were for sleeping in, and there was no lolling on top of them during the day. Patients lay in their bed or sat in the uncomfortable chair by its side. The ward sister ran a 'tight ship'. Various tests were done before I was taken on a trolley to a theatre, where I was given an injection into, I think, the sympathetic nerve in my neck. Nobody had explained to me beforehand either what they were going to do, or why the procedure was being done. Nor did I learn the reason for the strange things that happened to me, and, I recall, that never was I asked to describe in my own words in any detail, what my symptoms were.

I was lying on my back in the little operating theatre, and it was quite frightening when the needle was suddenly stuck into the side of my neck. Why was this being done? A few seconds later my left leg suddenly shot involuntarily into the air and I couldn't bring it down for quite a while. It simply stayed stuck straight up in front of me. Why had this happened? Would it come down again? Was something else going wrong with me? All these thoughts flashed through my mind until I realised that gradually the pain was receding from one side of my head to the other. It was bliss. I stopped worrying about my leg stuck up in the air; I was so pleased that the pain had so swiftly and easily disappeared. I thought this indicated that they had found what was wrong with me and there would be some treatment to give me relief. Eventually my left leg came down to lie naturally next to the right one, but it was a very strange experience. The pain soon returned in my face, however, and I developed a constant dull, but insistent, pain in a small area in the lower part of my spine; it hung around for quite a long time after I had returned home, but eventually disappeared. Whatever had been injected had strange effects, and I am sure that shortly after the injection in my neck I felt as if something had hit this area in my spine very abruptly. Nobody offered me any explanation about this entire procedure.

I was wheeled back to the ward and waited impatiently for the results of the other tests, especially the last investigation. A day or two later a very bossy staff nurse came up to me as I sat by my bed and handed me a bottle containing a hundred little white tablets and told me to take one three times a day. The nurse told me that when they became ineffective something else would be prescribed; I could go home immediately! I was stunned for a moment and could not understand why I was being summarily discharged with no explanation. I was obviously a disappointment to the professor, who I presumed had thought that the tests would confirm his provisional diagnosis of some illness he was teaching his students about, and I had not come up with the goods. I felt that I had disgraced him, and was bitterly disappointed. I never saw him again. Perhaps he was 'using' me to teach his students that my symptoms were not indicative of, say, a brain tumour, and had nothing to do with helping me. Why couldn't someone have explained to me what they were doing and why, and then have the courtesy to gently tell me why they could not help, not simply throw me out with a bottle of pills.

I was given no information about the reason for any of the tests that were done, or the results, but eventually I figured out that the injection in my neck was probably some form of local anaesthetic to see if there was any blockage in the sympathetic nervous system. Because the pain receded, it meant that there was no blockage. I assume that they were expecting to find some pressure possibly indicating a brain tumour, but I was never told. I came to realise that no blockage meant no diagnosis; no diagnosis meant no treatment. My leg shooting into the air? The pain in the bottom of my spine? I wish I knew!

I was shattered by the suddenness of my abrupt discharge, and the formality and coldness of my dismissal. I felt that I had been wasting the doctors' and the nurses' time, taking up valuable space in the ward, and that the staff thought I was a malingerer, a liar, or a fool.

I think attitudes have changed since then, doctors recognise that they haven't got all the answers, and now realise that there are many painful conditions they don't understand and at present cannot treat. But I still think that they find it difficult to deal sensitively with such a patient, who needs some understanding and encouragement to soldier on.

I felt that nothing could be worse than the medical limbo I appeared to be in, and when I arrived home I went to pieces for the first (and only?) time in my life. I think I did little but sit feeling downcast and weepy for a few days until I regained some composure and strength to cope once again. I had had such high hopes. I don't know what my children thought about me during that short period. I had to keep going for their sake, so I took the little white pills prescribed by the hospital. They didn't appear to give me any relief, but at least they did not have any adverse effect. I don't know what the name of the medicine was; no patient's information leaflet came with it from the manufacturer then. They were simply little white tablets in a little brown bottle. Instructions – Take one tablet three times a day. Prescriptions were handwritten, and who can read a doctor's handwriting? How times have changed!

We are now informed of all the details of any medical or surgical procedures we need, including any risks that may occur as well. When prescriptions are given we now know the name of the drug, and the accompanying leaflet gives us details of the drug, why it is prescribed together with a long list of all the possible side effects. Grumble as we do about the NHS, but in many respects it is brilliant in comparison with former days, although I think that patients may feel more like customers, or even mere statistics today.

I think I always had a positive disposition, or maybe I was just a fighter, but I couldn't give in. I had two children to bring up and a husband to care for, and parents for whom I felt some responsibility. I was sure that somewhere there was a key; someone must be able to give me some relief even if no actual cure. Unlikely as it may seem, I think (I hope) that family life soon became reasonably normal once again. One of my sons used to say that he 'always knew when mum was especially bad because she made a lot of jokes then and laughed a lot'. I think this was probably true. I don't know how I would have got by otherwise. I did try to hide how I felt, and put on an act of brightness when I felt most desperate or when other people were around. (I think I still do.) I didn't want to burden Maurice, my children, or my father, with my intractable pain. It was generally an unspoken subject in the household, and talk of its existence was banished. My husband believed that I was my own worst enemy because I did not allow people to see how severe my pain was. They could not realise how bad I felt when I put on such a cheerful, laughing front. When asked how I felt, my stock reply used to be 'All right, thank you'. I considered this to be a safe, truthful reply. 'All right' has a very equivocal meaning, so I felt that it could be taken in whatever way the hearer wished – 'everything's fine,' or 'things are passable'. However, this façade meant that when I did occasionally say how ill I really felt, people could not believe that I was as bad as I stated and perhaps thought I was exaggerating. I may be wrong in feeling this, but that was how I understood the reaction.

Chronic pain is a difficult condition to live with, and an almost impossible condition for non-sufferers to comprehend. It is difficult to understand the problem if one has not experienced it. I wish there was a support group for people with intractable, undiagnosable pain! I guess such people are usually 'putting on an act' – our own little drama – by trying to live a normal life, be like everybody else, and not give in, give up or complain when we are actually enduring intolerable pain.

Chapter Twenty

A DIFFERENT APPROACH

A year or two later I was told of a homoeopathic doctor in Buckinghamshire, who had successfully treated some very difficult cases over the years. After his retirement from general medical practice this doctor had been concerned that in his professional career he had been unable to deal with the cause of many of his patients' illnesses; he felt he had only, at best, helped to relieve the effects, i.e. the symptoms. He had not found the key, by that I mean the cause, which would lead to a greater understanding and possibly the cure. He had investigated various unconventional forms of medicine - long before the term 'alternative' or 'complementary' was used. He came to the conclusion that the homeopathic approach, with its emphasis on the whole individual, proved to be the most successful in treating difficult cases. Consideration of the inherited disposition of the patient to certain groups of diseases appeared to provide the answer to the question as to why some people were more likely to suffer from certain diseases, and possibly why they were so difficult to treat successfully. In his new (post-retirement) practice he needed to know not only his patient's symptoms, but also their disposition, what food they liked and disliked and also what their parents and grandparents had suffered from, and many other aspects of their personality. The remedy had to match the patient's personality and disposition, past history, inherited factors as well as present symptoms – often quite hard to do – in order to choose the most suitable homoeopathic remedies.

This form of medicine has been so despised, indeed, now dismissed, by many in the medical profession. However, I don't think a theory should be rejected just because it has as yet no clear explanation – or even proof. But who am I, an untrained, elderly lady, to comment, when many brilliant scientists and doctors refute any evidence of the effectiveness of homoeopathy? And yet others have found a strong case for its effectiveness.

I was prepared to try anything that might help and so wrote to the late Dr. Lawrence and he agreed to see me. My husband took a day's leave from work and drove me to the Thames-side village in which he lived. His wife ushered us in to meet a delightful elderly gentleman with snow-white hair and rosy cheeks who led us to his large book-lined consulting room. I believe the late Dr. Lawrence was in his early eighties when I first saw him, and he still had a busy private practice. He was a good advertisement for his medical skill, as he looked the picture of health himself. He had a very soft voice and a precise manner in speech, but a gentle, thoughtful approach to his patient; he wanted to hear every detail of my life history as well as my medical history, together with what I knew of my parents' and grandparents' medical history – which was very little. He seemed very concerned for me, and I felt confident that he would really do all he could to help me. He seemed to understand that I had kept going with difficulty. He considered that I had inherited a predisposition to nerve-related disease from my mother, and that her mental condition may have some connection with my neurological pain – nowadays one might conclude that 'it's all in the genes'.

He prescribed various homoeopathic remedies, and after some time my general health began to improve. A number of other symptoms that I had taken little notice of slowly disappeared. A neighbour who didn't know of my problem remarked on how much better I looked recently, and that I had more colour in my cheeks. She told me she had felt concerned about me, but didn't like to mention how ill she thought I had looked. She said she was pleased to be able to mention it now that I seemed so much better. I soon had more energy, and generally felt better, although my face pains grew only a little less severe. Nevertheless I was confident that in the end he would find the total answer, but, sadly, I have learned that having faith in a treatment does not necessarily make it effective. And yet, with years of hindsight, I realise that I must have had more relief with the homoeopathic treatment than I had appreciated at the time.

After a while I began to feel really well in myself. I guess that there were not the side effects that make many mainstream drugs almost impossible to cope with. The gentle homoeopathic treatment seemed to be helping me constitutionally without my actual awareness. Dr. Lawrence was very tenacious, and tried various different remedies. Yet still the pain in my face, my jaws and teeth really troubled me; my teeth felt like burning metal in my mouth and made my jaws ache. Dr. Lawrence thought that I had some wisdom teeth that could be causing the neuralgic pain in my face. I had not realised that I had any wisdom teeth until a dental x-ray showed three impacted wisdom teeth that had apparently never grown through the gums. I was recommended to have them removed. So once again I was in hospital, this time to have teeth extracted under general anaesthetic. They were apparently deeply and awkwardly embedded, and it was thought that they really could be touching a nerve and causing my problem, so I was glad to be rid of them. It was apparently very difficult to rouse me after the anaesthetic, but when I did come round I was immediately aware of unbearable pain in my face and could not stand the bright hospital lights. I think I was shouting and screaming the place down! The bright lights and the excruciating pain were driving me crazy. Ice packs were put around my face, and I had to stay in hospital an extra two days. I always seem either to have to stay in hospital longer than normal because something has gone a bit amiss, or I am thrown out quickly because nothing at all can be done to help me!

Dr. Lawrence also considered that the mercury in the amalgam fillings in a number of my remaining molars could in some way be the cause of my symptoms. Mercury is part of the amalgam that has been used for tooth fillings for many years. I had a lot of fillings, most of them dating back to shortly before my second son was born, when the NHS provided free dental treatment for expectant mothers. Regular dental check ups did not occur in my childhood. One only visited a dentist when you had toothache, and that usually meant a filling was necessary, or worse still, an extraction. (My first memory of going to the dentist was when I had raging toothache when I was quite young. My father took me to the dentist, and I required a large filling in a molar tooth, but when I returned home the pain was so severe that we had to return. The dentist's solution was to remove the tooth. My father had to pay for the extraction as well as the filling. I can remember the episode well!) So many years later the remaining molars felt too long, like hot metal in my mouth, and I often held a finger between my upper and lower teeth when I was alone to hold my jaws apart and relieve the pressure. I also had a persistent burning sensation in my teeth.

The theory that mercury is the cause of a lot of nerve-related illnesses, including MS, was being considered in the 1970s. I don't know if it has gained ground over this long period of time, but many dentists now use ceramic fillings for preference, and some even have a mercury-free practice. I think the safer filling is now becoming the preferred one. My own dentist recently told me that he has had a few patients whose medical symptoms seem to have disappeared after their amalgam-fillings were replaced with ceramic ones. Not much was known about ceramic fillings in the 1960s, and I believe they didn't last long and were extremely expensive in their early years but they are much more durable and less expensive now.

I was advised to have these amalgam-filled molar and pre-molar teeth extracted and they were removed in 1968 under yet another general anaesthetic. Again I reacted badly to the anaesthetic, and the staff apparently grew very concerned when they couldn't rouse me. I think my body is so relieved to be temporarily unaware of the pain it endures when I am conscious, that it takes advantage of an anaesthetic, makes the most of the pain-free period, and protests strongly when consciousness returns! I was again in hospital for about four days. For some reason I had to go to St. George's Hospital in Tooting, south London for this procedure, and Maurice drove across London in the rush hour after work to bring me home. He had to leave our boys to get their own tea, and when we arrived back in the house we found the two lads sitting cosily in front of our little old television, tucking into baked beans on toast. I was greeted with the remark, 'Andrew's a smashing cook, mum!' Strangely enough, although this wonderful culinary achievement came out of a tin, Andrew grew up to be an excellent cook, capable of producing a delicious meal with nonchalance and ease. I think that my persistent battle with pain made our sons self-reliant and capable, and they are now both very competent in every way in their own homes. I feel I led them a terrible life, but I know I was always cheerful; I kept home life running normally, we always had proper meals, we did things together, had lovely times at Christmas, good holidays and I tried to conceal the pain when they were around.

Sadly, when I got over this awkward bit of surgery I found that there was no improvement in the pain. Physiotherapy three times a week was recommended by the dental surgeon, and I began a course of infrared treatment to my jaws and cheekbones at my local hospital. After each session I experienced greater pain, and by the end of the first week it was so extreme that I had to discontinue the treatment; it was aggravating the pain instead of relieving it. I remember coming home on the bus on a cold winter's afternoon shortly before Christmas with fiery, fierce burning pain in my face after my physio treatment. I was frantic with pain and went straight to the bathroom, and held my face in a bowl of cold water for as long as I could to try and reduce the ferocity of the pain.

I was pleased to be rid of the teeth that had given me so much discomfort, and to be relieved of the hot metallic sensation, but sadly the procedure did not relieve the pain. However, if the theory of mercury poisoning from amalgam fillings is correct, the damage to my nervous system would have begun early in 1958, when the dental fillings were done when I was pregnant, and the neuralgic pain began in June of that same year. The mercury in them could possibly have gradually disastrously affected my nervous system. I just don't know! It later became good dental practice to ensure that no mercury fragments, or even vapour, are swallowed or inhaled when old amalgam fillings are removed, and barriers are somehow put in place to prevent this occurring. These essential precautions were not in place when the teeth were extracted. Most medics dismiss the theory of mercury poisoning from amalgam fillings – but opinions on many things change with the years - e.g. smoking!

Dr. Lawrence was almost as disappointed as I that the extraction of these teeth had not been successful. I think I was a challenge to him, and he would have appreciated winning this battle; it would have been a personal triumph towards the end of his long medical career. I know that is how I saw it; it was a battle that I intended to win. I am sad for his sake, as well as my own, that together we were unable to make me well. With all his skill, he hadn't found the key.

In due course I was fitted with dentures. I felt so ashamed to be wearing these geriatric appliances before I my fortieth birthday, but these NHS dentures proved to be a disaster. I could not tolerate the plastic, and I could only wear them for brief periods. My mouth felt like a cavern of fire, and I frequently had to remove the dentures, tuck them up a cardigan sleeve, put them in an apron pocket, or pop them discreetly under a cushion at home. It became a family joke with the boys. 'Where are Mum's gnashers?' was often a cry just before we were going out for the afternoon. I couldn't remember where I had put them, under which cushion I had placed them, or where exactly I had been when I couldn't stand the horrid things in my mouth any longer, and there was a brief game of hide-and-seek, feeling inside my pockets or down the sides of armchairs and settee, searching on the carpet in case I had inadvertently dropped them, until there was a joyful cry of, 'We've found them!'

An amusing incident occurred as we were driving home from holiday the following year. As we drove along I was in a lot of pain, had little to distract me, and without thinking had removed my dentures and held them in my lap. We were held up at a level crossing for a while. As we sat waiting in the car for the train to pass through, I asked the boys if they would like something to nibble. Of course the reply was 'Yes', and, of course, what they wanted was in the boot. I hurriedly opened the car door, stepped out quickly, and was about to run to the back of the car before the crossing gates were lifted, when, as I put my feet to the ground, my little treasures, which I had quite forgotten, were sitting in my lap, slid with a clatter on to the middle of the road. I hastily picked them up from the tarmac with as much nonchalance as I could muster, clasped them tightly in the palm of my hand, and ran to the boot, when to my even greater embarrassment I noticed two young men sitting in the car behind ours roaring with laughter at my plight. I grabbed a tin of cookies and a couple of apples, averted my gaze, and dashed back to my seat with one hand clutching my dentures and the snacks in the other. I very nearly dropped the lot as I scuttled back to the car. (I think I would have reacted very differently today – laughed with them and dangled the dentures in front of them before returning to the car!) The two smaller, young men in our car nearly choked with laughter on their cookies and had the giggles for quite a while afterwards. This little incident has been etched on my memory for so many years. I continued to feel embarrassed to be wearing dentures during the next few years, and felt that people would think I had neglected to look after my teeth.

A year or two later I was able to replace the horrible plastic dentures with a rather expensive, well-fitting set, based on chrome cobalt instead of plastic. These were more comfortable, but sadly the massive tooth extraction was not successful in relieving my pain.

I wanted to get some sort of a job to help to pay for all the private treatment I had been having. Dr. Lawrence had kindly reduced his normal fee, but it was an outlay that we could ill afford, and I felt I was using more than my fair share of the family income on private treatment. I made all the economies I could think of to provide cheap, nourishing meals for the family, and in those days one could buy four herrings for a shilling (5p.) and breast of lamb was very cheap, but took ages to bone. Liver made another cheap nourishing meal – although I had to make a bargain with young Ian, who didn't like liver. If he had one small slice plus a generous blob of tomato sauce, he would agree to eat it, along with appropriate face pulling. We also had various vegetarian meals – cheese batter or curried eggs come to mind. There wasn't the variety of fruit and vegetables around that we have today and I'm sure we had more sweet foods and cakes than I would dream of preparing nowadays.

Growing up in the war made it easy for me to know how to economise and we always a home prepared and cooked evening meal, and I am sure the family always ate well. We always had a second course – a home baked fruit pie, a Bakewell tart, rice pudding or, occasionally Instant Whip, one of the first of the modern 'convenience' foods. I thought it was nourishing because I mixed it with a pint of milk, but the artificial flavouring was, apparently, detested by one of my sons, (but he only told me this many years' later). In former years children were not asked for their preferences, but ate what their mother had prepared for them. I made my own cakes and pastry, but was aware that the accompanying mixing, beating and rolling did nothing to diminish my pain. I had a very reliable dishwasher (my husband) and two pairs of willing hands with the drying up (two sons – I think they were willing; they took it in turns).

I did a little temporary typing work at home, but banging the keys jarred the pain and also gave me backache. I didn't want to do secretarial work because of this. Modern, light-touch computer keyboards were not yet invented. My hand tremor was such that I didn't think I would manage shorthand very well. It was frustrating to want to do something useful that would help with the housekeeping (I don't think that I thought of personal spending money) but which seemed prohibited by my wretched constitution.

I then thought that if I could clean my own home, then surely I could clean someone else's, so I answered an advertisement to clean twice a week in quite a large house in the neighbourhood. I cycled there on Tuesday and Friday mornings, and actually enjoyed the satisfaction of leaving someone else's home looking nice and clean and tidy, but it was really too much for me; lugging a very large vacuum cleaner around and scrubbing a tiled kitchen floor five or six times the size of my own small one didn't help at all. I had to give it up. I sometimes thought that if I had been born a 'lady' about one hundred years earlier, with everything done for me and with servants to look after the house, I might have been less likely to suffer incessant pain. I don't think I would have survived the triviality of life like that, but maybe I could have become accustomed to it!

Somewhere around this period a Ghanaian family moved into our road. We were near neighbours so I called to welcome them soon after their arrival, and we became friends. Regina and I occasionally had coffee and a chat together. A year or later we noticed there had been a sudden addition to the family, in the form of a seven-year-old boy. Their son Peter, a year younger than Ian, had been brought up by his grandmother in Ghana until he was seven, when he flew to England under escort to live with his parents, and to begin his junior school education. He became a pupil in the same junior school as Ian and went on to the same comprehensive school.

It was at this time that I noticed that the acute, sore, pulsating, pressure pain on each side of my throat was eased if I wore loose clothing. I began to realise that constricting clothing – high-necked jumpers, fitted dresses, waist-bands on skirts, roll-ons (which we wore in those days, with suspenders to hold our stockings up) aggravated my pain; any constriction of clothing, especially around my neck or waist, not only made the neuralgic pain intolerable but added to my susceptibility to collapse. Many years had passed before I picked up on this and began to wear loose clothing. I threw out any tight-fitting garments from my wardrobe, and only wore loose-fitting dresses for many years. This made quite a difference; it was a small, easily attainable relief that reduced the level of pain. I wish I had thought of it years earlier.

I hated shopping for these loose garments. Looking along the rails for the most shapeless, baggy dress did not make for a very exciting shopping expedition. It was sometimes made worse by well-meaning assistants showing me nicely designed, well-fitting dresses that I declined to try on. No doubt the assistant felt she was trying to improve my lack of taste and poor dress sense. I stopped wearing skirts because of the tight waistband, so loose dresses were my daily attire. Hardly anyone wears dresses nowadays except for special occasions and loose gowns seem as fashionable as fitted ones. Trousers were rarely seen then but now they have almost replaced the skirt or dress; shop assistants are almost non-existent today, and customers browse along the rails themselves. How different the shopping experience is today, with vast arrays of, mostly black, trousers, or very bright tops, buttons that are decorative but not useful and frills in funny places, but quite often I can't actually see anything that I want to buy!

The wearing of seat belts was made compulsory around this period and my GP told me that I was the first person he thought of when the law was passed. He realised that I wouldn't be able to bear the tight constriction around my body. He had no hesitation in granting me an exemption certificate before I had even asked him. I was one of a very small minority of the population granted an exemption certificate. I am now able to comply with the legislation, as modern seat belts are more comfortable than the first designs, but I still find my seat belt rather tight.

My general health had certainly improved with Dr. Lawrence's homoeopathic treatment, and there was some reduction in my symptoms with my changed style of dressing, so I began to hope I was really getting better. I was going to look to the future, think positively, and make some definite step forward. Perhaps a different life style might help to break the habit that my nerves had adopted. I needed to find the right sort of career, hopefully one that would fit in with my children's school holidays. I had enjoyed my period of leadership in Sunday school and the youth group at church many years earlier, and was very interested in my sons' education. I began to wonder whether teaching would be a possibility. I wanted work that was outside the home, but a job that would allow me to be at home during the school holidays. I thought that perhaps a different way of life would divert my nerves from passing on painful messages to my brain and would jog my body into behaving in a different manner. A shortage of teachers at the time and there was an appeal for mature students to enter the profession. 'Mature' sounded a bit like a type of Cheddar cheese, or an overripe pear. (I was then in my late thirties and considered myself still young. I still do in my mind, although my body does feel rather 'mature' nowadays!)

I decided to follow my new ambition by upgrading the rather limited education I had received during the war and see where it led. I enrolled in an English and also a French evening class at my local college of education, and enjoyed the stimulation of writing essays and reviving my little bit of French from years ago. The following year I enrolled in some daytime classes hoping to obtain the preliminary qualifications required before being offered a place at a teacher training college. Dr. Lawrence seemed somewhat concerned when he heard what I proposed to do, and I don't think he thought it was such a good idea, but I was already on the way. I enjoyed my studies, and the year passed by incredibly quickly. I took the plunge and applied for a place as a non-resident student at a teacher training college in Hertfordshire for the following year. After an interview I was given a provisional place to begin a three years' course starting in the autumn term of 1968 providing I passed my examinations in the summer.

I sat the exams and soon after the end of the summer term we were going on holiday to North Wales. I had requested that my results should be posted to my holiday address. We set off in the middle of August to Criccieth in Snowdonia, accompanied by my father. I am sure he relished this brief period when he was sharing daily life with us again as well as having a change of scenery. It was a return visit to Criccieth and we were renting an apartment right at the top of this delightful little town. From the large bay window in our sitting room on the first floor we could look directly down towards the castle and the sea. The owner of the house was a school inspector and he was pressing the authorities for the teaching of Welsh to be made compulsory in schools. It was largely a Welsh-speaking town and the assistants were all speaking in Welsh to their customers when I went shopping. This was our third visit to Criccieth, and as I write this passage I realise for the first time that we had three consecutive holidays in Norfolk when the children were small, and much later had three consecutive holidays in Wales when they were in, or approaching, their early teens. We had never visited any other resort more than once, but I think that Walcott in Norfolk and Criccieth in North Wales have very special places in our family's memories.

In the enjoyment of the beauty of Snowdonia I almost forgot about my soon-expected examination results and the prospect of teacher training college. We were determined to get to the top of Snowdon when we met up one day with some friends who were holidaying nearby. After a picnic lunch together we left my father sitting beside the two cars, looking at the scenery and having a snooze, while we set off up the Watkin Path with Val and Geoff, our two boys, and their two daughters, plus their two King Charles' spaniels. We enjoyed the scenery, the waterfalls, and each other's company as we strode along in beautiful sunshine until we noticed that the sun was no longer shining, the blue sky had become overcast. We hoped the clouds would pass, and walked steadily onwards and upwards until we reached the long ridge that stretches up towards the peak, which was now shrouded in mist, and heavy grey clouds had gathered above us. Not to be outdone, the youngsters plodded on, but we all had to be careful when we reached this narrow ridge, with the scree falling away to our left and a sharp drop to a deep, dark lake on the right.   We were so eager to reach the summit, and 'Mars bars at the top' the youngsters shouted repeatedly with determination, but Maurice and Geoff had looked at the ominous clouds gathering around the peak, had a few quiet words together and decided that as we would still have a long descent *down* the rocky path, it was unwise to continue *up*.   We had to agree, although the young people were disappointed and grumbled a bit as we turned our backs on the, now hidden, summit. Our descent was made in dull weather, with lowering clouds and threatening rain, which I supposed decreased our disappointment. It would certainly not have been much fun if we had continued.

My father was still sitting patiently in his deck chair at our picnic site, but getting rather anxious and feeling a little cold in the now gloomy late afternoon. The weather was becoming very miserable, with large spots of rain falling. It had turned very chilly after the warmth of the morning, and we were all disappointed by our lack of success, but my father was relieved to see us safely back, glad to get out of his picnic chair and was longing to be 'home' at our holiday flat and sitting in a more comfortable chair. Our two families returned to our respective holiday accommodation, where I guess that Val, as well as I, set about cooking the evening dinner for the family. There was no abundance of cafés, pubs or restaurants serving food for families in those days. We all met up a day or two later for a day by, and in, the sea, relaxing in the sunshine and enjoying each other's company. We wished the weather had been as settled when we attempted to reach the summit of Mount Snowdon.

Towards the end of the holiday I received some eagerly awaited mail that informed me I had passed all my examinations. I was very thrilled with my good grades, but I think the family took it all very quietly. We didn't celebrate in any way; everyone was too busy packing up as we continued our holiday, leaving North Wales and taking the ferry across the Irish Sea to spend a third week in a farm cottage in County Cork.

I had enjoyed my classes and my private studies enormously, especially English literature, French, human biology and religious studies. The latter subject I had studied on my own; with the aid of various concordances and several sets of old 'O' level exam papers to guide me, I studied the appropriate Bible passages required for the syllabus, which included parts of the Old and New Testament. My essay answers to the questions set in the relevant old exam papers were kindly marked for me by the R.E teacher at my son's comprehensive school. Essay answers were required, and quite a lot of reading and personally assessing the text was necessary before writing an essay-length answer from one of these old exam papers each week.

I learned a lot about writing essays in this way during the year, and the comments concerning my answers were very helpful. It was an unusual but challenging way to study, as I had no teacher or lecturer, but through my personal study and the meticulous marking of Ian's R.E. teacher I gained a Grade I pass.

I also learned a lot through my own study in the French class. I had only a minute smattering of French at the beginning of the year's course and when I bought the required textbook I found that even the first page was totally beyond my comprehension. I had a lot to learn in a year. The teacher wasted a lot of time showing off - I presume to the teenagers with whom I shared his French lessons - but for our homework each week he requested an essay in French, or ten questions on a long comprehension text to be answered fully in French, or the translation into correct English of a long paragraph in French. If it wasn't done, so be it. Passing the exam was up to the student.

I think my teacher may have given up on some of his students, who were resitting their exams, but I religiously did my homework. I fear that many didn't bother. He marked my answers in such detail and corrected my mistakes so carefully that I learned an immense amount from his clear correction of every error I had made. (Five years later I found I was teaching his delightful twin sons.) In my oral examination I tried to keep the conversation flowing with words with which I was familiar. It was perhaps not the best way to learn, but it all worked for me as my Grade 2 result revealed. But for the present, examination results were quite forgotten, except by me, as I quietly contemplated my first term at college. I still wanted to enjoy a further week's holiday exploring Co. Cork. in southern Ireland.

Where is the Key?

We were accommodated in a typical long, low-ceilinged, single storey farm labourer's cob cottage in a rather remote village near the sea. The accommodation was extremely basic in rural southern Ireland. The boys went up to the farm every morning to fetch our milk for the day, fresh from the cow. One evening the farmer appeared at our cottage with fish for our dinner that his sons had caught in the sea that day; they wanted to share their catch with their short-term tenants.

We drove to the Ring of Kerry, climbed up to the top of the remains of Blarney Castle where Andrew kissed the Blarney Stone. (He's been a very good conversationalist ever since!) We spent a day in the charming seaside resort of Ardmore with its ancient high round tower, and noticed the almost hidden remains of an ancient chapel dating back to the fifth century. We looked in amazement at the beautiful sculptures on the one remaining wall of a later church, which depicted detailed biblical scenes. Ardmore was altogether a lovely, unspoilt, peaceful place.

We found some privately owned caves quite by accident somewhere in the Knockmealdown Mountains. We noticed they were open to the public, although we were the only 'public' we saw that day in what was then a very remote area. We paid the farmer's wife and were each given a lighted candle to help us see our way as we descended into the caves. She guided us along a rough, uneven pathway through the huge caverns, avoiding puddles on the way, with large stalactites hanging down from the ceilings and thicker, stumpier stalagmites growing up from the caves' floors. We could only see them dimly by the light of our candles as we almost stumbled along, and my father soon decided he had gone far enough. He insisted that the family continued, and we left him standing on a dry stone and leaning up against a damp cave wall, holding up his candle. I don't know how far these caves extended inside the mountains, but we all retreated before we reached the end of the path. I think we had seen most of its secrets and were worried about my father standing alone, holding his candle. Supposing it had blown out? We were glad to see his little light shining in the distance as we carefully made out way back, with more daylight appearing with each step we took. The incident makes me think of the old children's hymn 'This little light of mine, I'm going to let it shine' from my early Sunday school teaching days!

As we were about to leave at the end of our holiday, our farmer landlord came to see us off, and invited us to 'take a wee dram' with him before we left. I realise that wasn't the phrase he used - we were in Southern Ireland, not Scotland, but it was something that indicated he had his own still where he brewed his own whisky, and he wanted to send us happily on our way. We declined with warm thanks; we had a long drive from Youghal in County Cork to Dun Laoghaire to get our ferry to Holyhead and then a very long drive before we reached the English county of Hertfordshire, and our home. It had been a long, varied and very interesting holiday. It was now time to think of study.

Chapter Twenty-One

I LOOK TO THE FUTURE

October soon came around, and with it the start of a new phase in my life, when at the age of thirty-seven I became a student. Each morning I had a short walk before meeting up with two other new mature students waiting for the college bus to arrive at 9.30 a.m. There was often a long, cold wait in the coming winter mornings, but the provision of these coaches made it possible for mature, non-resident students to undertake this teacher-training course in those days. Transport was vital; without its provision there would have been an even greater teacher shortage in the coming decade. There were few two-car families in those days and many of the students were without a car, so several other college buses picked up groups of mature students in different areas of the county. Sometimes we had to be very patient; the bus was often late whilst the kindly driver waited for students who arrived late at their appointed pick-up point. We all had two lives to lead, with families demanding attention, and until 9.30a.m. they had to come first.

Although I was friendly with the two fellow-students who waited with me each morning, I had not made any close friends in my new locality. I hoped that I might make some - or at least one - personal friend at college, but mature students came from a wide area, and we were all struggling to meet our commitments at home and at college. We hurried to the coaches after lectures each afternoon in order to get home as soon as possible and return to our other functions as wives (or husbands) and parents, and also to do our study or essay-writing late at night. There was little time for us to socialise during the day or develop even a slight friendship; an opportunity not given to mature students who were away from the college campus in the evenings. I think there were between eighty and one hundred mature students in my year group. This is only an approximation, drawn from my memory, but we were quite a sizeable group of men and women amongst a very much larger number of resident, all-female younger students.

However, in my second term I did develop a friendship with one of the younger students in my main study group. She came from Northern Ireland, had no opportunity to pop home for a weekend to see her parents and I invited her to my home on several occasions. I can remember Lesley's remark of appreciation when she commented on her first visit, with a big sigh, 'Oh! How lovely to be in a home again, and to be away from college accommodation and the lack of privacy'. I think she appreciated the hospitality I was able to give her during her college years, and it was very nice to have Lesley's companionship during our music course. She has since used her considerable musical talent and college experience to great benefit for her pupils during a long teaching career.

We have only met rarely since we both left college in 1971 but have remained in touch, and every year I receive a long letter from her, with news of her family. She is now retired herself, and yet I still think of her as a young student!

After a course on contemporary studies in the first term, we began our educational studies in earnest with a series of lectures on the History of Education, which I found interesting and not too demanding in its ensuing essay requirement. There was a period of teaching practice in each of the three years of my course, and I enjoyed my first teaching practice in a local primary school. My main memory of this TP was the pleasure I had in listening to the class teacher telling the stories of some of the ancient Greek myths at the end of each afternoon. Miss Wotherspoon was an inspired storyteller, and I was held spellbound as I sat at the back of the class in one of the children's small chairs. I had never heard any of these tales before.

She was also the music teacher in the school, had a lovely singing voice, played the piano very professionally and accompanied the singing for the school assembly. She was an old-fashioned teacher, one not really approving of modern methods. I think I was placed in her class because music was my main study at college, but I wasn't asked to take any of her class music lessons, nor was I required to play the piano for assembly, much to my relief, although I know I could have managed to accompany the school in the singing of a couple of hymns. I enjoyed the opportunity of teaching the children in this Year 3 (First Year Juniors in my day) class of children. I also learned a lot from this teacher about how to handle a class of mixed aptitude junior school children, how to get the children 'on your side' and how to keep class discipline without sounding like an army sergeant! However it was all quite stressful and was certainly not an 8.45a.m. - 3.45p.m. job, but far more demanding of one's time, patience, creativity, and required many other talents and abilities.

Sometimes I was up well into the night finishing my preparation or writing up assessments of the lessons I had taken. One evening I wrote honestly about the difficulty I had had in keeping one little boy under control in my maths lesson. George would insist on walking around the room and annoying other children. I had hoped for some advice from my teaching practice supervisor, but when he next came to the school to observe a lesson, he read my self-assessment, and told me that in order to keep everyone's attention I must make the maths lesson fun, but he didn't tell me how to do this in a large class of mixed ability 7-8 year olds, with maths text books (Alpha for the brighter ones and Beta text books for the average or less than average) and a syllabus to get through. These large textbooks certainly didn't give an impression of being fun – quite the opposite. But, can everything in education – or life for that matter – be fun?

The three-week period of teaching practice was at the end of the second term, and was followed immediately by the Easter holidays. We had three weeks to recover, but also only three weeks to catch up on all the jobs that needed doing at home.

On the first day of the following term the students in each of the five mature student education groups met outside our personal tutor's study. There were about twenty students in each group and our tutor called us in one by one and gave each student a personal, private assessment of our teaching practice. I was aware of where I could have done better, and knew of my shortcomings, but I also knew that I had got on well with the children (except George) and my lessons seemed to have gone as planned – although I wasn't very good at drama. I had never 'done' drama or taken part in any form of acting in my life – although I soon realised that being a class teacher requires a certain degree of acting ability! There had been no preparation for teaching drama at college, but my teaching practice supervisor happened to be the drama lecturer! Everything was supposed to come from personal inspiration and creativity at that period. I awaited the interview with my tutor with hope and expectation mixed with feelings of self-doubt. I grew more anxious as I heard a number of my fellow mature students – especially, I have to say, the men amongst them – saying how wonderfully they thought they had done, what a terrific success their experimental music lessons had been, how one man's practical music session had the children 'eating out of his hand', or how someone else's practical maths experiments had been 'spot on'…etc. etc.

I was so relieved to be told at my interview that I had done very well, and that my tutor was well satisfied with my efforts, but I still wasn't given any help in how to deal with the small 'Georges' I would no doubt come across when I began my teaching career! I noticed that some of the bragging students were rather quiet after their interviews and seemed somewhat subdued. I wonder why? One even left and was never seen again.

I had chosen Music as my main study because I thought it might help me to get a job in a local primary school when I had finished my course. There was usually a shortage of music teachers in schools, if only to play the piano to accompany the hymns that were an important part of school assembly in those days. We began our main study in the following term, and I soon found that out it was geared to raising the personal level and ability of each student, not aimed at primary school children's needs. I enjoyed my piano lessons, and appreciate that my piano playing improved tremendously. Singing lessons were a bonus, although I found it embarrassing to do my singing practice at home. I studied the history of music, gained a little understanding of Sibelius' Fifth Symphony and did some work on harmony – which apparently I had a flair for - and composition, but this was all designed to improve my personal standard, and not geared to teaching children. I felt that it was not really the reason I was at college. I would have loved some practical help and ideas on teaching music in junior school, but the course was almost entirely for personal advancement.

I had a weekly piano lesson with Mr. McKay Martin, and got to work on Mozart's Sonata in C major. He must have taught me well, as I can still play parts of it on the rare occasions when I find the time to play the piano and I can still remember the correct fingering. (I seem to have spent most of my spare time 'playing' the computer keyboard in recent years.) During the following two years at College I had singing lessons with Miss Roberts but I have no memory of the song I had to sing for my Final, only that it was by John Ireland. I also had to sing an unaccompanied folk song. During the next two years I spent hours practising one of Bach's Two-Part Inventions and struggling with Debussy's 'Arabesque' for my Finals and suffered considerable shoulder ache as a result. I fear that the latter piece of music was rather beyond my ability to perform well.

I was relieved when the first year came to an end and I could have a few weeks at home to recover, have a little domesticity, time with the family and a chance to assimilate all the new things I had met with in the previous academic year. In the summer term there had been short courses of lectures on sociology and demographics. In the second year of the main Principles of Education course we had a series of lectures about the theories of a number of well-known educational psychologists, which I found very interesting. This was followed in our third year by a number of lectures on the philosophy of education. It was all interesting, and entailed a lot of reading, absorbing, and writing of essays, but I still longed for more practical, timeless or modern, help on how to approach different subjects, what to do in art, how to teach music in primary school, ideas for P.E., what methods were now used to help with the teaching of reading and maths etc, but this didn't occur. Those students who had opted for the Infant age group did have sessions on the teaching of reading, and I presume that it was expected that by the time children had reached the Junior stage they would have mastered the principles of reading. New maths and metrication were just coming in to the classroom and also into daily life, but children still had to be taught the 'old' arithmetic to get by in day-to-day life. When a request was made for more practical assistance with the art and skills of particular subject teaching one lecturer told us that 'we are not here to give tips for teachers'.

My second teaching practice lasted for a month and I was in a large fourth year (Year 6) junior class but I don't remember any interesting incidents worth retelling.

My husband and I began to look for a larger house during the summer vacation at the end of the second year at college. The kitchen and the third bedroom at our existing home were very small and our sons were growing older, and thus larger. We wanted to stay in the area, and had already looked at several houses, but found none of them to be suitable, or in our price range, when Ian came home one day after a cycle ride around the local streets, and announced, "I've found the house, mum!"

"Oh! Where?" I laughed, thinking he was joking. But he looked quite serious as he said he had seen a house in a nearby street with a 'For Sale' board outside; he thought it looked bigger than the one we had and he was sure we ought to buy it. I knew that this road had quite a lot of detached houses that were worth much more than we could afford, so I told him that we couldn't possibly afford to live in that road, and laughed it off. But he assured me it would be just right for us; he was twelve years old. No, he didn't become an estate agent!

The following day my husband made a detour on his way home from work, and walked down the street to give the outside of the house an inspection. I had already done the same, and felt rather excited by what I saw. It had promise. We contacted the agent, and went to view the house. There was an enormous elm tree at the pavement end of the front garden, which made the house look very dark and rather forlorn. Nothing had been done to the house since it was built in 1939/40, and yet the inside pleased me despite a number of drawbacks. The kitchen had its' original, deep porcelain sink, a wooden draining board, with no fitted cupboard beneath, an old-fashioned walk-in larder, no kitchen units, just a cupboard, and an ancient solid-fuel boiler set in one corner. But the kitchen itself was much larger that our existing one.

The reception rooms were larger too, and had wood-stained floorboards with a carpet square covering the main part of each floor; the hall, staircase and landing had rather sad-looking fitted carpet. The two main bedrooms had old-fashioned fireplaces with chimneybreasts set in the inner walls, and there was a small built-in cupboard in the corner of only one bedroom. Our existing   property had built-in wardrobes in both main bedrooms, but no such thing in this unmodernised house – and we had given the nice wardrobe that went with our bedroom suite to my parents when we first moved. A very ugly, bulky, 1930s-style, fireplace dominated the dining room, but a more modern, 1950s style, had been installed in the front reception room, which was the only modern improvement that had been made since the house was first built. The house had the advantage of four bedrooms. I felt that if and when my father grew unable to care for himself, we would easily be able to accommodate him.

Large cherry trees in the back garden of the house adjoining brought heavy shade on to the lawn when we first saw the house on a summer evening. All in all it looked somewhat depressing, but the location was right and it was much more spacious and looked well built. Although this house looked rather uncared-for, we could see that it had great promise. Because of its need of upgrading it was within our price range. We felt we could make a lot of improvements, so, with some uncertainty, we put in an offer to the agent, and went on our summer holiday to the Lake District.

When we returned we found that the sale had been withdrawn, no advertisement appeared in the paper and the board was removed, so we thought someone else had had their offer accepted, and our growing anticipation of moving suddenly subsided. But a few weeks later the house reappeared on the market with a different agent and a substantially reduced price. We were quick to act, our offer was accepted, and we thought we would be in our larger property by Christmas. Not so; the present owner had lost his offer on his hoped-for property; he couldn't find a suitable alternative property to purchase during the winter. We had had an offer on our house. Would our client hang on? We had grown more confident that this was the house we wanted, and our lady buyer was similarly keen to purchase our house.

This much-delayed house purchase dragged on through most of my third year at college, and we didn't move until the May the following year. This was perhaps a good thing, as I didn't have the distraction of the actual move until after I had finished my final teaching practice.

However, we had a double 'whammy' at the start of this third teaching practice. Andrew had developed glandular fever soon after Christmas while in the Fifth form at his school, and was not fully recovered when my teaching practice began at the beginning of February. He was still very poorly, and had been unable to go to school for quite a while and his '0' levels were approaching. We were anxious about him, and particularly so in view of his earlier childhood medical history. He still had to have an annual chest x-ray and a medical check-up at Clare Hall Hospital.

Then, a few days after I had begun my final teaching practice Maurice came home from work, put his briefcase down on the kitchen table, looked terribly worried as he announced that deHavilland engine company and the aircraft company were both bankrupt, the petty cash was being counted up in his office, and he was likely to be out of a job within weeks – and we were in the middle of an upgrade house purchase! I went off to my teaching practice the following day with my son's illness, plus home and future worries at the forefront of my mind throughout the day.

I was glad that I was, hopefully, about to start earning, and feared that maybe I was going to be the main financial support to the family. I can well understand the feelings of so many in the present (2010) credit crunch, with job insecurity, or sudden job losses. The bottom drops out of your world. Very soon, however, we were relieved to learn that both the aircraft and the engine companies were taken over by H.M.Government for a while, and Maurice still had a job. The deHavilland engine company was subsequently merged with Bristol Siddeley for a short period until it became part of Rolls Royce Ltd. and was named the Rolls Royce Small Engine Division.

Where is the Key?

Hawker Siddeley acquired the De Havilland Aircraft Company at the same period until it merged with British Aerospace in 1977, but both British Aerospace and Rolls Royce sites closed years later. The old de Havilland airfield, where the Comet made its first flight, and the Rolls Royce test beds, where the Gnome engine was developed are now Hertfordshire University Campus, a Business Park and a lot of housing. Certain buildings have retained the name de Havilland, but the famous name of de Havilland seems to have been quite forgotten nationally.

The worrying clouds passed; Maurice's job stabilised; Andrew recovered from glandular fever and our patience over our house purchase was at last rewarded. The sale was completed, and we moved into our new home during the spring half-term holiday preceding my finals. It was also immediately before Andrew's '0' levels too, so the week after we had moved in he and I spent most of our half-term holiday sitting in the garden revising for our respective exams, which I found very frustrating when there was so much to be done indoors. Ian was happily making the shed at the bottom of the garden into his private den. Full marks to him for finding the house and bringing it to our notice.

My revision paid off, and when the results came out I found I had gained a Merit on my teaching practice and in my main study, and was one of only six mature students in my year who received a Distinction in the Principles of Education examination. My revision had paid off! I had worked hard, well into the night sometimes when an essay needed to be finished and handed in on time. I think I wanted to prove to myself that I could be a good student, and that the limitations of my basic wartime education could be overcome. Many of my fellow mature students were a little younger than I and had had the benefit of not just a longer education, but had been to a grammar school. They had taken their matriculation or even an inter-BSc examination before they came to college, so I was very pleased with my results in view of only receiving what used to be called a 'senior school' three-year education.

I can't honestly say that I enjoyed the three years at college. The history of education, sociology, educational psychology and philosophy of education courses were interesting, but I felt that the lectures didn't add much to that which was already in the list of set books we had to read. I took massive notes of all the lectures, but after reading the books required for each essay I felt that I could have done them solely by reading from the set books at home. However it was quite a good feeling sitting in Hall for our lectures, and every Friday afternoon all the students gathered for our College Meeting, where the principal and all his staff were sitting capped and gowned on the stage.

The reading had been interesting, the study intense, and I truly enjoyed writing (or rather typing, on an old portable typewriter) my essays. But I felt the course was not sufficiently geared to practical aids in the classroom, teaching methods, or techniques of teaching. Sadly, I didn't meet a personal 'buddy' with whom to make a lasting friendship, apart from dear Lesley who lived so far away.

We did have a few practical sessions in our maths course. In our first year all the students had to make (or get our husbands to make) a set of wooden shapes in three colours, one large and one small set, one thick and another thin, in circles, squares and triangles; I think that made forty-two blocks in all. It took hours for my husband to saw and shape, then paint all these pieces in red, yellow and blue for me to use in a single practical maths session at college. They were called Dean's Logical Blocks.

I tried to make use of my set of Dean's blocks in the classroom when I began teaching, but there seemed little opportunity when I was trying to get the children through the set maths books each year. Did I find them useful when teaching? The answer must be, 'No'. I left them in a cupboard when I gave up teaching. They may possibly be used nowadays, but education was still quite formal in the 1970s with no classroom assistant to help with any practical, group or individual work.

Students were also asked to do a project on a chosen subject in maths and some were then asked to take a seminar on it. One chose the Golden Section. I seem to remember that my chosen project was on Fibonacci Fractions, which I found very interesting. They might catch the imagination of children in the strange number pattern, where each number is the sum of its two predecessors e.g. 1, 1,2,3,5,8,13 etc. I was fascinated to learn that this often occurs in nature, but I have forgotten all the details. It was most unlikely to be of use in a classroom, but I know that it took hours of study.

Another student was greeted with loud laughter when she announced the subject of her seminar – 'Sets'. Everyone misheard (?) and thought she had said 'sex', and were hoping for something interesting! But we had no lectures or seminars on how to deal with sex education, or how to handle a possible case of child abuse, or indeed, what to do if the teacher was physically attacked. I don't think that sex education was mentioned in Junior Schools in the 1970s.

The Presentation of Teaching Certificates ceremony was arranged in the autumn in Hertford, but by then I was too busy with my new job and home commitments to go to the event, and thus had no part in any official ceremony. I now regret this, as it had been three years of very hard work, and I should have allowed myself the pleasure of recognition. My teaching certificate arrived in the post.

The first thing we did at our new property was to have the huge, but ailing, elm tree cut down in our front garden and the bole removed. Most of my first month's salary paid for this big job! The blaze of light that its removal brought into our lounge gave me a feeling that I was going to love this house. Dutch elm tree disease had already begun to rampage through the country, so there was no sadness at the loss of the very old, malformed tree. Its' removal made such a difference to the external look of the house and also to the light within. It was the first of many changes that, year-by-year, as we could afford it, made the property and the garden into what I still consider to be my lovely home. I cherish it more as the years pass, and hope I don't have to leave it. The following year our next-door neighbours had the cherry trees cut down; they had become too large for their garden, and their removal allowed so much more sunlight into our back garden.

My face-ache had continued throughout this time, and I had a few very bad patches, but the distraction of hard study helped my mind to concentrate on my work and ignore the pain. On looking back to that period I think Dr. Lawrence's homoeopathic remedies must have helped me more than I appreciated at the time. I also think his note of caution when I told him of my ambition was perhaps a wise one and should have been heeded.

Our family holidays seemed to be coming to an end this summer, as Andrew was on a school exchange visit, staying with the family of a German boy from Worms who had spent a fortnight with us the previous year. Ian was on a school visit to Holland, staying with a Dutch family. Maurice was busy removing the bedroom fireplaces, and redecorating the bedrooms and I did jobs in the house. We fitted in a brief holiday in Malvern, where we enjoyed some walking in the Malvern Hills and going to the lovely Malvern theatre.

Chapter Twenty-Two

TIME TO TEACH

Hertfordshire County Council found placements for new teachers. A new member of staff was required at the school at which I had done my first teaching practice, and when I had my interview at County Hall I was told that the head of this school would like to have me on his staff. After an interview with him I was delighted to be offered the post of teaching a Second Year class (Year 4) in a two-form entry school. It was encouraging to start my teaching career in a familiar setting in my home town. I said to myself that 'life begins at forty' and I was sure that this new career would be fulfilling and in some way would be healing. I was looking forward – with a little trepidation - to new experiences, with the responsibility of having the educational care of thirty-six boys and girls for the coming year.

I found teaching very rewarding in the nineteen-seventies, without being burdened with all the exacting record keeping, new initiatives, tests and documentation that is required today. It was satisfying to see children's reading ability improve over the course of the year, to look at their artwork displayed on the walls of our classroom, to read the remarkable creativity in some of their poems and stories, and in their individual work on the topics we did together each term. Tests were set before Christmas by each class teacher to cover the work done during the autumn term after which I had to write my first reports. Towards the end of the summer term, external Bristol Achievement Tests were taken by all pupils throughout the school, together with a national standard reading test and class work tests set by each teacher followed by an end of year report. Test marking and report writing made a load of extra work, and are an even more burdensome task for present-day teachers. Despite the workload, I was enjoying my job, and was determined not to let my life be overruled by facial neuralgia.

Reading was very important in a mixed ability class of eight- nine-year-old children. When the standard reading test was done at the end of the school year, most of my class had a reading age that was above their chronological age of nine years, and a few had a reading age of 13+ at the end of their third year, when there were thirty-nine pupils in the class (Year 5). Many were avid readers and could read fluently, but a small group still had great difficulty in mastering the art. I am sure they were the ones who came from a non-reading home, who didn't get help from parents, who didn't do their required reading practice at home, were probably never read to and whose parents didn't come to any open evenings. However, neither would they have spent their free time texting on their mobile phones or playing computer games! They would have some individual help nowadays, and one or two would no doubt be considered dyslexic. Some would probably be given alternative approaches nowadays.

Where is the Key?

I would have been delighted to have a classroom assistant to help with reading and maths, in art and needlework lessons. I was usually still at my desk marking books, or climbing on tables putting artwork on display on the walls long after the children had gone home. Then I had to get home, cook a meal, and usually had more books to mark or preparation to do in the evening. It was more than a full-time job even then; I just don't know how teachers cope now. There was no room for a social life, little time to watch much television on the new TV set we had now been able to afford, and there was no time to read a book. Teaching is more than a full-time career.

I often think of my old pupils with affection and am always delighted to hear of the careers some of them have had. One gifted boy became an organ scholar at Cambridge University and is now the organist in a very large church in America. I remember this budding ten-year-old pianist having the honour of being asked to play the hymn for school assembly at the end of the Easter term. I believe that he had strong musical ambitions even then. Another, who was a very talented all-rounder at junior school, is now a consultant gynaecologist. Yet another is a doctor who was working in a deprived area somewhere in the heart of Africa when I last I heard of him; he was a very reserved, extremely polite boy who did the neatest of work in his maths book, but who found long multiplication rather difficult when I taught him in his third year (now called year 5). Yet another is now editor of a magazine in the USA and is a published author. I remember she had a wonderful talent for creative writing in her junior school. I would love to know what became of other old pupils; it is so interesting to hear of later chapters in their life stories.

On the last afternoon at the end of my first year's teaching my headmaster came in to the classroom as I was tidying everything up after the children had gone home, and congratulated me on my first year of teaching. I was so pleased to have his commendation because I had really found it hard work, and felt I needed a little praise. Teaching was yet another rather lonely job, just one adult in a room with thirty children or more for most of the day, with little time to spare at break times for conversation in the staff room. There was nobody to tell me how I was doing or where I may have been going wrong. My headmaster's comment gave me great encouragement, and enabled me to look forward to our first family holiday abroad.

We were hiring a caravan on the Dutch/German border during that summer, and intended to drive on into Germany and have a touring holiday driving alongside the Rhine, visiting some of the well-known Rhine towns. We took our Vauxhall Viva car across the channel on the ferry, with the boot crammed full with our luggage and some basic food requirements to stow away in our caravan. My father didn't accompany us on this holiday. After reaching Calais we had a very long drive through parts of Holland and Belgium before reaching Munchen-Gladbach, where we were hitched up to the caravan that was to be our home for the next two weeks. We thought that a couple of ex-RAF personnel had set up this company after demobilisation at the end of the war, hiring out holiday caravans in part of an old airfield on the Belgium/German border. My husband said they looked like ex RAF types! We were handed two caravan door keys. My husband put one in his purse which he placed in the inside pocket of his sports jacket (customary casual wear at the period – and very nice he looked too). He gave the other key to Andrew who put it in his purse and tucked that safely into the inside zipped pocket of his anorak.

We decided to pay a short visit to Cologne and I can remember my husband cautiously driving round the empty streets of Cologne on a Sunday morning, looking for somewhere to park a car towing a caravan. It was quite a problem. Eventually we found a spot and were able to spend a little time in this city on a very dull morning. My recollection of the cathedral is that it looked dark and rather dismal and very uninviting. I think that a lot of war damage to the city had still not been cleaned, restored or rebuilt in the early 1970s.

We found our first caravan site at Bad Gothenburg, but our car with its English registration number plate, and our caravan with its German one caused quite a bit of confusion when we first entered the huge caravan site. The manageress came out of her office, saw the caravan with its German registration and began to talk rapidly in German to my husband, assuming we were German. She couldn't comprehend why Maurice and I had blank expressions on our faces, or understand our gesticulations trying to inform her that we couldn't understand a word she was saying. It was incomprehension all round until our older son, who was sitting in the back of the car, suddenly realised there was a problem. He came to our mutual rescue and began to explain in fluent German that we were an English family towing a German registered caravan. There was utter bafflement for a few moments followed by a look of suspicion and a few questions, then, at last, came a request for our passports. (Andrew's German teacher would have been proud of his pupil's confident conversational German.)

We soon learned to make sure the camp site managers saw our English car registration number plate, and to have our passports ready before anyone tried to tell us what they wanted us to do or where to go. I don't think that many people brought an English car across the Channel and towed a caravan with a foreign registration then.

The caravan had fairly basic accommodation for four people. As I was the only female I slept in what I am sure was intended as a child's bed at the kitchen end of the caravan. My strongest memory of our first night in a Rhine-side campsite was our very early awakening due to the sound of the engines of the barges moored at each side of the river. At crack of dawn there was a sudden, slightly muted, but rough-sounding roar all along both banks of the river. Barges had moored for the night, and their engines were warming up as early morning breakfasts were being consumed before the huge barges began their journey again, either to Rotterdam and the coast, or for the long voyage inland. Either way, the engines' rumbles soon turned into a combined roar and the subsequent noise was more than enough to stop any further sleep. It was a great disturbance. When we got up we found that the weather was more sombre than the previous day, with a heavy mist over the Rhine, making the whole scene look very dismal.

The boys took on the responsibility for winding the caravan legs down or up when parking or on leaving a site, and they fetched the water to fill up the water container at the back of the van. They quite enjoyed the responsibility (at least I think they did), winding the legs down to support the van when not on tow after our arrival at a new site, and winding them up from the ground when we left. Maurice did the driving, and I did the catering, and maybe a bit of navigating, but I am sure that my husband had the greatest task. We travelled a long way on this holiday; he had never towed a caravan before; had never driven on the right-hand side of the road before and was unfamiliar with our route. We discovered that our Vauxhall Viva was also a bit underpowered for the task of towing a caravan uphill on the autobahn. Altogether I think he did extremely well, and I wish that he was still alive to read this (belated? - I can't remember; I hope not; I don't think so) commendation.

Toward the end of our first day we reached the Rhine-side town of Boppard, and parked in a pleasant campsite alongside the river. We went out for dinner in the evening. I think this was the first time our two sons had a glass of wine; they were both in their teens. A bottle of wine with a meal was an unusual occurrence in those days, usually indicating some special occasion. Our celebration was that we had got started on our adventure and felt we were coping. A terrific thunderstorm suddenly developed as we were about to return to our four-wheeled-home after our meal; we were unprotected, and Maurice rushed to the caravan, snatched up umbrellas and his camera, and sloshed back to where we were standing outside the restaurant on slightly higher ground. The rain tipped down heavily, straight as long needles, and the campsite was soon waterlogged. It was impossible to wade back to our caravan, and many campers were seriously concerned that the legs of their caravan would give way and it would float off down the river. The thunder crashed, and sudden flashes of lightning lit up the entire landscape on the other side of the Rhine. It was spectacular, and we forgot the flooded campsite, the pouring rain and our damp feet as we watched this powerful electrical display in the hills on the far side of the river. Maurice took some unusual photos of the landscape, lit up solely by lightning, which picked up the headlights of the cars driving up the hill on the far side of the river.

Time passed by, the thunderclaps became rumbles and as the storm gradually eased away and then ceased at last, we were able to take off our shoes and paddle back to our caravan. We were relieved to find that the flooding hadn't reached the door and our little 'home' was dry inside. It was very late when I climbed into my rather cramped bed and got off to sleep, only to be awakened a few hours later by the deep, throaty roar of the barges moored for the night alongside the river.

The following morning was sunny and although the ground was soggy the caravan was not floating in sloppy mud. We managed to drive away from Boppard and later in the day we arrived at Heidelberg, where we found a beautiful campsite on the banks of the River Neckar. The entrance to the camp required driving down a very, very steep slope – quite hair-raising I would think for a first-time driver with a caravan hitched on behind; my husband did it expertly, but I think he found it rather nerve-wracking. We had a very pleasant pitch by the edge of the river, and he was glad to be able to drive out the following morning without towing the caravan – especially up or down that steep entrance - as we explored the city and its surroundings. We hoped the weather would now be kind to us. We stayed a second night and had another day of sunshine, and returned to our rather idyllic-looking campsite beside the river. There were no barges moored alongside the River Neckar to wake us early the next morning, and we looked forward to another sunny day. But the following morning was dull and cloudy, and then - it rained.

The 1972 Olympic Games were being held in Munich at the same period that we were on holiday, and the weather forecast on our portable radio told us that there was a heat wave in the south, so we decided to abandon our plan, leave the river and drive further south to the Black Forest in search of the sun. We left Heidelberg in drenching rain, and got on to the autobahn. Maurice was soon enduring the feeling that he hadn't quite enough pulling power in the Vauxhall Viva engine. Pressing on the accelerator whilst travelling in low gear up the long hill in driving rain made him acknowledge that the lorries behind us, also in the slow lane, were understandably impatient with our underpowered car. My husband was stressed at being hooted at when his Viva engine couldn't do any better. He decided to pull off the road at the next lay-by to let the lorries go by; we would have a break and a bit of lunch. The boys got out, wound the legs down and brought in some water to boil a kettle and make some tea. I fried some eggs and bacon on our little hob, and together with a tin of baked beans we sat eating our lunch to the accompaniment of thunder and lightning once more, with a deluge of rain beating noisily on to the roof of the caravan. We could just about hear the radio giving us news of the fine weather and heat wave in Munich. The storm was soon over, so we set off, driving in that direction, hoping to find better weather further south.

The heavy lorries had gone, and soon the sun began to shine fitfully, reflecting on the wet road surface and before long we saw clear blue sky ahead of us. We still had a long drive before we found a sign leading to an accredited caravan park. We were not sure exactly where we were, but were just relieved to see a signpost to a caravan site. It seemed to be in the middle of nowhere – I guess it was; it was somewhere in the middle of the Black Forest. However, the camp looked very pleasant with widely spaced camping spaces in a large, open, grassy area. It was mid-afternoon, but there were one or two people about. The camp manager came out of his office; we exchanged 'Gruss Gott' with him. He had recognised our English Vauxhall, had noticed our English registration plate and he politely asked Maurice for our passports.

My husband reached over to the back seat for his jacket, and then remembered he had left it in the caravan after we had had our lunch. His jacket had our passports in the pocket and also the key to the van. The moment of annoyance quickly passed; there was no need to worry; Andrew had the second key. He turned in his seat to ask Andrew to go and unlock the caravan door and get our passports from his dad's jacket pocket, but when Andrew felt in his anorak pocket, and then hurriedly began searching *all* his pockets – there was no purse and so no key. Where was the key? He couldn't find his purse anywhere; it contained the caravan key and all his holiday spending money. For a moment we were shocked into silence. What could we do? We tried to think where Andrew might have lost it, and after a while he said he thought he remembered putting it on the top of the water carrier at the back of the caravan while he wound up the legs after our lunch stop in the lay-by on the autobahn. He might have forgotten to pick it up again and it could have travelled behind us, still on the top of the carrier for a while before falling off onto the road; or, equally possible, it slipped off as we drove away from the lay-by. He could even have left it at Heidelberg. (Oh! don't I know that feeling nowadays. I put something down, usually my glasses, and then can't remember where I put them.)

There was consternation all round. But whatever, and wherever, the caravan was locked, the key was lost; we were locked outside, unable to produce our passports. (Like the kitchen door, the caravan locked when you shut the door.) I dread to think what the site manager thought of this crazy English family with a German registered caravan, and no key to enter it. He seemed genuinely concerned for us, however, and appeared to understand our predicament and went off to speak to another camping family, who might have some tool that we could use to prise open a window.

I think he believed our story. We must have looked an honest family. (Perhaps a similar incident had previously occurred with another family?) We felt so helpless and didn't know what to do. Eventually, Ian came to our rescue, and we discovered his talent for burglary. Somehow or other he fiddled with the large spanner that had been offered to us, and managed, very slowly, to prise a fanlight window open just enough to enable him to push it down, squeeze his body through and jump down into the van. The opened window seemed so tiny, and to this day I don't know how he managed to ease his, admittedly slim, body through it. Once inside he was able to open the door and came out flourishing our passports. All the onlookers on the site cheered. We had caused quite a bit of consternation – and eventually, entertainment. Maurice was able to produce our passports; we were allotted our parking space with laughs from our fellow campers, who probably thought 'these mad English'. We were so grateful to Ian, who got us out of a terrible dilemma.

The campsite manager informed the police of a lost purse containing money and a key somewhere on the autobahn or in a certain lay-by, but no purse was found. We were still short of a key, and on our return along the other side of the Rhine we stopped off at Bingen and found a shop where we were able to get a key cut, and were thus able to return our van with two keys.

Before we reached Bingen we drove to Worms, to visit the host family with whom Andrew had stayed the previous year. We had tea with Eckard, whose English was quite good, and his mother, who spoke no English at all. As Andrew was the only member of our family who spoke any German, there was quite a bit of translating being done by Eckard and Andrew. We were shown over their huge house, which included a large games room and their own private cinema. No wonder Andrew had enjoyed his visit to Germany so much the previous year. I gave a thought to our modest semi-detached house and the tiny third bedroom that Eckard had slept in when he stayed with us before me moved! I wonder what he thought, but he seemed to enjoy his visit.

We left a little later, and Eckard, who had recently passed his driving test, led us to our caravan site a few miles outside the town. We said our farewells to this very nice young man. I was washing the dishes after we had eaten our evening meal when there were several hard bangs on the door to our caravan. We were a little worried, fearing that young louts might be attacking us, and I peeped through the window and saw a man waving to me with what looked like a large club in each hand. Maurice very cautiously opened the door a crack, to find a well-built middle-aged man, smiling broadly and cradling two bottles of wine in his arms. We didn't know who he was, but as soon as Andrew saw him there was a huge shout of recognition. It was Eckard's father, who had returned from work and was so disappointed at not seeing Andrew again or meeting us that Eckard had driven his dad all the way to our caravan site so that we could meet. We invited them in, and sat chatting all the evening whilst drinking his good German wine from the small, cheap tumblers provided with the van. (They were not, I would think, the kind of glasses he usually drank his wine from, nor where this successful businessman would normally be seen!) Eckard's father spoke a little English, but our respective sons again did exceptionally well in translating some of our conversation.

We enjoyed the rest of our holiday, but we were unable to catch up with the heat wave that was experienced in Munich, and altogether it was not the most successful of our holidays, ruined by the weather. This was to be our last family holiday. Our sons were growing up and it was not long before one was in the sixth form at school, and going on a trek to the North Cape, and the other was going abroad with his university choir on a concert tour in Spain. It was time for their mum and dad to spread their wings too.

Chapter Twenty-three

WORK AND PLAY

I was given responsibility for netball in the school during my second year of teaching, umpiring at inter-school netball fixtures and supporting the school netball team at the annual primary school netball rally. I really enjoyed coaching the girls, matching their enthusiasm with my own, and was very proud of their attainments when the head announced our successes (and sometimes our failures) in matches with other local schools. At the assembly following a match he always asked the netball team to stand up while he gave the result of the recent match and made some encouraging remark to the girls, which was followed by applause from the school. It made the team feel so proud to know they had represented their school and increased their desire and enthusiasm for future matches.

These extra-curricular activities added to my workload; netball practice was in the playground after school or in the dinner hour; matches with other local schools ended after school hours, and the annual rally was on a Saturday morning towards the end of the spring term. I now owned a second-hand Fiat 500 car, and in those pre-regulation days I would drive to a match with three girls squeezed in the back of this tiny car and a fourth at my side, while our school welfare assistant drove the rest of the team and our reserve. This was before seat belts were required or any school transport safety regulations had been brought in, and also before competitive sports began to be officially discouraged in schools.

We entertained an overseas student for a weekend during my second year of teaching. Our church had accepted responsibility for hosting a group of overseas students, giving them a taste of English home life as well as visiting an interesting city. My husband met Steve Tung at the station on a Friday evening and on the Saturday he and his fellow students in the group from London University were taken on a tour of the ancient Roman sites in St. Albans – the Roman theatre, the bit of the old Roman city wall, the hypocaust in Verulamium Park with its beautiful mosaic floor, and the Roman Museum. (The museum has been redesigned and rebuilt since then and is now a first rate visitor attraction, even more worth a visit, displaying some excellent mosaic floors, many Roman artefacts and interactive exhibits of life in the Roman city of Verulamium.) The students spent the Saturday evening with the youth group at the church, and the following morning experienced a traditional Anglican Church service with the local congregation.

Steve joined us for Sunday lunch at home before I drove him to the station after what I hoped had been an enjoyable weekend. As I was leaving the station I noticed a poster advertising an L.N.E.R. Society (London North Eastern Railway) excursion, with a whole day in Edinburgh on the **3rd May**. The date stood out so clearly, as it was our wedding anniversary. I took a second glance at the poster before I left the station, and as I drove home I pondered on the possibility of an unusual celebration of our anniversary. Maurice thought it was a good idea, and bought the tickets for the overnight train to Edinburgh on the Friday, 2nd May at 11.30p.m., returning at the same time on the Saturday, our wedding anniversary, arriving at about 7.30a.m. on the Sunday morning. All for £5!

It was already dark when a few weeks later we drove to Watford station on the Friday evening. An old LNER train arrived promptly on time. We had been given a compartment number with our tickets and after getting on the train we walked along the corridor until we found our compartment, which had the old-fashioned, upholstered, bench-type seats on either seat, normally seating four passengers each side. There was a sliding door opening on to the corridor and pull-down blinds at all the windows. We were the only occupants, which meant that we could lie down along the length of each seat, make ourselves as comfortable as possible, and sleep through the night while the train roared northwards. We didn't see any of the occupants of the other compartments.

The train slowed down at some point, and stopped for a while, presumably at points, before getting up speed for its journey north, and it was some while after this that our compartment door slid open, and a tall man burst in from the corridor. Where had he come from? The man slumped down on the seat nearest to the corridor. He slid the compartment door shut with a bang, and we immediately felt a little threatened. Had we misunderstood the limited occupancy of the compartment? The man put his feet onto the opposite bench (the one I was sitting on) and dozed off to sleep for a little while, fidgeting and slurring incomprehensible words from time to time. Maurice and I were sitting opposite each other on the window side furthest away from the corridor. We couldn't get out without walking past our 'visitor' if we needed to escape. Maurice slid his camera to the side furthest away from the new occupant of the compartment, and covered it protectively with his arm. We didn't dare drop off to sleep, and sat bolt upright looking at each other, not speaking, but eyeing our fellow-passenger cautiously from time to time. After a while he stirred; we felt even more discomforted when he roused and suddenly got up, and forcefully pulled down the blinds at the windows on the corridor side of the compartment, which shut us off completely from the view of anyone walking along the train. We were really frightened as he lurched across the compartment towards us and began to pull our blinds down, but Maurice told him politely, but quite severely that we didn't want the blinds down. He complied, with a shrug, as if to indicate that he thought we were mad: it's a night train, we're going to sleep, so why don't we 'draw the curtains' was what he seemed to be thinking. He sat down and mumbled and grumbled for a bit, and then he slid the door open and stumbled off down the corridor.

We heaved a sigh of relief, relaxed a bit and began to settle ourselves down, hoping to be able to drop off to sleep, but nevertheless, feeling troubled that he might return. I lay down along my seat, made a pillow of my handbag and tried to nod off. Maurice remained sitting bolt upright, still protecting his camera, on guard, but soon he too fell into a light snooze. My eyelids began to droop, and I dropped off to sleep too, when suddenly the compartment door slid open once again, and Maurice awoke with a start as a heavy lump thumped on to his lap. It was a real fright, but the man was standing with a couple of cans of beer in his hand – the third had been thrown into Maurice's lap. He proffered a can of beer to me, but I thanked him and declined, telling him that I didn't like beer. This must have been about one o'clock in the morning.

We were soon to discover that our fellow passenger was a 'gentleman of the road' with his own ideas of honesty, politeness and generosity. He had bought a can of beer for the couple of 'townies' that he had found he was travelling with. After his further alcohol intake – of *three* cans of beer - he became quite chatty, and although very tired, we had to respond. He asked us where we came from. I told him that we lived in St. Albans.

"Oh! I know St. Albans" he replied, "Oh yes, I've been to St. Albans – what a stuck up town that is; there's a park near the station isn't there?"

We replied that there was.

"Yes, I once spent a night in St. Albans. I had settled myself on a bench in that park near the station, was fast asleep, when a stuck-up policeman appeared, woke me up, and made me move on. What harm was I doing, sleeping in the park? I had to clear out and walk the streets for the rest of the night. Stuck up city, St. Albans."

I was silent for a while after this, but eventually asked him where he lived, and he replied that he lived anywhere and everywhere.

His next question was, "Where's this train going to?"

I was bewildered. "Surely," I replied, "you must have known your destination when you bought your ticket. What station did you buy a ticket for?"

"Ticket? I've never bought a ticket in my life. I'm a man of the road, and I travel everywhere. I don't buy tickets. Where's this train going to?" He spoke rather belligerently.

I told him that it was an overnight train to Edinburgh, due in at Waverly Station at 7.30a.m.

"I've never been to Edinburgh," he replied.

"Then why on earth are you on this train?" I was really puzzled.

"I was in a pub, when I thought about me mam in Middlesborough and decided to go and see her. I hitched a lift along the road and then saw this train going north, so I hopped on."

"But it's not stopping at stations going north, and it doesn't go anywhere near Middlesborough."

"Oh, I'll know where to get off. It'll slow down somewhere around there."

I have often wondered why the train slowed down and stopped at what we had assumed were points. Could the driver have known about this man of the road? Might it have been an arranged stop, or did our visitor take advantage of a temporary stationary train going north? I will never know.

My husband and I were by now silent, totally bewildered at this seemingly harmless rogue, who had offered us a drink, complied with our request to have the blinds pulled up during a night long journey, had not used a word of bad language, but who appeared to have no concept of honesty.

There was silence for quite a while; our friend nodded off to sleep again, and soon began snoring. Eventually Maurice and I both dropped off to sleep too, through sheer exhaustion, although I think we were both sub-consciously alert for any undue noise or movement. An hour or two later our fellow traveller woke up, and as he roused, so did we. He began to grow talkative again and asked us what we did. When I told him I was a teacher, he began to question me on what I actually taught. Then he thought a moment and said, "I went to the best school in England". He sounded just a little cynical, but he repeated what he had just said rather reflectively, and then added, "Yes, the best school – at the expense of Her Majesty".

It was, of course, a Borstal institution, and we learned that in his youth he had been sent to several. He told us a little of his childhood, that his father had been a policeman who was very strict, and the more he was repressed the more he rebelled. He told us he had escaped from his first Borstal, and then from his second. I think he had escaped from the third, and had been on the run ever since. He said that the stronger the security had been, the more he was determined to get out. I don't think he was 'on the run' because of a crime; he had just dropped out of society.

He spoke quite fondly of his mother, then told us that he never swore in front of women, and wouldn't dream of swearing in his mother's presence. When our journey was over we realised that we had not heard a word of swearing, or obscene language throughout our, mainly sleepless, night.

I asked him if he had a fixed home of any kind, and he told me he slept anywhere, and when he needed money, he got a job. He pulled out a £5 note from his top pocket, and said, "I owe no man anything; I pay my way". (I don't think he considered that he should have paid for his train ticket!) "I have worked in some of the best hotels in London – but I wouldn't eat in one if I were you." (I am sure conditions in hotel kitchens have improved since the 1970s!)

I became very curious about this man, with his confidence, and gentlemanliness, combined with his largely unrecognised dishonesty. How did he keep clean I wondered?

He pulled a razor from his top pocket, and said, "I shave every day, and when I need clean clothes I go to an all-night launderette".

We were relieved that he hadn't produced the razor earlier on! We were beginning to understand that we were not at physical risk, nor, indeed - we hoped - of being robbed. We dozed off to sleep again whilst vaguely aware of the speed of the train as it raced northwards through the night. Our companion disappeared again, but returned once more, and began to test my competence as a teacher by producing a box of matches and doing puzzles using matchsticks, which he laid out in certain patterns between us on the seat. I was not all that competent at intelligence tests in the middle of the night whilst moving at speed, but I was challenged to try and solve his puzzles. I seem to remember my Uncle Bert doing similar tricks with matchsticks when I was a small child.

After a while I remembered that he had told us that he was going north to see his mother in Middlesborough. I asked him, "When are you thinking of getting off the train?"

"Oh! It's too late now. The train was going too fast when I wanted to get off. I've never been to Edinburgh. I'm happy to stay put."

The rest of the night passed without comment or incident, and we had an all-too-brief period of silence and sleep. It was quite light when I began to sense the train was slowing down a little. Our companion of the night suddenly jumped up from his seat and said, "Well, I'll be off now".

"Where to?" I asked in all innocence.

"It's time I was off", was his simple reply, and with that he slid open the compartment door, politely said, "Cheerio. I might see you tonight", and left us. We were relieved, and very thankful that nothing untoward had occurred, that we had not been robbed, attacked or worse. We had seen no attendant walking along the corridor during the night. But not again tonight, we thought. Please not a return visit!

Our train reached Edinburgh on time, and as we walked along the platform at half-past seven in the morning for our day in Scotland we were assailed by the wonderful smell of bacon and eggs. We made our way to the station restaurant and took our places in the queue for a full English breakfast – in Scotland! We had almost reached the checkout when we noticed a tall man standing a little further back in the queue. It was our companion of the night! We had no idea how he got off the train, but there he was, as large as life, queuing up in the cafeteria. My husband immediately offered to buy him his breakfast, but he refused, telling us firmly he always paid his way.

We enjoyed our freshly cooked breakfast, and soon set out to explore as much of Edinburgh as we could in about twelve hours. I was already in quite a lot of facial pain, and I can remember sitting for a while in Waverley Gardens wondering how I was going to get through the day. I had been talking half the night, and my jaws were already hurting like mad. But an excursion is an excursion, I had never been to Scotland before and I was not going to spoil the day, but wanted to make the most of it.

First of all we went up on to Carlton Hill and in the early morning sunlight we had a wonderful view across the city. Then we made our way to Edinburgh Castle, which, even in the spring sunshine looked rather dour and forbidding. We walked along Prince's Street and then down the Royal Mile and found our way to Holyrood House where we had an interesting guided tour. After getting a bus back to the city centre we found it rather difficult to find anywhere to have a meal on our wedding anniversary. Edinburgh seemed to have rather posh, expensive restaurants, for which we were not suitably dressed, or rather rough-looking establishments. We ended up at a Kentucky Chicken restaurant, where we were served chicken that appeared to be undercooked. The meal was altogether only memorable for its disappointment. It was not the best part of our wedding anniversary expedition. We were very tired by early evening, but our train didn't leave until 11.30p.m. We had time to kill, and we finished off our day by walking part way across the Forth Bridge before taking a bus ride to the station. We found our train waiting, and were able to rest for a while in our compartment before our departure at 11.30p.m. Our visitor of the previous night did not reappear and we had the compartment to ourselves for the journey home. It was a memorable weekend in more ways than one!

It was back to school on Monday where normal class activities included art lessons. When we had a painting session, all the water had to be obtained from the cold tap in the large old sink in the boys' toilets. During the dinner hour I went to the boys' toilets to fill a large jug with water and carried it into the classroom and filled the jam jars I had set out on the children's desks. When home time arrived, I had to wait until the boys' toilets were empty before going in to check that the paint monitors had not created too much of a mess while emptying and washing out the jars, and annoyed the caretaker. Then I washed the paintbrushes in the old sink and generally tidied up before leaving for home. It was a messy performance in an old Victorian building, without adequate cleaning-up facilities.

I heard a ring on my front doorbell one afternoon during the next summer holiday. My ex-neighbour and Ghanaian friend Regina stood on my doorstep; I hadn't seen much of her since we had moved. I had been too busy. I thought it was just a friendly call, but before I had time to ask her indoors, out came her request, 'Sheila, will you have a third son for a year?' Regina was returning to Ghana with her husband and their young daughter who had been born in England. They wanted Peter to remain in England in order to sit his GCSE exams the following summer. To hear her request, 'Sheila, will you have a third son for a year?' was quite a shock! We did have a spare bedroom, so it was difficult to refuse, but would I be able to cope with full-time teaching, a 'third son', as well as my face pain during the coming year? How would Ian like to have another teenager living in his home? My husband and I discussed it, and found the request difficult to refuse, so we asked Ian's opinion, and had decided that if he felt unhappy about it, we would tell Peter's parents that it was not possible. Ian's reply was commendable: 'If I was in Peter's position I would be glad if I could stay here'. So Peter soon became part of our family for the ensuing year.

He had not lived with an English family before and was used to knocking on the door of a room at home and getting audible permission before he entered. I think we were not nearly as strict as his parents. He had a huge appetite; apparently enjoyed my English cooking, and Peter and Ian seemed to compete with each other as to who could eat the biggest dinner or the most potatoes every evening. He spent Christmas with us, and really had a good time. As he finished his Christmas dinner I remember him sitting back in his chair, giving a big satisfied sigh, before rubbing his hand around his stomach, then saying, "Mmm! I have never eaten so much; I have never had a Christmas dinner like this". There was tremendous excitement later on in the evening when we played Pit. I don't think he had played family games before, and he was almost overwhelmed with his frantic enthusiasm to be the first to shout, 'Corner'. Party games were always a part of our Christmas evening festivities.

He settled in very well, and did his homework up in his bedroom every evening, although we often heard strange sounds emanating from his room. It was a long while before I discovered that he was continuously rolling a ball across the floor while he was supposedly studying. He loved football, and found study hard. I think he had been used to having his homework supervised and his work was monitored very closely, but I had my own homework to do in marking work and preparing lessons. He was a sports and fitness fanatic, and I think he spent more time using his chest expanders than doing his French and maths! I only discovered the chest expanders when he was packing to go home to Accra the following summer. He was certainly quite a big fellow when he left us, had had his teenage growth spurt and was really tall and broad-shouldered. His parents would see a great change in him after that year of separation.

He took his turn with the drying up after our meals, but was a slow mover in the kitchen when we were all scurrying around trying to clear the breakfast table, get the washing up done, and rush off to work and school in the morning. He returned to Ghana when he was sixteen, but after his English education he may have found it difficult to settle in his own country and now lives in the USA, working in the film industry, sometimes going on location and has had parts in a number of films.

We took 'our third son' on a day's excursion after his GCSE exams were over. We toured part of Kent, visiting the Roman villa at Lullingstone, having a guided tour round a privately-owned stately home, and after tea in the garden we gazed across the Weald of Kent as the day drew to a close. This beautiful house is no longer open to the public. My husband and I happened to revisit it some years later, and enjoyed one of the last public tours of the house that were given, whilst the contents were actually being photographed for the sale catalogue of a big London auction firm. We were told by our guide that the beautiful old porcelain figures and ornaments, together with the china that had been in the family for generations had already been sold. There was no heir.

Peter had not seen much of beautiful England during the years he had lived here. He told us he had learned about the Weald of Kent in geography, but he had never seen it, and had no mental picture of what 'the weald' really meant or what it looked like until we had the long view from the garden of the old mansion. 'Oh, that's what they meant by the Weald of Kent!' he exclaimed. He had been very busy during the year with homework, sports and Saturday morning maths coaching, and this was our only opportunity to give him a day out to see a little bit of England - both history and beauty, we hoped - before he returned to his home country. We drove home via Tunbridge Wells in the late evening, and stopped to walk down The Pantiles, and drink some of the spa water. It was fish and chips for supper that evening. He had had a tiny taste of England. I wonder whether he remembers it.

I helped him pack all his belongings, his treasures and his chest expanders, plus all the items that he had been requested to take home to Ghana with him. He received many letters from his mother in the weeks leading up to his return, consisting mainly of lists of items he had to bring home in his luggage. There were quite a few shopping expeditions to do – buying everything from underpants to jellies to deodorants!

He said farewell to his friends as soon as the term was over and we drove him to Heathrow. As his cases were already tightly packed and bulging I had to stuff his anorak pockets with the heavy jellies and deodorants, and then zip them up. The luggage was already overweight, but even a massively heavy anorak would still pass as hand luggage. There were no intensive search or security measures in the mid-nineteen-seventies. Maurice and I found it strange to find we were the only white people to be standing at the not at all busy check-in before the Sunday morning flight to Accra. It made me realise what it must feel like to be in the minority.

We settled down to a slightly less hectic life at home, although the day after Peter left we were expecting the builders in to knock down the dividing wall between the sitting room and our dining room, to remove the dingy, old-fashioned tiled fireplace and replaster the wall. Our home was gradually improving. Maurice had installed new kitchen units, and we now had a modern gas-fired boiler. When the alterations were complete and our new living space was decorated we had a lovely light and spacious through-room, which made an enormous difference to our home.

Peter had gone home, Andrew was in Spain and Ian was on his way to the North Cape when Maurice and I set off for Gatwick to begin our summer holiday in Austria. The 'high' places always attracted us and our hotel was built halfway up a mountain in Landeck in the Austrian Tyrol. But mountains bring much rain, and we saw a lot of that on this holiday. I think the tour operators had difficulty in thinking of places of interest to take visitors, as many of the scenic ones had their beautiful scenery blotted out by mist, clouds and torrential rain. (We found over the years that our summer holiday frequently seemed to be dogged by bad weather.) We had a few fine days, spent a wonderful day in Innsbruck and managed to reach the top of a few of the local mountains – once we had ascended part way up in a cable car! We were not mountaineers, just mountain walkers, wearing appropriate boots and keeping to the footpaths that were not always clear, but were marked by large red circles painted – but sometimes faded and hard to see - on to rocks every half mile or so. It was quite a thrill to reach the mountain peak, each one in Austria surmounted by a huge wooden cross.

Chapter Twenty-four

A FRIENDSHIP VIA A HANDBAG!

The mountains still drew us and we arranged a holiday in Switzerland in the summer of 1979, spending two weeks at a resort on Lake Lucerne. As was not uncommon in our holidays – the weather was unsettled. We had an excursion to the top of Mount Pilatus, where my holiday record reminds me that our transport was on a cogwheel electric railway, reputedly the steepest in the world. During our slow ascent I got into conversation with a young lady sitting next to me. Her mother, sitting opposite her, had pointed to a crocheted handbag sitting in my lap, and then said something to her daughter, who interpreted to me that her mother was admiring my handbag and thought the hand-crafted crocheting was very good. (I had actually bought the bag at Marks and Spencer's, and had always been hopeless at crocheting!) Through this comment I began a conversation with the young lady, who I learned lived in Leiden, Holland, and had just finished her first year at Leiden University. I asked her if she had been to England, and on learning that she had not, I began to wonder whether I should ask if she would like to have a holiday in England and stay with us. She was reading Classics and I explained that she could get into London easily from St. Albans and would enjoy visiting the British Museum. I leaned across to my husband and suggested that perhaps we could invite her to stay for a week or two the following year. I think he probably thought I was a little crazy to do this when life was a struggle already. I am not in the habit of inviting unknown people to stay in my home and I find it quite amazing that it should have entered my mind.

I learned that the young lady's name was Gerrie. When we reached the top of Mount Pilatus, and the awful noise of the cogwheel railway had ceased, Gerrie introduced us to her parents, and also to her boy friend, Marcel. I hadn't realised that the young man sitting next to her on the train had anything to do with my new acquaintance. We exchanged addresses, and Gerrie suggested that we should get to know one another through correspondence until her summer vacation the following year. As a classics student, the British Museum would interest her, and she was old enough to enjoy the sights in London, and we would take her out at the weekends, which would be a treat for us all. I was still suffering constant pain. I explained to Gerrie that I suffered from 'headaches', and she told me that her mother had frequent migraines, so I felt she would understand if I was not always at my best

We shook hands and said our farewells, and began to walk around the mountain peak, but the views from the top of Mount Pilatus were obscured by thick mist, and the journey in the cogwheel train is remembered more clearly than any of the mountain top views we should have had during this entire holiday. August is not the best month in which to visit Switzerland. The best weather we had was on the day we gave up trying to see views from the tops of mountains, and spent a day by the lakeside at Weggis, when the sun shone constantly. I had a very long swim, almost half way across the lake and back, easy swimming, accompanied by another guest from our hotel, chatting from time to time as we swam, sometimes in very cold water (in greater depth of water or deeper water churned up by the lake steamers) and at others in very pleasant temperatures. It is still a delightful memory.

On our arrival back home an envelope containing a long letter from Gerrie, thanking me for the invitation, telling me a bit about herself and her boyfriend, both undergraduates who were so thrilled at having the opportunity to visit England. I hadn't intended the invitation to include Marcel, but on consideration, Maurice and I agreed that it would make things easier, as we would not have to feel responsible for Gerrie's safety in London; she would have her boyfriend as escort. Andrew was now working and had his own flat, so we had two spare bedrooms. Some while later we had further correspondence from Gerrie saying that 'it is essential that Marcel and I have separate bedrooms, as we are neither engaged nor married. We have wanted to have a holiday 'together but not together if you know what I mean' for a long time and are so thrilled with your invitation. It was an answer to our prayer'. I began to feel that my spontaneous invitation was a moment of insight, and looked forward to their arrival, and was pleased to feel that I was doing something useful away from the classroom.

We met these almost complete strangers at Victoria Station, only known through handbag, a chance encounter, and a year's correspondence, but almost immediately there seemed a close bond. They had a great holiday, we enjoyed their company and took them out at the weekends, and when they left to return home it seemed as if we were saying good-bye to family, and I realised how much I enjoyed having someone of my own sex in the home. I had lacked female family all my life. We kept in touch and they visited us again in the two following summers, by which time they were engaged to be married. We were delighted to receive an invitation to their wedding the following year.

We took our car on the ferry to Holland in 1984 and Gerrie and Marcel spent most of the following day - the day before their wedding - taking us around Leiden and The Hague. They even found time to take as to Maduroarma in the late afternoon, and as we walked around this amazing scale model of the capital city the lights came on and the insides of the accurately modelled buildings were lit up. It was fascinating and very impressive.

Their legal wedding ceremony was held in the Town Hall, a very impressive building, but the celebrations began earlier in the morning at the

Where is the Key?

Reception hall, where all the invited guests gathered for light refreshments. The bride and groom appeared briefly before leaving in their chauffeur-driven, florally decorated car to the accompaniment of waves and cheers from the guests. After a while a coach drove up, and all the relatives and guests piled into it and we were driven off to the Town Hall. We didn't go inside, but lined the pavement and the steps, and cheered the bride and groom as they stepped out of their car and went in, and we all fell into line behind them. It was an impressive start. This ceremony was followed immediately by their wedding service. The church was just across the road, and as my husband and I reached the doors, a lady stepped forward (who we found out later was the Best Woman) and handed us an English translation of the whole service. We were the only English guests, and someone had taken a lot of trouble to translate it all so that we could understand the service. We were so touched by the kindness of everyone. The church was full with all their university friends as well as the guests and when the long service had ended everybody waved the bride and groom off for a little break while all the guests piled into the coach again and returned to the Reception hall, to await the bridal pair, greeting them with balloons and streamers. All their friends were invited to the first Reception, when the cake was cut and everyone had cake and wine, presented the bridal pair with gifts which were unwrapped there and then and everybody was kissed twice on both cheeks. The Best Woman (there didn't appear to be a Best Man) was standing to one side making a rapid and careful list of each gift and also the giver, tidying up wrapping paper and piling up presents. She had a tremendous responsibility throughout the day, with so many different aspects of the wedding to organise. There were many different customs from our English weddings.

Eventually many of their university friends said their goodbyes, and the main Reception began with the relatives and other invited guests. It was all very informal and friendly, and when everyone was fully satisfied and toasts and speeches were over, an open space was made in the middle of the hall, Gerrie and Marcel took front seats and the entertainment began. There was some dancing, with Gerrie looking radiant in her beautiful dress, before various amusing skits we performed by Gerrie's brothers and sisters and friends on aspects of their home and University life, and amusing poems had been composed and were read out by other guests. Eventually our turn came!

We had received a letter from the Best Woman a few weeks before the wedding, asking us if we would perform a little sketch, or recite a poem or perform in some way, offering it as a gift to the bride and groom. We were horrified at first; how could we make fools of ourselves; we couldn't act; whatever could we do? (I suppose we could have made up a sketch about my handbag and how we first met the bride and groom half way up a mountain? That didn't occur to me in 1984!)

Now was the time to see whether we were 'up for it'. We had hoped that the evening would pass before our names appeared on the list of performers. But no, after a while we were introduced, and all the guests sat back to see what this English couple would do. We had decided to sing two English folk songs, comparing the hills and valleys of England with the flat landscape of the Low Countries. Gerrie and Marcel had shown us the 'hill' in Leiden the previous day. It was like a pimple with a windmill on the top. We had already decided to sing 'Sweet Lass of Richmond Hill' and a second song about the ' Down in the valley below'. We sang them unaccompanied, with my husband putting in the harmony while I sang the tune. We raised a laugh in our introduction by contrasting the English hills and valleys with the flatness of the Dutch scenery, and I think we were thought to be very brave to sing among such a large company, but yet unaccompanied! I had typed out the words of the songs and rolled the paper up in a scroll tied with ribbon, and handed it to the bride and groom after we had sung, and discovered that this was the custom that had been done by all the other performers, so I was much relieved. The reception ended at midnight; everyone had a very happy time, and everyone was still sober. At that time English wedding receptions were still about as formal as mine had been twenty-five years previously and this was a great contrast, much more fun, much more relaxed, and, best of all, the bride wore her wedding dress from morning till midnight – and looked entrancing. Likewise, Marcel wore his very smart wedding attire throughout the day but probably discarded his jacket and tie as the evening wore on!

Gerrie and Marcel spent Christmas with us a couple of years later, and on a further short visit they stayed overnight whilst on their way to a holiday in Canada taking with them their four-month-old baby son. Baths were not common in Holland; everyone had a shower. Marcel had been much taken with our bath when he first visited us. He sometimes knocked on the bathroom door when Gerrie was having a bath, asking her 'are you all right in there?' with a mischievous twinkle in his eye. He wanted to give his baby son a bath while staying with us, and had brought his bathing trunks so that he could sit in the bath and bathe the baby! There was always fun and laughter when Marcel was around.

Now I must go back in time and return to school in 1979 when I had a third year class when the autumn term began after our holiday in Switzerland. I really enjoyed the more advanced work they were able to do. I made a book of some of the poems they wrote that year, and I wish I had kept it. Many of the children treasured their topic books and really tried to do their best work in them, which contained class teaching, but also included lessons in handwriting, poetry, creative writing and artwork, a bit of science sometimes, all based on the title of the topic. The children had the option of doing additional work from their private study, based on the current theme. Some of these topic books were really exemplary and a pleasure to read through, and were taken home with pride at the end of term. I wonder if any ex-pupils still have them.

The children didn't have set homework every night, but I wrote twenty spellings on the blackboard early every Monday morning, which they wrote down while I took the register and collected their dinner money. They were expected to learn how to spell these words at home by Friday, when we had a test. A star was given to those who had spelt all the words correctly, but I also awarded one to those children who had a higher score than the previous week. This encouraged the weaker children to achieve some success, and to try harder to achieve a higher score the following week. If they had only eight words right one week, but their previous week's score had been seven – they had a star, but they would need to get more than eight correct spellings in future in order to earn another star.

The class also knew that they should learn their tables at home, as I was likely to spring a tables test on them – with a little warning beforehand! (My times-tables still come in useful and are an invaluable piece of number-work to have firmly stuck in one's memory.) Apart from learning spellings and tables and doing some reading practice, any additional homework was voluntary work on their topic. All this sounds very old-fashioned, and education is very different now, far more structured; set homework is given from a very early age and parents are far more involved.

The children worked hard in those days too, and most of them were enthusiastic and keen to do well. With the exception of their topic work, which was done in loose folders, the class worked in traditional exercise books. I often think of the amount of paper that must be used on work sheets for many of present day lessons. I wonder whether a sheet of paper, used once, might appear less important to some children than if they were working through an exercise book in which they could look back, be reminded of what had gone before, and feel proud of it, or learn from it, or try to do better. To me a work sheet seems less important than an exercise book and must use (waste?) an enormous amount of paper.

There were usually one or two disruptive children in every class; some would now possibly be labelled as suffering from attention deficit disorder. It's a good expression, and certainly describes a certain kind of behaviour, but I never had a child in my class who was rude to me, or kicked or slapped, or who swore. I can remember one boy with a rather insolent stare, another who couldn't sit still without kicking or sticking his foot out to trip somebody up. There were many who were talkative, when a classroom in those days was supposed to be quiet. The funniest 'naughty boy' I can remember was in my second year of teaching. I had told him to redo a piece of work as it had been very carelessly done. He snatched his book from me, slouched back to his seat, slammed the book down on his desk, and shouted out, 'Knickers!' I could see that the class was on the verge of bursting into laughter and then going out of control, so I thought quickly and replied coolly, 'Yes, Dennis, we all wear them in some form or another'. The laughter changed, and they were laughing with me instead of with Dennis and at me, and it soon quietened down. We didn't have a riot and a pleasant atmosphere resulted. There were problem children, some children from broken families, but these were certainly in a minority. I can remember one boy coming up to my desk on a Friday afternoon to tell me that, 'My mum's going to marry my dad tomorrow'. Another boy had overheard this statement; he looked at me in utter incomprehension. I had to try to tactfully explain to him how this might sometimes occur. The school was in a mixed catchment area, which included a large estate of what used to be called council houses, where most, but certainly not all, children came from two parent families in stable home environments. How society seems to have changed since that period, when the norm and the expectations were of a settled family life with two – married - parents!

The autumn term at school always passed too quickly; so much had to be crammed into it, and soon Christmas festivities were upon us, but I am sure they were much less frantic than nowadays. Each class had an afternoon party a few days before we broke up for the holiday. The children brought in food, cakes, sandwiches, sausage rolls, the usual things, and I hid all the packages away in a cupboard until the dinner hour, when I prepared our classroom for the party. First of all I moved the desks to the walls, and then laid out all the goodies the children had brought in on dinner plates, ready for the afternoon. In my class, whether it was second or third-year juniors (Year 4 or 5) we played traditional games - pass the parcel, blind man's bluff etc. - before the feast began. I think everyone enjoyed the good fun and the party food; but there was always quite a lot left over at the end of the afternoon. I gathered it up and put it into cake tins and hid them a cupboard on top of the maths books.

The following morning I told the children that if they worked really hard we would stop ten minutes before playtime, and have a quick 'morning party', with a game and the rest of the food instead of going out into the playground. You could have heard a pin drop as they tried to impress me with their industry during their maths lesson, while I hurriedly sorted the food out in a corner so that each group of tables had an equal share.

End of Christmas term presentations by the school were very low key when I first started teaching in 1971. During my first term I was told that each class must choose a carol from a different country, and rehearse it to sing at an end of term carol concert. Each teacher rehearsed his or her class, and the children memorised the words of their carol before performing in front of the parents at an evening concert. And that was it! No big presentation requiring many rehearsals, no dressing up.

Three years later a new school was built for us outside the city centre. Our headmaster had retired and we had a new head teacher. When we moved into our new building we found the classrooms had carpeted flooring, which made a much quieter environment. Instead of the old desks in which the children put their exercise books, textbooks, and personal belongings – but also rubbish – in, there were groups of tables. The classroom looked much more informal. There was a separate area with a large sink, big enough for a group of children to use for practical work, which was shared with one other class. I no longer had to go to the boys' toilets for water for flowers, and washing thirty-odd paint brushes! It was a much nicer classroom, but the school must have been designed for much smaller classes, the children were very tightly packed in, and the practical area would have been of more value as part of the classroom. The school cleaner once commented to me that 'if only the school had been built even a metre wider all round' and I couldn't have agreed more.

I was rarely off sick during the years I was teaching, although there were a number of occasions when my husband pleaded with me not to go to work after I had had a very bad night. I would not allow this pain to ruin my life and prevent me from being a useful member of society. I don't know how I did it but for so many years I hope I have put up a cheerful carefree *persona* (if that's the right term to use) that prevented other people from being aware of the constant severe pain I suffered. Although I didn't 'do drama' I think I must have been a pretty good actress!

Some time later I was referred to yet another specialist, who considered that I was suffering from ME, which was *then* called Royal Free Disease. I was advised to have a month's complete rest – lying down for 23 hours of the day, and having one hour of activity - and after this month was over I was told to rest a lot and take life easily for another six months. I always connect the annual Trooping of the Colour on TV to this period in my life, as it was the first day of my enforced rest. I lay on the settee watching the ceremony on a beautiful sunny Saturday, longing to be out in the sunshine somewhere, anywhere but having to lie down. It was a very difficult period, as I am by nature an active person, and enforced rest was not in my 'rule book'.

I felt I could not leave my headmaster or my class with the problem of my lengthy absence, and was reluctant to allow neuralgia to force me to give up my job, but it was becoming almost impossible to read a story to the class at the end of the day, as the pain in my jaws, my cheeks and throat was so intense. It was unfair to leave my class with a supply teacher for an unknown period, or my head teacher, and the rest of the staff, in limbo while I 'rested' at home. One teacher's absence puts an additional burden on the rest of the staff. I also realised that I would be ill advised to carry on teaching full time.

Job-sharing had not appeared on the scene then, but two fully committed half-time teachers would have provided the class with more than 100% teaching time and would have been very good value for the school and the local education authority. I could have managed that, but if a head teacher lost a full-time teaching post at that time he would never get that full-time position guaranteed from the LEA again. I was on sick leave at home for the last part of that summer term, before being advised to take early retirement. Having to give in to this painful ogre was a great sorrow to me. I felt I had lost the battle. It was a very difficult time. I didn't feel able to say good-bye to my class and felt that I had let them down. How could I explain to them why their apparently fit and healthy teacher could no longer be there for them? I had left so abruptly and mysteriously, that I felt almost under a cloud of suspicion. I subsequently felt that if I had not seen this particular consultant I would still have been working. It really upset me. All the preparation for my career, the satisfaction of teaching, the enjoyment of my responsibility for netball, all suddenly taken away because the pain had beaten me into the ground; I felt really depressed and rejected and dejected. The days seemed so empty, as I thought of my class, abandoned in the middle of an exciting topic on the History of Ships. I had lost the battle of not allowing this wretched pain to interfere with and overrule my life. I rested, but it made little differerence.

Chapter Twenty-Five

WHAT A LIFE!

It seemed as if I was in limbo, and inwardly I felt a complete failure for quite a long time. I wasn't ill; it was a 'condition' not an 'illness'. I was in good physical health. It was so many years ago, but I suppose I still feel that I failed. It was a severe wrench to be forced by pain to take early retirement when I was enjoying my work so much. It was rather like a sudden bereavement. The next year or two passed by slowly, until a neighbour recommended a naturopathic doctor to me. I first saw him a week before Christmas. He put me on to a very strict diet: I was told I must have no sugar or anything containing sugar, no coffee and no flesh. He also prescribed a herbal, lime-flower tea from the naturopathic pharmacy in his surgery and urged me to eat brown rice. The tea was quite pleasant to drink and was supposed to be very calming to the nerves, but I detested the brown rice.

The diet was supposed to reduce the acidity level of the body and so make less demand on the nervous system. Omitting coffee was no problem, but I had already ordered a turkey, had made my Christmas cake, mince pies and Christmas pudding. I cooked the dinner for the family and my father on Christmas Day, and ate just the vegetables with cooked brown rice. I served the pudding and mince pies but didn't eat any and ate some fruit. We had visitors the following evening and I was unable to share in the turkey pilaff or eat the desserts I had made. Altogether it was a very difficult Christmas, but I was determined to stick to this diet if there was any possibility that it would bring about even a little relief.

This doctor gave me a memorable analogy about pain, likening the nervous system to a washing line and that the medications I had been prescribed over the years had made my 'washing line' sag, and thus weaken, by keeping it unnaturally down, deadened with all the drugs I had been prescribed for many years. I could understand his analogy. My monthly consultations with this doctor were very brief, and as winter changed to spring and then to summer Maurice and I turned the monthly drive to his consulting room in Berkshire into a subsequent afternoon's outing, by spending an hour or so in one or another of the beauty spots along the Thames after I had seen the doctor. I remember the beauty of the changing colours of the tree-clad Chiltern Hills as we drove home alongside them the following autumn. His waiting room was always crowded with patients, but we all seemed to go in and out of his consulting room pretty rapidly.

I soon got into a vegetarian way of life; I ate cooked brown rice, made nut roasts and lentil flans, and began to enjoy a different way of eating, but my face pain seemed to become worse. (A year or two later I found that I was intolerant to any form of beans, and most wholegrain cereals including brown rice and wholemeal flour, so it is no surprise that my symptoms became even more severe.)

The next phase added to my treatment was to have what was called a 'dry day' every three weeks, in which I ate three servings of cooked brown rice and nothing else throughout the day. I was also forbidden to have anything to drink. In the evening I had to wrap myself in a sheet, then a blanket and go to bed. The treatment was supposed to draw out uric acid and other toxins from the body which would be absorbed by the sheet, and that this procedure would eventually bring relief from pain. The day was absolutely awful, and I shudder even as I type when recalling those platefuls of cooked brown rice. Ugh! I think it worked better with rheumatic pain, as the neighbour who recommended me to this doctor had been much helped by his treatment - although please don't try it! These 'dry days' were awful, and after a while I noticed that an itchy rash appeared around my wrist after each 'dry day'. I told the doctor that I thought I was allergic to the brown rice and he changed my 'meal' from brown rice to three slices of unbuttered wholemeal bread three times during the 'dry day' every three weeks. I struggled to swallow this dry bread but found it impossible to do so without any liquid to accompany it. I chewed and chewed it and almost gagged as I tried to swallow it. I felt really ill, shaky, and dizzy, with increased pain, as the day wore on.

Nevertheless I kept up this treatment for several months, until I began to get a widespread itchy rash all over one buttock the day after the horrible 'dry day'. I told the doctor that I thought I should stop, and that there was something in the brown rice and wholemeal bread that made me worse. He replied that he was sure that *'somewhere there was the key that would unlock the door'* to my pain. I gave up my vegetarian way of life, which I don't think had suited me, with its emphasis on whole grains, pulses and nuts, but I remembered the phrase; I am still looking for that KEY. Naturopathic treatment had certainly not been a success for me.

My father had lived independently since my mother's return to hospital in 1963, and had continued to visit her every three weeks for the following nineteen years. It must have been very difficult for my parents to find much to talk about on these visits. My mother had such a restricted life that she had little to tell my father, and he had little news for her. He led a very quiet life, and his main interests were his grandchildren, Maurice and me, his TV and his enjoyment of pottering around in his garden. He sometimes drove to Dunstable downs and sat in his car watching the gliders, but his social life was limited to his weekly visits to us every Sunday. He loved reading my holiday diaries and on our return from every holiday I made it a priority to write my record and paste in all my pictures, maps and postcards, as he spent an entire Sunday afternoon looking at all the pictures and carefully reading every word of my record. I felt that in a sense he had a vicarious holiday after our return home each summer through reading these detailed memoirs. I continued this habit after my father died, and now have several books full of description and pictures of many, many lovely holidays, which bring to mind many half-forgotten memories and mental pictures whenever I find time to read from them.

My father drove my mother to tea at our home on one Sunday afternoon, collecting her from her villa in Shenley, but it was thought unwise for her to visit my father's new home in St. Albans. I think she assumed he still lived at Kenton. My mother and I were walking around the garden on one of these Sunday afternoons, when I spotted my next-door neighbour. I called out 'Hello' to her and then introduced her to my mother. Winnie starting talking to my mother and it was lovely to see them chatting away together so naturally for a few minutes over the garden fence. They might have known each other for years. I hope my mother enjoyed this bit of normal domesticity in her long-term institutional life, and I much appreciated my neighbour's kindness and the total absence of any stigma in her attitude. I believe that our old neighbours in Kenton were equally friendly towards my mother when she was home. The stigma that is frequently attached to mental ill health disappears when you get to know the person and normality appears alongside compassion and understanding.

My mother was occasionally taken for an escorted week's holiday in the summer to Weston-super-Mare, but she didn't appear to enjoy this change of scenery very much, telling us afterwards that the ladies were left sitting on the seafront – sometimes when it was raining – for entire mornings, so my mother said. Of course, they had nothing to do, no family with them to take them for a little walk along the promenade, have a deckchair on the beach or look around the shops. These ladies were not used to making even small decisions. The only occasions on which I heard a little grumble from my mother was after these annual holidays.

I feel I must mention that there were *no* long corridors anywhere in Shenley Hospital. People always seem to associate psychiatric hospitals with long corridors! Shenley Hospital was opened in 1934 and comprised a number of separate, two storey buildings, each of which comprised four villas or wards. There were, I understand, about 2,000 patients accommodated in the hospital. They were well built of good brick, had no long corridors, but had large sash windows, a large sitting room, a dormitory and a dining area. I don't know how the patients were treated in those early days in the 1930s and 40s, and just hope that my mother did not suffer the assaults and hard conditions that apparently were common practice before anti-psychotic drugs were developed. I do believe that she had courses of ECT, about which I knew nothing until television programmes revealed often disturbing programmes and pictures.

The villas were set in very spacious grounds with beautiful old trees in which the patients, and their visitors, could walk, and for the period Shenley Hospital had a modern approach to the care of the mentally ill. When visiting my mother after my father died we occasionally took her out for a little drive, but she seemed happiest, more secure I think, back in hospital. We invited her home for the day at Christmas but she said that she preferred to stay in her villa. I think she became quite nervous at the thought of leaving her known environment for any length of time. There was a large patio outside my mother's villa, which overlooked the landscaped grounds, and when we visited in the summer we occasionally found her sitting outside with a number of other residents. She seemed to be getting a little frail, but she still looked the most able lady amongst those sitting around her. There was not a sign of conversation among them; they just sat there; but what would they have to talk about? They were probably all sedated or just living in their own little world with nothing to talk about and nothing to do. They were all elderly and they saw nothing of the outside world to promote conversation. There was a good side and also a bad side to becoming institutionalised; the patients were comfortable and cared for, but had nothing to do, nothing to contribute, and no stimulation. I think there is little difference between my mother's villa, except its size, and the care homes many end their years in nowadays.

My father had always been slim but he grew painfully thin during the early months of 1982. He had a small appetite but had always enjoyed his meals, especially Sunday dinner with us, and his eyes always sparkled at the sight of strawberries and cream – especially the cream! Over the years he had eagerly accepted the little plastic boxes of goodies that I gave him before he returned home after a day with us, which would help him with his catering during the following week. It became obvious that he was failing in health during the summer of 1982. He had lost his appetite, and the little treats no longer interested him.

He accompanied us on a visit to our son shortly before he became ill, and was very listless throughout the day. We overtook a group of cyclists as we were driving home, and my father, who was sitting in the back of the car, suddenly said, 'In my mind I feel I could join them, but my body won't let me!' He had enjoyed his years of cycling when he was younger and his spirit hadn't aged, but his body was failing fast. (I now have a similar feeling: in my mind I still feel young, but I know that I can't do all the things that I used to do.)

Only a few weeks after his comment in the car my dear father became critically ill and was admitted to hospital. I drove him to the hospital in my little Fiat 500 car, and as he walked down the steps of his bungalow, I think he had a sense that he would not return to his home. I stayed with him for a while as he was settled into the ward, and returned to see him in the evening. It was only the second time he had been in hospital in his life. (The first occasion was before I was married, when he had an accident when on his Minimotor - a motorised bicycle - and a policeman 'phoned me at the office to inform me that my father was in Wembley Hospital having fractured his skull. I had to wait until the evening visiting hours before I was able to see him, and found him half-sitting up in bed in a hospital ward with his head covered in bandages and suffering severe concussion. It was a great shock. I had never even been in a hospital until that evening. He was in hospital for a month.)

As I got out of the lift in St. Albans Hospital in 1982 I was once again very shocked when I saw my father, this time on a theatre trolley, being wheeled at that very moment towards the lift I had just exited. The porters told me he was on his way to the theatre to have major surgery. I had not been informed of this beforehand, and if I had arrived only a few moments later, I would have been unable to speak to him before he was operated on. I asked if my father understood what was about to happen to him. I was informed that he been told. But he was almost totally deaf. Had he understood, or even heard, what a nurse had told him? Did the staff appreciate how very deaf he was? He was presumably able to sign the consent form, but I very much doubt that he had heard or understood what was going to happen to him. Deaf people don't like to have to admit that they can't hear.

The porters waited a few moments while I spoke loudly into my father's ear, trying to explain to him what was about to happen, but this was rather difficult in a public space. I was able to hold his hand very briefly and give him a kiss before the porters hurried into the lift with my father on the trolley. I am glad that I arrived before he had the anaesthetic and that I was able to speak briefly to him. He survived the operation, and was very poorly, although lucid, when I next saw him. A day or two later he sounded very aggrieved as he told us in a very weak voice, 'They have made me walk round the ward; it's too much for me....too much'. I'm sure it was too much, but I can appreciate that, medically, the staff wanted to get him moving a bit. The nurses called him 'Percy' but I think that he would have preferred to be spoken to as 'Mr. Brook'. He had not been called Percy for many years, and belonged to a more formal age. His staff had called him Mr. Brook and his neighbours had addressed him similarly. I don't think my mother gave him any name when he visited her. 'Mr. Brook' was more familiar to him than 'Percy'. He couldn't understand why a young lady whom he didn't know should address him by his first name, saying, 'You're doing all right, Percy aren't you?' when he knew he wasn't, and he didn't like to be addressed in such a familiar manner by someone he didn't know!

Now everyone seems to be called by their first name, whether the person is known or not, and it's often the people you know the least who are the ones to use a first name. (In another age we used to call it our Christian name.)

My father lived for a week after his cancer operation, but suffered from acute heart failure at the end. He was nearly eighty-eight years old. I think it was a mercy that he did not recover from this operation; I think the problems of coping with a stoma at his age and with his frailty would indeed have been too much for him. There comes a time when enough has been attempted to retain life. Independent living, which meant a lot to him, would not have been possible. I think he had had enough of life's struggles, and was glad to be at rest. He had had a hard, lonely life, with a lot of trouble to bear. Queen Victoria was still alive when he was born; he remembered being taken to see the procession at her Golden Jubilee when a very small boy. He had lived through five monarchs, two world wars, had experienced the loss of his father when he was seven, and then the death his firstborn daughter, and had borne the absence of his wife in his daily life for nearly fifty years. He had experienced great pleasure and pride in his grandsons, and had always taken an interest in their lives. He never complained, and always appeared cheerful. I never knew what his innermost thoughts were, and dearly wish I had understood his loneliness and loss when I was younger. I wish too that I had asked him about his childhood, his forbears and his war service in the Orkneys. My mother appeared quite indifferent to the news of his death and never spoke of him afterwards.

Chapter Twenty-six

TRIUMPH AND DISASTER!

Not long after my father's death I was loaned a book about food allergy, called 'Not All in the Mind', by a Dr. Richard Mackarness. I believe it was quite a controversial book at the time, but it made me wonder whether my symptoms could be related to food intolerances. I remembered the effects of the brown rice! I had tried so many conventional and also alternative treatments, but had not considered my diet. As a child I was expected to eat everything that was put on my plate. I enjoyed my food, enjoyed cooking, and I think I was resistant to the possibility that food could play any part in my problem. What might be causing this pain, I thought? What vitamin deficiencies might I have? I knew that Vitamin B was supposed to be essential for healthy nerve function and wondered whether I could be deficient in this vitamin. So I bought some wheat germ. I sprinkled a little over my breakfast cereal and shortly afterwards I was beside myself, screaming with pain in my face, and literally banging my head against the kitchen wall to try and 'knock out' the pain inside it. For a little while I went berserk, ranging from one side of the kitchen to the other, not know what to do to ease the awful pain, and then flinging cold water over my face. My husband was at work and I didn't know what to do, where to go, or who to turn to.

After a while the immediate extremely acute pain had subsided, my screams and tears had eased, and I wondered whether it could be possible that the wheat germ had aggravated my symptoms. I threw it away and stopped eating my homemade wholemeal bread, and almost immediately found I had a little less pain. I used to make my own muesli, and realised I developed severe, sore pain in my cheeks and jaws a short while after eating my breakfast, so I stopped eating oats. I began to think that at last I had found a key; it hadn't totally unlocked the door, but I felt it had opened a little crack. The pain began to lessen in severity, with brief episodes of extreme pain when I had eaten a certain food. I decided to organise my diet so that I could lead an ordinary life without continual torture. I didn't mind what I was going to have to eliminate from my diet. I would do anything, so long as I could be free from pain. Within a few weeks I had found a number of foods – wholemeal bread and anything made with wholemeal flour, rice, oats, stone fruits, beans, peas and lentils, chocolate, some green vegetables, most kinds of fish and strawberries - appeared to cause, or increase symptoms. I eliminated these foods from my diet and soon I was feeling free from pain after so many years - it had worked! I could hardly believe it. It was marvellous to get up in the morning and then enjoy a pain-free day.

A new life soon began. I hadn't played tennis for years, but I met a lady who would like a game of tennis, and so we played singles once or twice a week throughout the summer season. We weren't very good, but we had both improved by the end of the summer, and it felt wonderful to be able to use my racquet without painful consequences; I was over the moon! The following spring a flyer was put through our letterbox, asking for new members at a local tennis club. I joined as a midweek member, and relished the opportunity to enjoy myself without the continual neuralgic pain that had dogged me for so many years. I played tennis in this lovely small tennis club with a number of different partners for the next eighteen years until I was in my early seventies.

I joined a ladies choir and sang with them for many years. We rehearsed weekly and gave concerts at the end of each term to various day centres in the district. A little later I joined a folk dance group and a keep fit class. I was utterly free from pain for about three years and was really enjoying myself, but also feeling the deprivation of so many foods I had eaten for most of my life. It was so difficult when I was invited out, and I felt I was a nuisance and a bit of an oddity.

After a lengthy period of strict elimination I yearned for the foods I used to eat, and thought it would be safe to try to introduce them back into my diet very gradually. What a delight it was to be able to eat some of the problem foods once more! However I found that I could not tolerate wholemeal bread, porridge or rice and found I still reacted badly to a number of fruits and vegetables, when my cheeks would suddenly begin to ache and my neck would throb. After some time I found a very itchy patch appeared in the palm of my right hand a day or two after I had eaten certain foods, and open eczema patches gradually developed along all the lines of this hand. This appeared to confirm that the additional pain I had soon after eating one of my 'dodgy' foods was due to an enhanced sensitivity to it. I had to be careful. It seemed that the effects of the food eventually showed in my skin. The itchy patch became a good guide, which helped me discern the foods I still needed to avoid. (Strangely enough, I no longer get an itchy patch of eczema developing in my palm, but I still get adverse reactions to a number of foods.)

I was urged to share my experiences and wrote a book. I called it **'I Found the Key'**. I thought it could possibly help others in similar circumstances. It took a long time to write and before I could attempt to get it published, I began to suffer entirely different, but still painful, symptoms elsewhere in my body. I had typed this book in the mid-1980s on an old portable typewriter, sitting on a metal-pillar typist's chair, which had a hard, unupholstered seat.

Towards the end of a period of typing I began to notice a cutting pain in my left crotch. (I don't know a better term for where the top of the inner thigh joins up with the bottom of the pelvis – it was right through this area.) At first I only noticed it when I sat down during an evening, when reading or watching TV, but then this cutting pain forced me to stand up for a few minutes and have a wriggle. The pain then disappeared for a while. I couldn't understand it; I had had more than enough of pain, and I refused to admit to myself, let alone to anyone else, that there was anything wrong.

But I began to feel disheartened as I felt that **the key,** which was central to my story, was slipping from my hand. I could not attempt to try to get a book published that ended with the triumph of my freedom from pain, when pain had begun to occur elsewhere. The typed manuscript - I had no computer in those days - was pushed into a drawer, not forgotten, but neglected for years.

I hid my dismay, remained positive, and decided to write another book, one that might be of help to people who had found that food intolerance was involved in their undiagnosed or untreatable pain, or other not-yet-understood health problems. A lady who suffered from a similar kind of facial neuralgia to mine had heard about my experiences and got in touch with me. She still suffered with pain in her teeth and jaws, and she also had frequent acute panic attacks. She had found that her symptoms could be controlled, or at least helped, through a very strict diet. Her diet was very limited, monotonous and difficult to manage. A recipe book might help people like her.

I enjoyed cooking, and was not going to allow my restricted diet to add to the other restrictions that my body, or my nervous system, still forced upon me – loud noise, tight clothes etc – and I began to devise a collection of recipes for soups, main dishes, drinks, cakes and biscuits etc. that would help people to cope with food intolerances. These recipes grew into a book, and I entitled it 'Eat Well With Your Allergies'. I typed it out on my old portable typewriter, still sitting on a hard metallic typist's chair. Typing recipes was not nearly as straightforward as typing a script. It was really difficult to do. I noticed that after I had been sitting for a while at my typewriter my groin pain was worse, but I made no connection. I just didn't want to acknowledge, even to myself, that I had pain again.

When it was complete, I showed the typescript to the chief dietician at the Royal London Homoeopathic Hospital, who had agreed to vet it. She looked through the recipes, gave her approval, saying in a letter to me that she thought 'that the recipes are excellent and will be very useful to people on
restricted diets'.

I submitted my book to one or two publishers, and soon a well-known publishing house accepted it for publication and, for a first-time author writing a book with restricted public appeal, I received quite a satisfying advance payment. I had used the traditional system for the weights of all the ingredients to my recipes, as grammes and kilogrammes were not in common usage in the U.K. in the 1980s, but I was asked by the cookery editor to go through the entire book adding metric weights and American 'cups' to every recipe, as the book was also going to be published in America and Australia. This was a bit daunting but as I worked my way through the recipes, working out all the relevant alterations, I began to be very excited at the thought that my book would appear in bookshops 'over there' and also 'down under'. Although I had taught metric weights to my class at school, all my recipes were in pounds and ounces. It was quite a task to convert every ingredient in the book into grammes and also into American cups and half cups. Soon after I had done this I was told over the 'phone that the cover had already been designed and the cookery editor hoped that it would not be long before my book was on the shelves of bookshops. Wow!

We were at the beginning of an earlier recession in the late 1980s, but it was a tremendous shock when I was informed over the telephone just a few weeks later that in an editorial conference that morning it had been decided that certain areas of publication must be cut, and books in the cookery section were among the first to be dropped. I soon received a letter of confirmation from the cookery editor in May 1989 accompanying the return of my typed manuscript, saying: 'Dear Sheila, Just to say that I do hope you are feeling better – anything that makes sitting for some time painful and uncomfortable is not only inconvenient, but very depressing as well – so I really do sympathise…this has meant a great many manuscripts falling by the wayside, I fear. Yours sincerely…' It was kind to have this sudden news softened by her sympathy, but it was an upsetting shock, especially as I had been told that it was so close to the printing press and publication.

I now appreciate that cuts – like job losses, and large companies failing - happen very suddenly in an economic crisis, and that a specialist cookery book was likely to be at the top of the list at such a time. The advance payment I had received when they had accepted my work made me feel that my book was worthy of publication and gave me some tangible reward for all my work, but I had really wanted it published in order to help people. I wasn't bothered about royalties, which I knew were only worth considering if you had a best seller. But perhaps my book would have been a best seller? It was just another failure.

Throughout this period of preparation, typing, excitement and then dismay, the cutting pain in my crotch was becoming ever more severe, but I didn't want to know about any renewal of pain, and I suppose I was in some sense in denial. It was some time before I admitted to myself that I must see my doctor. I simply detested the thought of having to go the doctor again. Medical science seems unable to do much for neuralgic pain. I was prescribed some pain relief tablets but they did not relieve. Rather, the pain was growing in intensity, and when I returned to my doctor, and he came into the waiting room and saw me sprawled on the floor, resting my weight on one buttock, he took me seriously and gave me a very strong painkiller, told me I had 'a little trapped nerve' and suggested that I 'kept walking'. I was used to quite a bit of activity one way and another, and did as he suggested. For a while I could not sit down at all and was forced to kneel at the table to eat my meals, until, I suppose, I developed some tolerance of the intolerable! The painkillers adversely affected my bowel function and the pain spread right through the groin to my 'nether region,' and eventually to the organs within my pelvis.

We had a five-door Honda Civic Shuttle car but for quite a long time I could not sit in the car seat. If I needed to travel anywhere my husband had to open the hatchback door, push forward the backs of the rear seats to enlarge the boot so that I could lie out in the back of the car. We had not bought a hatchback car for this purpose! It was very uncomfortable and insecure spread out in the boot with no upholstery and no support. I felt like a suitcase, or a sack of rubbish for the tip!

I returned to my GP who was by now very concerned for me, and told me that I was suffering from perineal pain. 'Oh Sheila, you don't deserve this' he said to me kindly. I agree! But what was perineal pain? I had never heard of it, and he didn't explain; it is just a medical term to describe neuralgic pain in what I politely called my 'nether region'.

People sometimes ask me if I have seen a doctor! I have seen so many. I was referred to a gastroenterologist many years ago who examined me and said, 'I expect you know that there is nothing I can do for you?' At my shocked expression he referred me to my local hospital's pain clinic for a nerve block. The pain consultant said he 'wouldn't dream of doing a nerve block as there were too many nerves involved; I wouldn't be able to find the right one'. He advised me to have treatment for my food allergies, but I could only get this at a small, specialist private hospital. Another consultant dismissed the idea that food allergies had anything at all to do with my pain and totally trashed the allergy treatment I was having, making me lose faith in it and give it up – it *was* very expensive and appeared to be necessary for ever, but the vaccines I had injected myself with every day had helped me to eat a greater variety of food than I can now tolerate.

Doctors seem to ignore the aggravation in symptoms caused by food intolerances, and are not concerned with the difficulty of coping with dietary limitations. When showing one doctor a list of the foods I could not tolerate, his only response after glancing through the list was to comment on how he could not possibly live without mango! He couldn't empathise with the limitations of my diet, or consider that the many foods I couldn't tolerate might cause deficiencies or imbalance in vitamins, mineral, essential oils, or other nutrients, or that my diet may contain insufficient fibre and certainly lacked green vegetables! He gave me no advice. I have to try and work that out for myself. Interesting food adds greatly to life's pleasure, but my enjoyment of cooking has been tested beyond the limit when trying to create a varied diet within the boundaries of what my gut will tolerate. I cannot cope with it, and am pretty sure I now eat some foods that subsequently aggravate my symptoms in various ways.

I had a hysterectomy at very short notice in 1996 because an x-ray had shown a lump pressing on the rectum. It was thought that the painful pressure I could feel inside me might be cancer. It wasn't, and was only an old fibroid, which I had been told some years previously would shrink as I aged and would never require surgery! I have seen osteopaths, homoeopaths, but only one naturopath. I have had acupuncture and relaxation therapy (when I couldn't relax because I was so much more aware of pain when lying down with nothing to do but imagine beautiful scenes). I have had cognitive behavioural therapy with a very kind and thoughtful psychotherapist who felt that I was already doing everything possible to help myself with activity and diversion.

I have to say that all the alternative therapists showed great concern and were more understanding than some of the orthodox doctors I have seen. I don't think any of them have 'ripped me off' and were all trying their best to help me.

With time I have learned to live with pain, and am able to sit for longer and try to ignore my pain or disguise my feelings in front of other people. Long distance holidays became impossible as I couldn't sit for lengthy periods in the car or in an aircraft, but my husband and I continued to have holidays nearer to home, right up until the summer before he died. We sometimes stayed in a hotel but more frequently self-catered as it meant less worry about the food, and it was quite fun to make a home for a week in various cottages, apartments and farm conversions. We have stayed in a converted milking parlour, a converted pigsty, a coach-house an old almshouse and an ex-fruit-packing building – all altered very tastefully and turned into well-equipped holiday accommodation for two people – first-class 'recycling' of property! Most cottages or larger properties cater for more than two people, so we usually found ourselves in unusual holiday homes. They are now so well equipped, attractively furnished, and with comfortable beds. However, it is rather nice to be catered for, and we stayed in hotels when we were able to go abroad.

Chapter Twenty-seven

A SPANISH HOLIDAY

During the past fifty-plus years I have only had about four or five holidays that have been free from pain. My father had died before he could read the record of our holiday in Spain, when I had no pain and we had no anxiety. We felt that a great burden had been lifted from our lives.

In 1983 my husband had some holiday leave that had to be taken before the end of the financial year, and so we decided to have an early spring holiday in Rota, on the bottom tip of the southwest Spanish coast. The hotel had a large, open-air, unheated swimming pool set in spacious grounds amongst all its other sports facilities. I have always enjoyed swimming in the open-air, but had never done so in March. It was the end of the Spanish winter, and I think the other guests thought I was mad to swim in such cold water, but the sun was shining and the water looked so inviting. It was extremely cold when I managed to immerse myself and began swimming in the cold water. It was essential to get moving, and I didn't intend to quit and make a fool of myself in front of the other guests walking under the palm trees. Several other brave souls, including my husband, were soon tempted by the sight of the sun sparkling on the beautiful clear water and joined me for a brief dip. I guess we were the first bathers of the season. I hadn't had such a cold swim since I was a child, when, mainly out of bravado, my friend Joan and I used to go to our local open-air, unheated pool on the day it opened each spring. I guess the temperature of the water in England on the first of May was comparable with that of the pool in Spain in the last week of March.

Rota was a traditional Andalusian town and we had several walks around the quiet residential streets, looking at the small patio gardens that could be seen behind a variety of intricately designed, beautiful wrought iron gates. Many of these private paved gardens had fountains in the middle, which must be very cooling in the hot weather. Rota was a small fishing town with an attractive old harbour. We were told that there was a large NATO base somewhere outside of the town, but there was no evidence of it, and no servicemen were to be seen in the quiet streets. The long sandy beach was almost empty in this out-of-season period, but there would be a very different scene a few months later. From the terrace of our hotel we could look right across Cadiz Bay, where the Battle of Trafalgar took place in 1805, and Nelson's famous victory over Napoleon secured our safety from French invasion.

We had an interesting excursion to Arcos de la Frontera, one of the 'white towns' of Andalusia, with whitewashed houses that stood out clearly on a jagged hilly promontory. The high tower and the ruins of an ancient fortification looked very dramatic against a vivid blue sky. We were told that in the 7th Century B.C. the Phoenicians, 'the sea people', first settled on this rugged headland that became Arcos. Much later it was inhabited by Arabs, then later still reconquered by the Spaniards. Our guide told us that the church was built on the site of a Visigoth fortress, ruins of which left its landmark, set on the very edge of a rocky precipice. History comes alive in such surroundings. We found that Arcos, along with many other towns along the rough mountainous area that forms this ancient natural border, have the suffix 'de la frontera,' as the border changed so frequently with conflicts between the Arabs and the Spanish. As the Spanish moved forward across the land, each mountainous reconquered village became the frontier – hence 'de la frontera' was added to the name of several of the white towns.

The following day we visited another of the 'de la frontera' towns, with very narrow, stepped, deserted streets, and many whitewashed, flat-roofed white-painted houses with tiny windows. It looked much more Moorish than Arcos, and there was utter silence as we walked around the little town in hot sunshine during the afternoon siesta period.

On another day we hired a car and drove to Cadiz where we treated ourselves to a tour around the city in a horse drawn carriage. The driver pointed out all the important buildings as our horse trotted around the main streets, and told us the history of the city in quite good English, but he spoke too fast for me to remember any of the details while we were on the move, and the horses' feet blurred the sound of his voice. We just enjoyed the drive and the experience. It was an easy way to see the city, especially as Maurice had not been feeling well; perhaps the cold bathe on his first day had upset his stomach?

We drove to Ronda, a breath-taking town, with an amazing bridge that crosses a deep, deep gorge dividing the modern city from the ancient one. We wandered down the old streets, taking in the atmosphere as we visited some of the old baroque churches and saw the outside of an ancient Arab bathhouse. The ravine made a natural division between the two eras; the new city looked far less interesting.

In another city we watched a row of huge old palm trees being pruned as the spring season approached. A very long ladder was propped up against the thick trunk and the old lower leaves were being hacked off. Huge sprays of date flowers had already appeared in higher branches, which, together with other sprays already laden with tiny dates, made us appreciate the origins of the dark, mature, sweet dates we eat at home.

Between these excursions we were able to spend some time on the beach, sunbathing in temperatures that were not likely to harm us, but not swimming in the sea, which was far too cold. Instead we strolled along its' edge on the beautiful long stretch of soft, clean, golden sand that curved round the headland in the distance, to the accompaniment of the gentle sound of the waves lapping near our feet. The air temperature was around 22 degrees, very pleasant, comfortable but not too hot. I swam several times in the hotel pool, and thought the temperature of the water grew a little warmer as the days passed by, but I didn't even dip my toe into the sea.

We saw an advertisement on the board of a small tourist agency for a day trip to Tangiers. The shop was often closed when we were around, but eventually we found it open, and booked the trip. We were to cross the straits of Gibralter on a new hydrofoil. We had not dreamed that we would set foot in North Africa when we booked this early holiday in Spain! A hydrofoil made it even more exciting, especially for my husband who had had some involvement in the early development of the hydrofoil. We left the hotel at 6 a.m. It was very blustery, cold and still quite dark as we stood outside the deserted little tourist office, and discovered we were the only people from the town who were waiting for the coach to take us to the port of Tarifa. At last a small minibus arrived and we found we were among a group of Americans who were staying at another resort. We had a two-hour journey to Tarifa, a small port right on the tip of southern Spain, and the nearest point to Tangiers on the other side of the Gibralter Straits. We had a lot of fun on the coach with the Americans, who kept asking us to repeat phrases. 'Oh, your English! we *so love* your accent.' they laughed. They were so amused by our, very ordinary, southern English speech. The problem was that their American accent was so strong that although we spoke the same language Maurice and I had difficulty in understanding what they were saying to us. I can't honestly say that we reciprocated a love for their accent, but the banter all helped to pass the time on the long rickety, bumpy drive down to Tarifa. The minibus was not well sprung, the engine was very noisy and the road surface was not all that good.

A strong wind nearly blew us over as we stepped off the coach. Were we mad to be crossing the Gibraltar Straits on a day like this, we pondered? As we gazed at the beautiful new hydrofoil at the port side we noticed that there appeared to be some dispute amongst the crew. Eventually we were told that the sea was too rough to make the crossing that we had so looked forward to on the hydrofoil. The crew refused to operate in this strong, gale-force wind. In a way we were relieved; I don't think anyone fancied the voyage in that lovely vessel with such a gale blowing, and we began to think we had made this long coach journey for nothing. We were told that the tourist office should have informed us that the trip was cancelled; but the tourist office was always closed! We had all paid, and we were there, at Tarifa, waiting at the water's edge.

After some delay we were informed that we could board the ferryboat, which we understood would make an unscheduled stop to pick us up and would arrive shortly – which meant another wait. The wind was terrific, but the sun was now shining briefly, although heavy clouds blew across the sky and sudden heavy showers descended on our little party of would-be passengers. When the boat arrived we were surprised to find it was full of yet more Americans. I think we were the only English couple on this day excursion.

We didn't know where it had come from, but once aboard we were again surprised to find how large it was, and were told it would take ninety minutes to cross to Algiers. We were tipping and dipping before we were even out of the harbour and soon huge white-capped waves were all around us, whipped up by the gale, as the Mediterranean fought with the Atlantic Ocean. We couldn't stand up on deck, and everyone rapidly settled for inside, although my husband managed to stay on deck for a very brief time, busy with his camera. When he was almost blown over and the wind whipped his camera strap from off his shoulder as he was taking photographs, he realised it was too dangerous and that personal safety came first, but he had managed to get some fantastic pictures, and cling on to his camera, before he was forced down below by the strength of the wind.

Before long the clouds had blown away entirely and the sun shone brightly in a vivid blue sky. It was turning into a beautiful day and soon dolphins were spotted swimming and disporting around the ship. The gale also lessened and the sea became a little calmer. Everyone came up on deck when there were shouts that dolphins could be seen, and they put on a grand display and had an appreciative audience to watch the show. We were all on the lookout for fresh groups of dolphins, cheering when they suddenly rose up from the water and their gleaming black bodies curved gracefully as they dived back in to the swirling sea. It was a wonderful experience and a lasting memory. Soon someone spotted the coast of Morocco on the horizon, and the city of Tangiers shortly appeared. Everyone is so well travelled nowadays, but it was still a bit special to be able to set foot on the African continent way back in the 1980s.

Once on land we were immediately caught up in the hustle and bustle of Tangiers. We stood and watched the water-sellers with their camel-hide bags bulging, trying to sell scoops of water to passers by. We noticed tiny little women sitting, half hidden at the back of miniscule shops, with the lined brown faces of their husbands standing outside trying to attract customers to buy something from their meagre display of goods. It was all so colourful but we could also see so much poverty. We were divided into groups before being escorted by local guides through the fascinating Old Medina. We were instructed not to stop, but to keep walking behind our guide, and not to attempt to buy anything as we sauntered in the heat through the narrow streets.

Lunch was included in our tour, and before long we were seated at low tables, whilst a group of very tall men sat on a very small stage, playing Moroccan music on traditional Moroccan instruments to entertain us as we ate our Moroccan lunch in a traditional Moroccan restaurant. I found the huge pile of couscous on my plate rather overwhelming but it was great fun talking to our American fellow travellers over our meal, and their friendliness added quite a lot to my enjoyment of the day.

In the afternoon our charming Moroccan guide escorted us on an interesting coach excursion through the old colonial part of the city. We had a short stop at the coast on the outskirts of Tangiers, where we looked down from the cliff tops at the two different colours in the sea, where the incoming Atlantic Ocean met up with the out-flowing Mediterranean Sea. There was a distinct difference in the colour, with one swirling dark blue sea meeting up with another, lighter, almost turquoise blue.

Our final visit was to a carpet shop, where we all sat around the walls of a large, lofty, carpet-lined room. Tiny cups of apple juice were handed round while samples of carpets with varied patterns were displayed to us, each being flung to the floor with an accomplished flourish. Each pattern apparently had difference significance, and was from a different area. The sales patter was intense and one or two Americans were tempted to make a purchase, adding an exotic rug to their souvenirs. All this display and sales talk went on for quite a while; it was very hot. We had been up for hours and many pairs of eyelids began to droop. I'm sure that a cup of tea was at the forefront of most people's minds. But we were not released yet; there was more to come as, on being ushered at last out of the carpet saleroom, we found we were shown into another large warehouse-type tourist shop. There we had to remain until our guide turned up – I think he had gone home for his afternoon siesta! We were stranded there for so long that we began to fear we had been deserted, and I'm sure we were left there until every last person who could be tempted to buy a souvenir had opened their purse. (Nobody carried bottles of water around with them in those days, although I am sure we were all dying for something to drink, but it was uncommon at that time to see anyone walking around with a plastic bottle of water, taking an occasional slurp from it.)

Eventually, the doors of this huge emporium were flung wide open, and as the afternoon sunlight burst through we realised how dark it had been inside. But also, almost bursting through the doors with the sunbeams, were dozens of young lads, who were begging, shouting, with arms extended and palms up, pleading with us to buy their wares. They stayed just outside the doorway, preventing us from passing through it; it was like getting free from a swarm of bees. They were not intimidating, many of them were laughing, but they were most persistent and a real nuisance. It was doubly troubling as none of their goods was desirable or useful, but I wondered later on that day whether their supper depended on the cash they brought home. It was worrying to see how necessary our cash seemed to be to their existence. They followed us to the coaches, and kept bouncing on to the step as we waited – a long time – for the driver to appear - was he still having his afternoon siesta? My husband and I happened to be sitting in a front seat, and I had brought a flask of tea with me, and as we drank our cup of lukewarm tea, one lad tried to persuade me to exchange our empty flask for one of the kaftans he was trying to sell. I think it would have been a poor deal for both parties. What use would an empty Thermos flask be to him, and what would I have done with a caftan? Our flask of tea was almost a lifesaver to us on many occasions when we were on holiday or out for the day.

We arrived back at the port to board our ship at 5 p.m. We had seen quite a lot in six hours, with a very varied tour and an excellent guide. There was still a lot of the day left, but we were tired and went under cover as soon as we boarded the ferry to buy some refreshment and then have 'forty winks'. I snoozed for a little while, then woke up and could still see the coastline of Morocco to our right (port) side. I kept looking, waiting for the ship to make its way to the open sea and begin to cross the straits back to Tarifa, but we were still hugging the coast of North Africa and the boat seemed to be heaving and the engines labouring. I began, silently, to wonder whether we had boarded the wrong ship; I hoped we were we on our way back to Tarifa. It was nonsense, of course, and eventually the ship turned to starboard and headed out to the open sea. The ferry had hugged the coast of Africa for quite some while before heading out to cross the Straits back to Spain because of the strong gale, but at the time I couldn't think where we could be heading when I could see the mainland for such a long time. I think the ship was moving slowly against a head wind. After a while, another huge hunk of land appeared through the window and seemed to block out everything else as we sailed alongside; this mountain of land seemed so near to the ship, and I suddenly realised that we were sailing past the island of Gibralter. We had not gone past Gibralter when we sailed from Tarifa in the morning. No sooner had the island disappeared than we found we were returning to an unknown port. If our knowledge of the Spanish coast had been better we would have realised immediately that we would shortly arrive at the port of Algerciras. The ferryboat had made an unscheduled stop to pick us up at Tarifa in the morning, but sailed directly to its designated port of Algerciras in the evening. How were we to reach Tarifa to get our coach back to Rota? Nobody had told the few additional passengers in the ferry of the alteration in our programme, but the agents had been informed, and we were mightily pleased to see the old minibus waiting at the dockside. The driver told us that the port of Tarifa had been closed because the wind was too strong for any ships to berth there. We quickly set off and had an even longer coach journey home, and it was very late when at last we arrived back to our hotel, where everyone, staff and visitors had gone to bed. My record of this holiday tells me that our journey home from Algiciras was 158km. What a long day, but what memories!

Our hotel had tennis courts, which I didn't use, and horse riding was also available. I had never even sat on a horse, but thought I would give it a go, and had two, one hour, sessions. I felt so high up when seated. I am sure my horse sensed that I was a complete novice, and he kept stopping and eating grass at the side of the lane. As his head went down, I felt I was being drawn down too, and I had great difficulty in getting my horse to lift his head and 'get a move on' – but not too fast, please! Eventually I did manage a cautious walk/trot along the beach, which was rather nice. However, I felt I would stick with my tennis, folk dancing and exercise class, and didn't feel inclined to add horse riding to my activities when I got home, but it was an experience; with a few more lessons I might have been hooked!

We had one last adventure before the end of this holiday, which began with a two-hour bus journey, mainly on an almost empty, post-rush-hour motorway, into Seville. It was rather a dull day, but we viewed the cathedral, where Christopher Columbus is buried, and which was a mosque at some period in the past, and the twelfth century minaret can still be seen sitting atop the cathedral tower. We walked around the Reales Alcazar (Royal Palace), marvelling at the beautiful architecture and mosaic decoration, then walked round the Palace Gardens. We wandered round the Plaza deEspana and through the Jewish quarter. Many of the streets were lined with orange trees, laden with small Seville oranges. I think they were only used for decoration in Seville and not for marmalade. Only the English eat marmalade!

This was our last day in Spain, and as we were walking down a narrow street in the latter part of the afternoon a youngster on a small motorbike came zooming down the street and snatched my handbag from my shoulder. I was so shocked; I thought I had been hit, and a few seconds passed before I realised that someone on a motor scooter passing through the narrow street had wrenched my bag from my body. I saw the motorcyclist as he accelerated away, and started rushing after him, shouting, 'He's got my handbag'. Nobody took any notice; he whizzed round a corner, and I knew my bag had gone. Fortunately it had little in it. Just a book I had brought with me to read on the bus and a purse with a few pesetas left inside at the end of a holiday.

My husband had a very good camera hung around his neck, and while we were waiting at the bus station to return to our hotel, we noticed a man hanging around behind a pillar; he kept peering out and looking at Maurice and bobbing back again when he saw we were looking at him. We felt sure that he was planning to snatch my husband's camera. There were not many people around, and we both felt very uncomfortable and threatened, and were extremely glad when the bus appeared, and we were able to have a safe journey back to the hotel.

In conversation with other guests at our hotel, we heard that five visitors had been robbed during the two-week, out-of-season period we were staying in this not very busy hotel. A watch and a handbag had been snatched from a small group as they walked along a beach into Rota, another lady had her watch snatched off her wrist as she was sitting in a garden in Cadiz, a wallet was stolen, and at the end of two weeks I lost my handbag. How sad, in this beautiful country! We had not then had a countrywide crime wave in the towns and cities in our own land. It was shocking to us then, but sadly theft seems almost commonplace in Britain now.

It was a wonderful, pain-free holiday, and thankfully we were unaware of the cloud ahead of us with the development of an even more disabling neuralgic pain that would descend on me a year or two later.

Maurice had the first of three pacemakers fitted in 1986, to deal with the acute arrhythmia that had first affected him very seriously two years after this holiday. Until his retirement two years later he had been in charge of quality control for the instrumentation of a new engine that was being developed by Rolls Royce in conjunction with Turbomeca Aircraft Company in France. This required frequent flights to Toulouse Airport for meetings with their company team in Pau. Although stressful, Maurice really enjoyed this last project in his career, which was completed after his retirement. The engine was named the RTM 322 and was installed in the Merlin and Apache helicopters, as well as in its French counterparts. I suppose that RTM stood for Rolls Royce and Turbo-Meca. It was not such an intriguing name as the Gnome, or the Goblin. I wonder how many – or indeed, if any - new British aircraft engines have been developed since that period? He had worked at de Havilland and Rolls Royce engine companies from the start of the development of the small jet engine, and had forty-nine years service with these two prestigious companies. The name de Havilland has a long history going back to the very early development of aircraft by Sir Geoffrey de Havilland, who founded the company in 1920, designed the World War 2 Mosquito aircraft and subsequently the ill-fated Comet.

Chapter Twenty-eight

A TRIBUTE

My mother had led such an uneventful life but she, like my father, really enjoyed hearing about our holidays. She didn't read my holiday diary (I don't think she could see very well) but she liked us to tell her where we had been. She always came out with one of her comical comments after anyone in the family told her of their activities: 'You do get about in your tea half-hour' was a frequent comment after we had been anywhere interesting, and her little saying became a family joke. We always smile when we think of this and have warm memories of her. I can't think when anybody had a thirty-minute tea break, but it certainly used to be customary for office, shop or factory workers – and teachers too, officially - to have a definite tea break of around fifteen minutes during the morning and afternoon.

If I told her something – to her – unbelievable, my mother's favourite remark was, 'You're up the pole, my girl!' or, 'My 'godfathers!' We often have a chuckle when we remember her favourite phrases. Our visits were always pleasant; we enjoyed her company and were very fond of her. She once asked me if I would buy her a new corset. I really didn't know anything about corsets, and didn't know where to buy one. After some difficulty I found a very helpful shop; I explained what I wanted, and with some assistance I made my purchase. On my next visit I gave my mother the corset and explained that I wasn't sure whether it would fit her, as I didn't know anything about corsets. She responded with great surprise and a firm reproving voice, 'You don't wear a corset? You'll be in for trouble, my girl. You'll see!' I suppose lack of a corset or any confining garment is part of the reason why 'older' ladies nowadays have trouble with a 'tum' that is no longer flat! Words of wisdom from my mother – but I don't think I could wear a corset!

My mother sometimes spoke of a friend she had in another villa. I never met her, and I don't know how my mother knew her. One day we heard that this friend, whose name I have forgotten, had died. I don't think my mother made friends with anyone else during all the years she was in Shenley Hospital, and yet she was a friendly person.

It was always helpful if I had plenty to talk to her about, because she began to ramble a bit if I didn't have some news to keep the conversation going. She always took it very calmly when we told her that one of her relatives had died. Her comment was always, 'Oh, another one gone', and she never showed sorrow. (I believe that a possible side effect of her medication is to deaden emotional response.) Her mind sometimes wandered if our conversation flagged and she would say that she had seen her sister Ada (my aunt), or her brother-in-law Bert (my uncle) in the grounds of the hospital, and could not accept that they had died some years previously. She had probably been thinking about them as she sat alone with her thoughts. As far as I could tell she had nobody with whom she appeared to chat, so it is quite possible that she might talk aloud to her relatives, even though they were not there (not necessarily a symptom of madness). However, very occasionally she appeared to hear a voice, seemingly speaking to her from over her shoulder, to which she would reply. I was with her on one occasion when she suddenly turned her head sharply over her shoulder and said in a loud, shocked voice, as if speaking to somebody behind her, "Oh don't say that!"

"Say what?" I queried.

"Don't say you wish I was dead; don't say that," she replied, still looking over her shoulder. She wasn't addressing her reply to me, but to some unknown voice coming from within.

My mother-in-law had been widowed and moved to an elderly care home in our locality. The initial slight pain in my groin area had become so intense that when visiting either my mother or my mother-in-law I had to either stand or sprawl on the floor. I would sit for a few minutes after greeting one or other of them until I could bear it no longer and gradually slid off the softly-upholstered chair in the villa at Shenley to sprawl on the floor, and did the same when visiting my mother-in-law, to the astonishment of them both, as they could not understand the nature, or the severity, of my, what I then called 'under-carriage' pain. It was probably quite improper for a lady to be sprawling on the floor in their generation. They did appear to be quite shocked.

This pain seemed to have become yet another of those hidden, unspoken-of conditions that does not receive compassion or understanding and is very difficult to treat. In quite different ways, my mother and I were both suffering from 'unmentionable' health conditions, which could not be talked about in polite society. And yet we both suffered intolerably, my mother with her loss of freedom, and me with my constant pain.

I had a telephone call one day to tell me that my mother had had a fall, had fractured her hip and was in the Royal Orthopaedic Hospital in Stanmore. I was very concerned and drove there immediately. I don't think it could have been a severe fracture, as she didn't seem to be in any discomfort and seemed quite happy in a ladies' ward. I think she saw the episode as a bit of a holiday! The next time I visited I asked one of the other patients in her bay of the ward if everything was O.K. 'Yes, she's fine,' the lady replied. 'She entertains us in the evening by singing all the old songs!' I had not heard her sing since I was a small child, but had grown up with my father singing all the 'old songs' when he was doing little jobs around the house. I would love to have heard my mother singing some of those early 20th century songs.

On visiting his grandmother some years after he had started work one of my sons mentioned that he had bought a new car. She seemed quite interested, and when he visited her a few months later, her first remark to him was, 'How's the car going, dear?' She had remembered him telling her of his change of car from his previous visit, and wanted to know about its performance. Her question was very typical of my memory of a similar greeting that was exchanged when we visited our relatives when I was very young. A car was not reliable in those days; it might break down. Cars were usually serviced at home by their owners, and the usual greeting when we met my aunt and uncle was, 'And how's the car going Bert?' – or Percy.

Her memory was good in many respects. She didn't appear to have any difficulty in recalling the relevant words when in the middle of a conversation, (as I frequently do nowadays!). She would listen with interest to whatever family news we were able to tell her, could hold a conversation with us, although she had little to contribute as she did nothing, but she remembered details from our previous visits, and she certainly did not suffer from dementia. But if I tried to remind her of incidents when she was at home when I was little girl, she could recollect nothing at all.

My mother's afternoon cup of tea was poured from a canteen-sized pot, with the milk already added, and I would watch her drink it from an institutional green china cup sitting on a green saucer but, thankfully, not poured into a plastic beaker. I recalled that for so many years my father was present when she was given her afternoon cup of tea, but he was never offered one. Apart from those few months at home my parents had not even been able to share a cup of tea together for so many years. The thought led to an idea…

One day I asked the Sister if I could bring in afternoon tea for my mother, and if I could have the use of a little table. Sister took us into one of the small rooms at the side of the dining room on our next visit, where we found a small table and three chairs. Maurice and I carried in two large holdalls containing a large flask of hot water, a couple of tea bags, a hand-embroidered tablecloth, three serviettes three cups, saucers and plates from my parents' best tea service, some dainty sandwiches and some homemade cake. I found my mother in the lounge and brought her to the little room, and she sat down at the table. I popped a teabag into the flask then spread the cloth on the table. She was quite bemused as I began to lay the table with her own china, the pretty serviettes, the sandwiches and the cake. I couldn't really bring a teapot, so I had to pour tea from a flask, and add milk from a small medicine bottle, but apart from that it was just like the afternoon tea she would have had years ago at home.

It was quite moving to see my mother drinking tea from one of her own (probably a wedding present in 1920) best teacups. We did this on several occasions and it was a very happy time together. I wished I had thought of the idea when my father was still alive. On one occasion she said, 'Oh, it's like a young Christmas every time you come!' On the next occasion another Sister came into the room and tried once again to get my mother to acknowledge that I was her daughter, but she replied, 'I don't know who she is. I had two daughters and they took them both away from me. I don't know who she is, but she's my best friend.' I realised I couldn't ask for more. She obviously enjoyed the little tea parties, but after a while we found that the room was not available.

Her medication appeared to have dampened her nerves to a level where she didn't become animated, or excited, or really interested in any mental or physical or social activity, but this might just as easily be caused through old age, lack of stimulation, and the effect of spending more than half of her life in a mental hospital.

I didn't know how to give my mother a treat as she grew more aged. She had no needs, and no space or privacy for anything personal, but I sometimes took in some strawberries and cream in the summer, or a chocolate éclair. She enjoyed fruit yoghurts and I sometimes took in a pack of four. I took a spoon with me and she ate one while I was there, and the rest were put in the ward fridge, hopefully, for her to have another day. When I next visited she had no recollection of being given even one of the yoghurts. Was this a lapse of her memory, or had someone else had them, I wondered? But there was a reluctance to enquire in case there were unpleasant consequences for the patient. Communication was somewhat difficult with the staff in the latter years, whose command of English was limited, and I often found it difficult to understand what they said to me.

My mother-in-law came to the hospital with us one Christmastime, and the two very elderly ladies sat chatting together as if they had known one another for years. They were both about ninety. How different life could have been; the two mothers might have been good friends. Mum was very good with my mother, especially as she had never been in a psychiatric hospital before and could have found the ward of elderly ladies a little disturbing. They had met once before when my parents had visited my in-laws at their home on the Essex coast during the summer in 1963 when my mother was living back in her own home. I wonder whether they went down to the beach? My parents had enjoyed so many holidays and day trips to the seaside in their old Austin 7 during the 1920s, and I can remember some seaside holidays in our Ford 8 when I was very young. A few seaside scenes are among my most vivid early memories of us together as a family. Schizophrenia, like so many mental illnesses, destroys almost everything that makes life worth living, and yet, my mother always seemed content.

Where is the Key?

My mother was transferred to another villa in her final years. This villa was for very elderly patients who required more care and assistance with eating, with dressing, and in every way, and most of them appeared to be suffering from some form of dementia. My mother, however, was not demented, could eat her meals and dress herself. She just sat, quietly thinking her own thoughts in her allotted chair near the back of the lounge. I felt that having nothing to do, nothing to look at, no aim, no conversation, living with companion patients who were well along the downward slope of a progressive age-related mental illness, would encourage the development of dementia in my mother. But it didn't. My mother was rational, really quite lively when we visited her, and her mental condition appeared to be kept very stable. I don't think this was an appropriate villa for her, but I was told the move was required for logistical reasons.

However, when visiting my mother a little later on she told me very quietly, very confidentially, and with a little embarrassment, that a young man was bathing her. She had obviously accepted this and realised that she needed assistance, but it must have been quite shocking for a lady of her age and generation to have a young man seeing her naked and helping her in the bath. It would be quite disturbing for anyone! A little later a young man approached us as we sat in the lounge, and introduced himself, saying, 'My name is Geoffrey. I am your mother's carer, and I help her in the bath'. I was so pleased that he had made himself known, and appreciated that my mother was a bit upset at having a man present in very personal, intimate situations. She was then in her early nineties, was quite stout, and probably needed someone strong to aid her. Geoffrey was very kind and gentle in his approach, a very nice man and a real carer. I'm so glad my mother felt able to confide in me her concern about having a man in the bathroom; I believe it relieved her of a feeling that this shouldn't be happening to her. She was, after all, born long ago at the end of the nineteenth century; I think she had felt it was wrong until I was able to reassure her, after Geoffrey had himself to me. It must have been awful for her nonetheless.

I think my mother would have been delighted to have her story told, and her expression of disbelief would have been one of her memorable little phrases! Perhaps her experience will produce some deserved sympathy and understanding for present-day sufferers from mental ill-health. I feel that I am now giving her inadequately expressed life a real value.

Most of the patients seemed to be seated a long way away from the television, although this was possibly their choice, but they were also far away from the full-length bay windows that brought natural light and sunlight into the room and which   overlooked the gardens. This was where the nurses and aides sat chatting to each other and glancing at the TV whilst keeping an eye on any need or problem that might arise with their patients. There appeared to be little attempt to communicate with them when I visited my mother in these latter years, but I realise I was not there all the day. She sat, along with many other ladies, at the darker end of the room well away from the windows. There were no other visitors, as I sat j-uncomfortably – beside her as we chatted. By this time I had learned to endure the pain for a while when sitting, but I always preferred a firm seat.

A year or so later we had an invitation from the ward staff to a Christmas party. My husband and I accepted the invitation and arrived on the Sunday afternoon, and found a festively decorated ward sitting room. There were bottles of drinks of all kinds, huge piles of chunky sandwiches, large cheese straws and sausage rolls with loads of puff pastry around tiny bits of sausage, all rather hefty stuff and not the kind of food that elderly people would really enjoy in the middle of the afternoon. There were very few visitors, but I had never seen quite a lot of staff who stood laughing and chatting together as they ate and drank, while very loud pop music was played. We tried to chat with my mother but the noise was too much for each of us; we couldn't hear ourselves speak let alone hear a reply and we had to retreat to a quieter corner. It was quite a big party and there must have been office staff and nurses and carers from other villas present. I am sure that the staff enjoyed the party, but I think most of the patients just sat and looked on, feeling a little bemused and looking a bit miserable. The party was more suitable for the staff than for the patients and there was no interaction between the two groups, but most of the patients were too old, and too removed from the present world to enjoy such a noisy Christmas celebration. The hospital was obviously running down, and I think all the elderly patients in wards throughout the hospital were taken along to this Christmas party. There were indications that the hospital was running down, and I guess these old folk would have to be cared for until they died.

In earlier years one of the staff nurses had always made a beautiful nativity scene in a central position in the ward, with shepherds, the angels, the wise men with their gifts, lots of animals, and of course Mary and Joseph, a crib with a little baby in it. I think that was a very thoughtful and more appropriate treat for the patients, which they could look at whenever they wished over the Christmas period, possibly remember what Christmas was really all about, and probably visited the scene several times. There was plenty to look at with so many individual pieces, and the whole scene was well worth spending time over.

As my mother became more aged I noticed that she seemed to have the same, very tatty, beige dress on every time I visited her. I asked her why she didn't wear another dress. I usually bought her a dress at Christmas, but she never seemed to be wearing one of her own dresses when I saw her, but always this dull, shapeless ill-fitting garment. For a while I assumed that she must have worn a different dress on other days and it was coincidence that I saw her on the day she happened to be wearing this particular, hospital issue, dress. After a while I felt it was too much of a coincidence and I asked my mother to take me to her dormitory, so that I could find a different dress for her to wear. Visitors were not supposed to enter the dormitories, but there was no member of staff around for me to ask permission so my mother and I simply walked along the short corridor together to where she slept, and I saw the huge room, full of narrow beds, where my mother must have slept for so many years. It was quite upsetting to know that such a very private lady had to spend her nights so publicly and with so little comfort.

There was a tiny wardrobe-cum-locker by the side of each bed, and I couldn't believe my eyes when my mother took me to her bed and I saw her little wardrobe was crammed full of horrible, unsuitable, mostly unwearable, charity-shop cast off dresses. They must have arrived at the hospital in plastic bin bags. I counted *thirteen* dresses that had been put on skimpy hangers and stuffed into her tiny bedside wardrobe. They were packed in so tightly it was almost impossible for me to drag a single dress out. None of the dresses was suitable for her age and many were not even her size. Most of them were unfit for anyone to wear. I was furious! It was not surprising that she had put the same dun-coloured, baggy dress on day after day; the little wardrobe was so crammed with these dreadful clothes that she could only manage to pull out the dress in the front – or most probably – she didn't hang it up at night as it was too difficult to push the other old clothes back far enough to make a space. Nobody seemed to have noticed that she had the same dress on every day. It was atrocious.

I looked through them all with difficulty as they were so tightly packed. I heaved my shoulder against them and managed gradually to drag them out and lay them on her bed. I found about five that could be wearable. One of these had no hem, so I took it home and turned up a hem to enable my mother to wear it. A couple of the outfits one could only describe as a joke, something for the two ugly sisters to wear in a pantomime. One was an outrageous frilly party dress: for a ninety-year-old lady to wear? I felt insulted on behalf of my mother. I took a huge armful of these clothes to the sister in order to complain, but there was no sister on duty; nobody seemed to be in charge or who would take responsibility for this really awful pile of old rags. I had to leave them on a desk and was told that someone would see to it later. I never had an explanation, but was told later by someone in authority that it was impossible for my mother to wear her own personal clothes; they would be lost in the hospital laundry. I had never been told that it was inappropriate to buy my mother her own dresses or cardigans but can understand how, even if clothes are clearly marked, some could go astray, but all my mother's nice clothes, whatever they were – dress, bed jacket, cardigan – were never seen again. Everything that I had bought for her had 'gone missing' – I wonder where? It appeared that unsellable charity shop clothes had been substituted.

She told us that as soon as we had left after visiting her on her 90th birthday her presents had been taken away from her. When we went to see her after Christmas, to see if she had opened, still possessed, or was wearing her presents, she told us that they were taken away as soon as she had unwrapped them. She didn't know where they went. On enquiry I was told they had to be sent for marking, even though I had always sewn a label in every garment we gave her, with her name and villa number printed in into the fabric in red, but they never reappeared.

At one visit my mother said to me in very conspiratorial tones, 'You don't know what goes on here at night'. I never actually knew to what she was referring, but I fear that night supervision was not always as good, or appropriate, or as adequate as it should have been, and, as she said, I had no idea of what might be going on. What could I have done?

Conditions had deteriorated in the latter years; there appeared to be fewer staff around; it was difficult to make out whom, if anyone, was in charge. It was difficult for me to understand what the nurses were saying, so it must have been even more difficult for the patients. And, did they talk to them? I thought fondly of Sister Brown and some of the, very formal, but caring staff who had been in my mother's villa years ago.

We had arranged a week's self-catering holiday in Deal in Kent in 1992, not too far away from Hertfordshire, and visited my mother just before we went away. I had not been informed that she unwell, but she was obviously not her usual self when we arrived, and I was told that she was on antibiotics for a urine infection. We sat with her for a while, and she didn't want to talk, and obviously felt very poorly. We discussed with the sister if we should cancel our holiday, but she seemed to think that the antibiotics would soon take effect. I gave her our holiday telephone number, and asked her to be sure to let me know if my mother grew worse and we would return home. We were not far away. I also gave her my son's 'phone number if he was needed urgently.

We set off, feeling a little concerned, but not unduly worried. I had had frequent urine infections over the years myself, and, although most unpleasant, they cleared up after a course of antibiotics. Although aged 96 my mother still seemed quite well. When we visited she always knew who we were, seemed pleased to see us, and was able to converse with us sensibly; she was certainly not suffering from dementia.

Maurice and I were self-catering in a converted almshouse, with the owner living nearby in a large house with its own swimming pool in the garden – unfortunately not for the use of those renting the holiday property. We didn't have access to a telephone; it was before the era of mobile phones, and we relied on the hospital being able to contact us via our landlady's phone.

Three days later, there was a brisk banging on our solid front door in the evening. On opening I found our rather haughty landlady standing outside in the dusk, saying that I was wanted on the 'phone. I followed her, assuming I would be taken into her house, but no, we went through a little, almost hidden, doorway, which led straight on to the poolside. I was then shown to a tiny room (which was actually a rather swish outside toilet) in which there was a phone - and also a shelf of books. On picking up the receiver I heard my son telling me that my mother had died. He had been contacted, presumably because the hospital had been unable to reach me, and had been told that his *mother* had died, and it had taken him a moment or two to realise that the hospital meant to inform him that it was his *grandmother* who had died. He had had quite a shock for a few seconds, thinking that in some way Shenley Hospital was in touch with him to tell him that *I* had died. We discovered that our landlady had been away from home for the weekend. Her 'phone may have rung, but remained unanswered.

I was so upset to find out that I had not been contacted earlier, and that I had not been with my mother in her last days, and especially, hours. She had been alone for so much of her life, and I had always intended to be sure that she didn't die alone. I dearly wish that I had been with her. I felt we should not have gone away; but she had soldiered on for so long I hadn't seriously considered her actually dying, neither, presumably, had the hospital staff. I think death sometimes creeps up on us almost unseen. You don't believe it's coming.

My mother died in the summer of 1992 aged ninety-six, having spent most of the years from 1931 in residential psychiatric care. She didn't have Alzheimer's, was mentally alert, coherent and was always polite to the nursing staff. When I first saw her in 1959/1960, the sister in charge of villa 4A, Sister Brown, told me that my mother was her 'head girl', and she knew she could trust her to run errands for her to another ward. Although still mentally ill at the time of her death, my mother didn't suffer from arthritis, never complained of a headache, and never suffered from a cold. She didn't know what physical pain was, and was not deaf, although her sight was very poor.

She had made a full recovery from her broken hip. She had another accident a few years before she died, when I was informed that she had had a fall. I drove immediately to the hospital and found her bleeding quite profusely from the back of her head. She was being attended to, and I was told that she had fallen over. She sat quite quietly as the nurse bathed her head, and made no fuss. The cut healed rapidly. She never told me how it had happened.

Geoffrey, her male carer, told me that my mother even said 'Thank you, Geoffrey', when he held a cup of water to her lips shortly before she died. She had shown little concern for my father as he grew into his old age, and she outlived him by ten years. She left no personal effects, no jewellery, not even an engagement or wedding ring. The hospital had no personal effects to hand over to me after her death. It seemed incredible. How different her life would have been if she had been born fifty years later when modern drugs might have helped her to lead a normal life. Although I was sad at her death, I was just so thankful that neither her physical ability nor her mental capacity had slowly been taken from her and that she had gradually declined. She made no fuss either in her life or in her death. She died of a urine infection, aged ninety-six. But what an incredibly sad, unfulfilled life she had.

My grief turned to anger when we returned home from Deal, driving directly to the hospital to receive my mother's death certificate, on which a doctor had written that the secondary cause of death was dementia. Whatever the name of her mental illness, she was not demented. I commented on this when registering her death, and the registrar urged me to query this secondary cause with the hospital authority, as it was felt at the registry office that too many deaths were being registered with dementia as the cause. I don't think you actually die 'of' dementia although you might die suffering 'with' it. It was an easy secondary cause of death for a duty doctor to give for an elderly patient in a psychiatric hospital who maybe he didn't actually know at all. But it is important to expose the inaccuracies if this distortion occurs nationally, and for a true secondary cause to be given.

We returned immediately to the hospital and I explained my concerns and the registrar's comment, and was immediately granted an interview with my mother's consultant. I had never seen this lady doctor before, but she looked at my mother's hospital records, which went right back to 1939, and agreed with me that my mother was not suffering from dementia, and her mental condition was not implicated in her death. She offered to issue a revised death certificate, but the death had already been registered. I felt it was a real dishonour to my mother, who had in a strange sort of way 'kept her sanity' throughout all the years of her psychotic illness, and had remained a real person right to the end of her life. I wish I had been there for her.

She had no friends as far as I know at the time of her death. She had had tough times in her childhood, and I am so glad that she and my father appeared to have had some fun and pleasure on the tennis courts and at the concert halls before I was born, and had holidays and excursions with my aunts and uncles in the 1920s. But it was such a short period in the early years of their married life. They were married in 1920 and before I was born in 1931 they had had a baby and lost her; I think my mother possibly suffered from some form of depression for a while after this bereavement. They had had the thrill of car outings, with trips to the seaside and elsewhere in the early years of motoring, and even a holiday abroad before I was born. What a brief time that was, filled both with sadness and happiness! I feel most of her life was so hidden, unknown, in the land of 'don't speak about it'. I wanted her voice to be heard, her strength of character to be understood and her uncomplaining acceptance of her restricted life to bring belated sympathy and understanding to my memory of her, with corresponding understanding for those suffering with mental ill-health and all those other conditions that seem to suffer from lack of compassion.

I think that given the limited understanding of mental illness during that period my mother probably had the best care available. I hope that with the ever-increasing understanding of mental illness, there is equally good, or better, care nowadays. There was something to be said for a really safe environment, for the patient, and for the safety of the public. But today, given appropriate treatment, supervision and support few people would have to undergo my mother's 'life-sentence'. When sectioning is necessary nowadays it is for a limited period, and can be renewed if needed. Patients are encouraged to get back to their families, or helped to live in the community if possible, but so often this doesn't seem to work. We are still looking for the key to cure mental illness.

I received a very touching little note from someone who I can only presume knew my mother in hospital. This lady did not give her address, but her name was Maria Kashinski, and she wrote the following note to me, 'I always admire your mother. She is an example of how to grow old. She is content; she never grumbles; she never says things about other people.' What a tribute! I never knew who this lady was, but she must have observed my mother and warmed to her character, and I have kept her little letter and thank her for it.

There were very few people at my mother's funeral, as hardly anybody knew her. I *was* very sad that nobody from Shenley was able to come; staffing problems meant that nobody could be spared. The nurses who really knew my mother had retired, but it had been her home since 1939. I think that she must have been one of the longest, and oldest, residents, and I really would have liked a representative to have been present.

The minister who took my mother's funeral gave her life such a meaning that I asked him for a copy of his address. I feel I must quote a few sentences from this: '...Lily's tragedy was not a private one, but one which touched Percy, who kept loving and visiting; and one which Sheila and her family lived with all their lives. I feel it is a tribute to the faithfulness of the different generations that there has been continued caring, when many families would just have written their loved one out of their life. Although Lily's life might not have been the sort of life to offer a great influence, it has certainly affected the family, and I believe, drawn out resources of love, patience and compassion, which have meant that, perhaps – in a way that she would certainly never have understood – she has indeed been an influence for good on others' lives, and for that we are thankful...A life such as Lily's poses questions which have few answers. I must be honest and say that I cannot understand how it is that a loving God allows such a great measure of suffering in the life of one individual. What I do know is that this is indeed a broken world that we live in, and that a life such as Lily's is a sign of that brokenness…'

Perhaps in the telling of my mother, Lily's, story, her life will become an even greater influence for good. In addition to telling my own story of the past sixty years, the second theme to my book has been to give some substance to my mother's secluded, unrecognised, life, and this has become the main theme in part of my book; the title is appropriate: Where is the key to the cause, and the cure, of mental illnesses? Will it ever be found?

Chapter Twenty-Nine

WE'LL MEET AGAIN

I cannot complete this story without writing about a very different chapter in my life. It began with a minor comment when my friend Beryl was visiting in the mid-to-late-1980s. We were chatting away, reminiscing as old friends often do, when one or other of us said, 'I wonder what happened to Joy?' Joy had been one of our school friends, the one who swooned whenever our maths teacher came into the classroom at Hendon Tech. I never knew Joy's address and once we had started work we lost contact, until I bumped into her in about 1950 while walking up Harley Street on my way home from work. Joy looked very elegant; was smartly dressed, with long dark hair and wore rather a lot of lipstick. She seemed very tall and elegant in her high-heeled shoes, composed, confident but still with a lively twinkle in her eyes. How much she had changed from the tomboy at senior school who skipped a needlework class to spend the afternoon romping around in the school grounds with a friend, before she was spotted by a teacher who saw them leaping over the air raid shelters! She sang well even then, and a year or so later had developed a beautiful singing voice in the madrigal group run by our maths teacher at Hendon Tech. I was so surprised when she told me she had just - or was about to be – married; it was so long ago, I can't remember which. I had not seen her since 1947 when we both left our commercial college to begin work at sixteen years of age. We chatted together for a few moments, but we were both in a hurry, and we never met again. Few homes had telephones then, public transport was difficult, and not many people owned a car, making it much more difficult to keep in touch with friends in those days. I had often wondered how life, and marriage, had turned out for Joy.

She remained in my thoughts after Beryl went home. What *had* happened to Joy, I pondered? She couldn't have had a humdrum life! Energy, humour and mischief were strong characteristics that I remembered. I got out an old photograph album, and looked at the school photo of our huge class of forty-six pupils in our first year at Chandos School in 1942. How had all their lives had worked out? I decided to send a copy of the photo to the local paper in Harrow, together with a brief article entitled 'Where are you now?' requesting them to publish it. I didn't hold out much hope of any response; forty-five years was a very long time since we had parted.

However, within the next couple of months I had heard from ten 'old girls' who had been in my class and who now lived in various parts of the country, from Jean in Dorset, to Vera in Bournemouth, Pam in Surrey, Dorothy and Gladys in Bucks, Sheila and Beryl still lived in Kenton and

Joan was in Ruislip, another Joan lived near St. Albans, Margaret and a second Sheila had moved to Hertfordshire. I was the third Sheila who made up the trio of girls with this name in our class at school. I was amazed at the response, but sadly I received no news of Joy. But I had received letters from girls (or rather, sixty-plus year-old ladies) some of whom had seen the article, but most had heard about it indirectly - a cousin had seen the article, or an old friend, a sister or even a bridesmaid who still lived in the area, had passed on the article.

We all wanted to meet up. My home was not far from junctions on the Al, the Ml and the M25 and was considered the best venue. It was also quite easy to reach St. Albans by train. We had our first 'Form 1A' Reunion in 1991. Apart from Beryl, I had seen none of these ladies since our schooldays, although I had the advantage of knowing who was coming as they began to arrive on the day. At each ring of the bell I opened the door, and as I greeted the lady standing on my doormat I tried to recognise each guest from my recollections of the teenage girl I had last seen so many years ago. Some were instantly known; they hadn't really changed at all, merely aged a little; others needed a lot of thought before I felt I could say their name with confidence. I led them into our lounge, and there was a lot of laughter as each person slowly, or instantly, recognised their old classmates. The room was soon filled with happy chatter we all began to remember little incidents from the past that immediately drew us together. Some renewed friendships that had begun when they first started school at five years of age. As lunchtime drew near we were still waiting for one guest, the other Sheila who lived in Hertfordshire, who had telephoned to say she had a problem at work but hoped to arrive shortly. So we delayed starting our meal, until a later call told us that she couldn't settle her work problem, and was unable to make it to the reunion at all. The photographer (my husband) was still on hand, waiting to take a group photo of us all before going out for a quiet pub lunch, leaving the ladies to their lunch.

He had taken a few informal photos of us as we sat and chatted, but had waited until all had arrived before taken a formal group picture. Our lunch was very delayed as we waited for my last guest to arrive and he could take his final picture. He thought his job was over, but nearly everyone else had brought a camera and he was asked to take a photo of the group on a variety of cameras. It had taken a long time, and we were all about to sit down at last to a very delayed lunch, when the empty place setting was noticed, and my guests insisted that Maurice joined us. He was reluctant at first, and didn't really want to be the only man amongst a group of ladies, but during the delay everyone had got t know him, so he agreed that he might be too late for a meal out; the empty place was tempting – as was the food. So he joined us and took more pictures while we sat eating and chatting over our meal and became really acquainted with them all. He poured the wine, sat with us for our first course and then helped to take the dishes out to the kitchen. As I carried in the desserts I saw that he had made a quick move to the kitchen sink. While we tucked in to our second course he donned an apron, and got stuck into all the washing up. Some time later he appeared with trays of tea and coffee as we still sat talking round the meal-table. The dishes were washed and dried and the kitchen had been tidied up.

Maurice had made such a good contribution to our first get-together, becoming not only our official photographer, but also our wine waiter and our living-and-moving-dish-washer for our future gatherings. After serving our tea or coffee when the meal was over, he entertained one or two husbands or relatives with tea and chat as they arrived to collect non-driving wives. He had not only got to know and become friends with all my old school-mates, but had also become indispensable to all our annual gatherings. We were all winners!

 He has been sadly missed at our reunions since his death a few years ago. He had been such an asset on the day for so many years and was a tremendous support to me before, during and afterwards. As well as all his acquired tasks on the day, he had helped me to prepare the table, brought extra chairs downstairs etc. and helped to clear up when our guests had left.

As we exchanged memories over lunch we frequently spoke of Miss Oyston, our old form teacher, as we commented on how much we had appreciated our education, especially the ethos of the school, and we felt had been greatly influenced by Miss Pike, our headmistress. We thought that although our secondary education had been brief and adversely affected by war conditions, it had affected our lives very positively. We raised a toast to Miss Oyston. Our meal was over, but we continued to sit around the dining table over our coffee as each one in turn briefly told her life story.

Vera had heard of my article through a friend still living in Kenton who had sent her the news clip. She told us that she had had a long and interesting secretarial career working for the Billy Graham Organisation. Vera had remained in touch with another old school friend, Gladys, and had passed the article on to her. Vera came up by train from Bournemouth for several of our subsequent annual reunions, but sadly she died some time ago.

When Gladys left Hendon Tech. she decided that (like me) she didn't want to spend her days as a shorthand typist; she wanted to have (also like me) a nursing career. Her father didn't approve (like mine) but Gladys went ahead, enrolled as a student nurse, and her father soon came to accept his daughter's wish. She spent some years nursing in England and then abroad, ending up in the Canary Islands, where she married a Danish count and had a family before making a career change and becoming a medical secretary. She returned to England after the death of her husband. She has a wonderfully sounding, double-barrelled surname and is officially a countess...but as Gladys says airily, 'Oh, that means nothing; they're two a penny in Denmark!'

Jean emigrated to Canada with her husband soon after her marriage, where she brought up her family before returning to England. She and her husband became hoteliers for some years, but now live in retirement in Dorset, enjoying frequent cruises. The first Sheila in my class became secretary to the director of an engineering company. She worked for the same firm until her retirement, and is still in touch with her late boss's wife. She married later in life but had no children, and sadly her husband also died some years ago. Sheila and Jean had been friends throughout their school years, sitting together from their first day at infant school. Their lives had been so different, one so well travelled and the other remaining in Kenton for most of her life, but they picked up their friendship immediately they met again at our first reunion. Sheila has now moved from the house in which she had spent her entire life into sheltered accommodation in Sussex.

Pam met her husband in the bank where she had worked. She had two daughters and now lives in Surrey and is very involved in the W.I. Margaret stayed on at Hendon Tech for a further year and took her Matric before doing secretarial work in a London hospital until she married. She moved to Hertfordshire with her husband where she brought up her family. She has been widowed for many years.

Dorothy married and moved from Kenton to Buckinghamshire, where she brought up her family of four children, but very sadly Dorothy died after surgery for breast cancer some years ago. She was still working, using her secretarial skills until she became ill. There were two Joans at the Reunion. One did a variety of training and work experience allied to cookery and cookery demonstration before she married, and was then employed as a draughtswoman at G.E.C. She had two sons, and now lives happily in retirement with her husband in Norfolk.

The other Joan became a shorthand typist at St. Dunstan's before having various secretarial jobs. She married and had two sons and later became a playgroup supervisor. She has been disabled with rheumatoid arthritis and diabetes for many years, and has been unable to meet up with us since our first reunion, but we keep in touch. She takes delight in her two grandchildren and, like me, has memories of many lovely foreign holidays before she became ill.

Beryl, my friend of over sixty years, trained as an officer in the Salvation Army and began her ministry in a small town in Yorkshire. She became a major (equivalent to the title of reverend) and worked in the Salvation Army training college and at the international headquarters doing secretarial and administrative work as well as assisting in the training of the cadets who would become S.A. officers. She had a period overseeing the S.A. community work throughout the country. After her official retirement she had a very interesting part-time job for a while in the S.A. family tracing service. She has not married but has a host of friends and still belongs to the

Salvation Army Hall in Oxford Street in which she grew up. Thus in our small group we have a countess and a major!

We learned later that the second Sheila (who couldn't be with us on our first reunion) also worked in a bank, travelling up to the city of London each day, and met her husband there. He very sadly died when their two sons were quite young, and Sheila brought up her children alone. She has had a long career with social services organising home care – an understandable reason why she had a problem at work and missed our first reunion. She has been able to be with us on all our subsequent reunions and is now retired, but still living in her family home in Hertfordshire.

A third Joan was added to our group a few years later; the Joan who had been my close friend when we were young and about whom I wrote in 'Child of the Thirties', but with whom I lost touch after we started work. I knew she had moved to St. Albans with her husband and family many years ago, but I didn't know her married name. I hadn't seen her since we were both sixteen, but I often looked at ladies' faces when I was walking through St. Albans shopping centre on our local market day, wondering whether Joan could be amongst the shoppers. One day I thought I recognised her; this lady looked very like my recollection of her mother. I hesitated. Was I being foolish? Might I be considered rude? I plucked up my courage, and looking straight at this lady, I smiled and said quietly, 'I think you are Joan?' She looked nonplussed for a moment, but as she looked at me she began to recognise me and exclaimed, 'Sheila!' We couldn't have changed very much to be able to recognise each other after more than forty years, in an unexpected meeting in a market crowded with shoppers. We stood and chatted and reminisced amongst the market stalls. Joan moved to St. Albans early in her marriage where she brought up her family and she often joins us at our annual lunches.

At our last meeting Joan told me something that I had completely forgotten. I mentioned to her that I couldn't remember how we first met, or how we became friends. She was so surprised at my lack of recollection, and told me that she had been unable to start infant school at the beginning of the term when she was five because she had scarlet fever. When her mother brought her into the classroom a couple of weeks later, she felt so shy when she saw the other children already settled in the classroom, but that I had spoken to her and said, "Would you like to sit next to me?" That's how our friendship began; I had no idea! We both lived on the 'wrong' side of Kenton Lane and were allocated to the collection of wooden buildings that formed the first Priestmead School in the area. The children on the other side of the road attended the new brick-built school. There was no choice at all in those days, and one just accepted the decision of the local education authority, which allocated children to the nearest school – that's just another of the countless changes that, as I have told my story, have impressed me; so many things that I would never have recalled if I had not written this book.

One other contact was made with an old classmate who now lives in Australia. The story of how Barbara got in touch with me is quite amazing. I can do no better than quote from the letter I received from this 'old girl's' daughter, who had returned to England as an adult and was living in the Harrow area when my little article was published.

Her daughter wrote to me in August 1990 as follows: 'Imagine my surprise on opening the Harrow Leader to see the photo of Form 1A Chandos School, and there was my mother's face. I instantly recognised the photo as it is the same one my mother has, although I have not seen it for years.........My mother lives in Melbourne, Australia, having emigrated with my father in 1950 to a small country town... She went into the local theatre group, and later became quite a prominent actress on both stage and television...acting in a variety of television serials.'

A few days later I received a long letter from Barbara, telling me that her dearest friend was Joy Coleman whom she had thought of many times over the years, but had not seen since she left school. (Joy is the girl previously mentioned and Barbara was her rebellious companion on that Friday afternoon!) Barbara's six-page typed letter on A4size paper was full of reminiscences of her schooldays at Chandos, with quotes from poetry she remembered learning and the words of a song we had sung. She also wrote of the tremendous influence she also felt that the school – via the teachers and especially our headmistress – had had on her life. Barbara had been the star pupil in our class in what would now be called creative writing, and she became a journalist on a local paper in England before emigrating to Australia after her marriage.

She gained a BA degree in professional writing and literature in Melbourne as a mature student and continued with her journalistic career. She telephoned me when she was on a trip to England a year or two later, and I arranged a mini-reunion at short notice with a few of our old Chandos friends who lived not too far away. It was great to meet her, but we all still wondered what had happened to Joy. We would love to know how life fared for Joy Coleman who lived in Stanmore. Barbara and I have remained in touch by email.

Chandos School used to comprise a girls' school and an almost identical but separate boys' school. It is now a large co-educational comprehensive school and has been renamed Park High School. The head teacher saw my little article and responded to it with an invitation to our group of former pupils to visit the school. Six of us were able to accept the invitation, and in October 1992 we met in the large school library.

We were served coffee by some very polite and confident Park High School prefects, and then given the privilege of an escorted tour round the whole school by the deputy head teacher, visiting some of the classrooms while lessons were in progress (a very special privilege), seeing the wonderful new additions to the school – the science block, music block. We were sad to find that our old form room was now used as a storeroom. My beloved gym had disappeared and was in the process of being replaced with a state of the art sports centre. It was so nostalgic to walk down the corridors, and stand in the school hall.

It was nearly lunchtime at the end of our tour, and the dinner tables were being set up in a manner that was familiar. We recognised the serving hatches where we used to queue up for our midday meal – some things never change! We turned to look at the stage on which Miss Pike had led our assemblies; what memories came back to us. As a small group of six 'old girls' we felt very privileged to have been given the invitation from the head teacher to have this tour and to see our old school in action.

Some of us had a further visit to Park High School in September 2009, on the 60th anniversary of the opening of the school, then called Chandos School. There was the opportunity of another tour, this time led by present students, around the greatly enlarged and modernised school where we saw the science block and an amazing new IT block, giving the present students a great education and the opportunity of a vast array of careers. In very many ways I envy them, but I continue to value the ethos I imbibed during the war at Chandos School.

When Chandos School was opened on the 1st September 1939, just three days before the start of the second world war, it was the most up-to-date, though not fully equipped, senior school in the district, with a modern 1930s-architectural style and well constructed buildings, but the facilities were tiny compared with those required for present day educational needs.

The secretary of the Chandos Old Girls' Association (COGA) read my little article and wrote to invite me to their annual reunion. I had forgotten that such an association existed until I was rummaging among old papers recently and found a handwritten letter from Miss Pike, my headmistress in 1945, saying how pleased she was to see 'my smiling face' at the Chandos Old Girls' Association meeting. It must have been started in 1945 immediately after the end of the war, and I guess I had attending its first, or at least one of its very early meetings, but I can't remember ever going there or knowing anything about it. I guess if I had continued to attend its' meetings I would have had more social links in my teenage years, but I think that after a day at college with homework to do, or later, after a day's work, I didn't feel like walking the mile and a half to the school after preparing our meal in the evening. Thus I had lost touch with what would have proved a social, friendly group who would probably have been drawn from the homes much closer to the school.

The COGA had totally faded from my memory. Perhaps this was another analogy with my mother who, because not seen, met, or spoken about, was completely forgotten. The brain needs frequent nudges or reminders before it develops a lasting memory.

However, I did accept the invitation to attend the 1990 annual meeting of the COGA, but I met only one lady who had been in my class; she is one of the two Sheila's already mentioned. Nobody knew of Joy. One member of staff was at the reunion who had taught at Chandos while I was a pupil, and I had a word with her and asked her if she knew anything about Miss Oyston. I was delighted when Miss Grimley told me that my old form teacher was still alive. Miss Oyston lived alone and she was sure that she would be pleased to hear from one of her old pupils. I guess they both sometimes wondered, 'Where are they now, and what did they do?' She gave me Miss Oyston's address and I wrote to her and told her how I had managed to get in touch with a number of my old classmates, and that we met up annually. I wrote that at our reunion 'Form 1A 1942' lunch there was a group of her old pupils who had thought of her, had talked of her and toasted her.

Some time later my telephone rang. As I answered it and heard a voice saying, 'It's Miss Oyston here'. I can remember that I immediately stood up straight and pulled my shoulders back as I greeted her! She told me what a surprise and great pleasure it had been to hear from some of her old wartime pupils, and how much she had enjoyed reading my letter. She said she remembered each one of us. She told me she was now crippled with arthritis and could not get out and about. At our next reunion we all signed a card for her and I enclosed it with a copy of the photo my husband had taken, and a lengthy letter giving her some account of what her former pupils had done with their lives.

We continued to send her a card, enclosed with a letter and a photo after our reunion every year until she died, and I also sent her a Christmas card from us all. She sent us a Christmas card for several years before she became too frail to write. Below the printed greeting on one card she wrote, 'With many, many happy memories of Form1A 1942-1943 from "Miss Oyston", beneath which she wrote 'Edith G. Oyston'. Children (as we were still called when at school) and young people were not told their teachers' forenames in my young day. We always wondered what E.G. stood for when she awarded a house mark for good work with her initials E.G.O, or wrote our reports in her distinctive handwriting. It seemed to put us in the category of friends when she let us know that her name was Edith. Her very strong, neat signature was retained well into her eighties, until her arthritis made writing impossible.

Her executor found my address in her address book after she died. When he informed me on the telephone that 'my friend Edith' had died, it was obvious that he had no idea who I was. When I told him that actually I was not an old friend, that I had not seen Miss Oyston since 1945 and that I was merely an old pupil, he was speechless for a few moments. He told me that as my name, address and phone number was one of the few in her address book, he had assumed I was a close friend. He asked me to come to her funeral, as he said it was unlikely that there would be anybody else there to represent her earlier years. I considered this and didn't think that it was really appropriate for me to attend, but he was quite pressing, telling me that she spoke so often of the wartime years when she taught at Chandos, and that it would be very much appreciated if I could attend. She had no relatives, and nobody else who would remember her from earlier years.

So my husband and I drove to the crematorium and found about ten other people there, who all knew each other and were old neighbours and friends of Miss Oyston. In her Christmas card addressed to 'the girls' in 1993 she wrote, 'I find life great fun – and I still meet a lot of very interesting people. We have long and sometimes heated political exchanges. I'm also glued to the TV for all sport programmes – except soccer. I've always played competitive sports'. I think she was bedridden by this time, and life in reality was very difficult and lonely for her, but I guess some of the people at her funeral were the 'very interesting' people she had written about on her card.

Her executor soon approached us at the crematorium, and introduced us to the minister who was going to conduct the service, who looked very startled when told that I was an ex-pupil. I think he found it hard to believe that this very elderly lady had still been in touch with one of her pupils from so long ago. As we spoke together he asked me what subject Miss Oyston had taught. I told him that she had taught us geography, English, maths and R.E. (Religious Education). At this he interrupted me, and repeated, "R.E? She taught R.E.?" I think this was quite a shock to him. "What did she teach you?" he asked.

I replied that I could remember learning about St. Paul's missionary journeys. Miss Oyston's interest in geography came into these R. E. lessons quite a lot! We had maps on which we traced Paul's journeys, and marked all the places where he stayed...I couldn't really remember much R.E. in it. We had to learn the Ten Commandments one year, and I told the minister that I also remembered memorising the chapter in Corinthians Chapter 13 that began with the words, 'Though I speak...' He sounded astonished when I said this. "You memorised 1 Corinthians Chapter 13?" he queried almost disbelievingly.

"Oh yes," I said. "I still remember most of it, and can well remember standing at the back of the class and reciting: 'Though I speak with tongues of men and of angels and have not love...love suffers long and is kind, it does not envy, it does not boast, it is not proud. It is not rude; it is not self-seeking.... Love does not delight in evil but rejoices with the truth. It always protects, always trusts, always hopes, always perseveres... (followed by the rest of the chapter, and ending)...and now these three remain: faith, hope and love. But the greatest of these is love"'. (The word 'love', meaning caring, selfless love, is now used, more correctly, in place of the word 'charity' that I learned using the Authorised Version of the Bible. I have used a more modern translation, from which I have quoted just a few of the verses.) We were awarded a house mark if we could recite the whole chapter aloud and with clarity of voice. I think the passage had quite an effect on how I have tried to conduct my life.

The minister looked absolutely amazed to learn that we had been expected to recite an entire chapter of the Bible from memory. He immediately excused himself and disappeared rather rapidly into the vestry. There was quite a delay before he reappeared and led us into the chapel, but when we were all seated and had sung a hymn, the minister began to give his address prior to the committal. What was his reading? The first book of Corinthians Chapter 13! He had had a few moments in the vestry to change his talk, and gave a very moving address, based on this chapter and aligning it with Miss Oyston's life and teaching career. I'm not sure that Miss Oyston would have expected her life and career to be linked with a well-known chapter in the Bible, but it was a very honourable tribute. I felt very privileged to have been able to attend my late form teacher's funeral. It has almost brought my life-story full circle.

I met her carer after the funeral and she told me that when Miss Oyston was bedridden she often asked her carer to read out to her the 'Chandos letters' she had received each year after our reunion. Her carer told me that Miss Oyston was a very lonely lady and that she derived great pleasure from hearing all about the lives of her old pupils during the war. Apparently she had kept all the letters I had sent her in a box under her bed, so I think those years were special to her as they were special to us.

Life has not grown any easier with the passage of years. Treatment for chronic, severe neurological pain is not very effective and most drugs that might have offered me relief in the past had side effects that made their use impossible. I often spent hours kneeling on the floor during the night playing Patience or doing a jigsaw puzzle, because the pain prevented me from even remaining lying in bed. Dawn was often breaking and my eyes were watering with tiredness before I crawled upstairs again and managed to drop off to sleep. My doctor then insisted that I took a sleeping tablet, and I have relied on one for a reasonable night's sleep ever since.

However, the introduction of Pregabalin a few years ago as the first specific drug for the treatment of neuropathic pain (what was formerly called neuralgia) does give some slight relief. It also has side effects – weight gain being one, and the other, of course, as with all painkilling drugs, is constipation.

I think my tolerance to pain has improved a little, and with the lessening of my ability to fight it has come a certain acceptance. I can sit for longer, especially if I am on a firm seat, such as my present typist's chair, or my firm car seat, but it is still exceedingly painful, and the pain increases as the day wears on, as does my ability to cope with it, and I think that the pain is actually becoming gradually more severe.

Various vague terms have been used over the years to name this condition – trapped nerve, perineal pain, functional pain, neuropathic pain, (pain for which the original cause has gone but the 'gateway' in the spinal cord remains open to pain receptors in the brain, which now has a 'memory' of whatever was the original cause). None of these words make it easy to explain to others, and their vagueness and uncommonness only seem to serve to make it appear odd or unreal to those who do not have it. The terms are simply descriptions of pain caused by hypersensitive nerves that have somehow become permanently switched on. It has been likened to the torment of trigeminal neuralgia, but is in a totally different, less accessible, and unspeakable (in polite society) area, where sitting or resting only aggravates. There is no easement.

These vague descriptions are now being replaced with the term 'pelvic pain' which covers any long-standing pain condition below the waist, within the pelvis, for which no organic cause can be found. I have often felt embarrassed at not being able to give a recognised name to my condition, and pelvic pain is easy to say, but is somewhat misleading, as it would appear to apply to the pelvic structure itself. I hope my 'structure' is still reasonably O.K. Those who fall within this description may try to keep up a bright exterior and maintain a calm, coping existence, but can feel isolated, lonely or misunderstood. I am told there are many types of pain that are as yet undiagnosed, cannot be successfully treated. They are all neurological, life-diminishing conditions, like ME and MS or autism, along with so many who suffer mental ill health, but we are no different in our humanity from those who have arthritis, cancer, diabetes, a broken hip or a broken arm, who usually receive sympathy, understanding and help.

It is difficult for those with unrecognised diseases or unusual symptoms to lead a normal life and 'keep going'. I am sure chronic pain sufferers tend to hide their symptoms as best we can (as if ashamed of them) by keeping cheerful, maintaining optimum interests and being as active as possible. I am still determined to 'keep going', but I sometimes wonder whether 'keeping going' in the early stages, not giving in, or not being able to take life easily, can make what might be a passing condition into a permanent affliction.

Distraction seems to provide the best relief, and by implication means activity of mind or body, which is fine, but, as I get older, also becomes very tiring. Any distraction I manage to have also has to be quiet, so any activity or pastime must be without loud noise. Constant pain is very exhausting, but rest, or any occupation where my mind or my body is not actively engaged is accompanied by increased discomfort. It's a no-win situation. There *must* be a key!

Tennis, folk dancing and the ladies choir are now long-distant, happy memories, but my weekly Fitness League and Medau Movement classes have been much enjoyed in recent years and the teachers kindly reduced the volume of the music that accompanied our activity. Swimming is becoming a regular activity that I can I do without any discomfort. I enjoy my garden and still do a lot of its upkeep. I always have a book or two on the go plus a jigsaw puzzle now and again in the winter, and find these, or an absorbing television programme, a slight distraction from the awareness of pain. I soon have to resort to sprawling on the floor while reading or watching TV, when I should be sitting in a comfortable easy chair. I love company, and conversation is an excellent distraction, but concerts, the cinema or a church service are all too loud. Public address systems have been a bad thing for me personally although I recognise their usefulness, but they are so LOUD. A recent attempt to go the cinema ended with an ambulance crew standing around me, as I had collapsed before the film even began. The overloud sound projection of the advertisements was too much for me. The ambulance wasn't necessary; I just needed to get away from the noise, but the manager's regulations demanded their attendance.

Chapter Thirty

FINAL THOUGHTS

I wish some of the consultants I have seen in earlier years had asked a few more questions and had discussed my condition with me rather than just reading the referral letter then ordering expensive tests to exclude cancer. I have told more than one doctor that I would have been dead long ago if I was suffering from a life-threatening disease as I have had the same kind of pain for so many years. They then seemed to lose interest and say there was nothing they could do. Might they not occasionally learn something new if they had been able to spend more time listening to the patient? Everyone is different. Might it have led to more help for future sufferers? – or even for me? It is so easy to forget symptoms when suddenly sitting in front of a consultant, a complete stranger, who doesn't want to hear the history but is anxious to get on wit his examination. I have often been unable to mention my other odd symptoms: that as well as the pain, I can't stand loud noise, that I collapse like an overcoat being dropped if I am exposed to any sustained loud, or abrasive noise; or if there is any restriction in clothing, especially around my neck; that I sometimes feel strangely unwell, the pain suddenly becomes even more severe, or I am overwhelmingly sleepy and weak if I have inadvertently eaten some food I cannot tolerate. This combination of symptoms might give a more complete picture, lead in a different direction or suggest some other help, or, at least, show a little understanding.

I fear that when I took the liberty of mentioning any of these symptoms years ago I appeared to get a look of disbelief, disinterest, and felt I was written off , and that I was making it all up. But I'm not. I throw off these incidents when they occur, and tell anyone involved not to worry, not to cart me off to A&E, that I will soon be O.K. again. Just remove the noise, release the tight collar, consider what I have recently eaten – just be kind and try to understand; I'm not making a fuss, nor am I showing off! I am no drama-queen, although I am in fact masking daily perpetual, throbbing, cutting, sore, internal pressure pain with a cheerful (I hope) calm exterior, which is a different form of acting! It is the only way of coping.

Many who endure unexplained conditions would, I am sure, understand what I am writing, and would also gain some comfort and strength if they felt there was some attempt at explanation, or sense of understanding their difficulties and what they were enduring day after day.

Doctors seemed to back away if they couldn't give a straightforward diagnosis for a patient's symptoms. But such a patient is a human being, a 'sufferer', who deserves as much – if not more - understanding and support as is given to someone who can be treated successfully. I think that there is now a different medical approach. I have found that consultants are more likely to accept patients' written information concerning their condition, and my GP even thanked me a while ago for 'the helpful notes', that actually saved her time, but enabled me to get across the points I wished to mention.

In referrals to hospitals many years ago I sometimes sensed a subtle change in a doctor's attitude once an enquiry was made about my family history. Although no comment was made to me about a possible connection between my earlier facial neuralgia and my mother's mental illness, I felt that I was in some way considered to be 'tainted' – or was it doomed? – because of her psychiatric illness. When I described the symptoms of my facial neuralgia, I sensed incomprehension (disbelief?), a feeling of helplessness, or a referral to someone else!

Mental illness is still a comparatively hidden and unspoken subject with a degree of stigma, or disgrace, about it, and together with neurological illnesses is not fully understood, so I hope that writing about my mother's mental illness, together with my own experiences with persistent, severe neuropathic pain, will help to bring more understanding and hopefully more research to find the keys that will unlock the doors to bring a cure for all these conditions.

Before the 1950s there was very little effective treatment for those suffering from any severe mental illness. My mother was among the early beneficiaries of chlorpromazine (largactil), which I think was the first of the new anti-psychotic drugs that were developed after the end of the war. These drugs are more refined and extensive now, but more understanding of the brain and the nervous system is still needed before a key to real cure for severe psychotic psychiatric illness is found.

Many years ago (in the 1970s) I remember the sister in charge of my mother's villa telling me that 'there is very little more understanding of the brain now than fifty years ago'. This was thirty years on from the arrival of the first antipsychotic drugs. The professional attitude to mental illness may have moved on quite a lot since that remark. Anti-psychotic drugs can control symptoms do not often cure. The side effects are often unpleasant, and if patients stop taking their drugs their symptoms are likely to recur.

Cancer was an unspoken word not so many years ago but nowadays it is an open subject in all its forms, and understanding and support is provided. Massive sums of money have been used in cancer research. Mental illness in one form or another strikes at quite as many families as does cancer, but I wonder what proportion of research money goes to mental illness or the various aspects of neurological illness when compared with that given to research on cancer?

Epilepsy used to be considered by some to be caused by an 'evil spirit' many years ago. Sufferers were often shut away, not spoken of, and sometimes forgotten, but now appropriate medication, along with help and support mean epilepsy is no longer an unspoken condition with stigma attached. But people, who live with mental ill health, pain,autism, or one of the many neurological diseases, may, together with their families, suffer in silence because of the stigma or simply the disbelief, misunderstanding or unacceptance that accompanies their condition.

Could any of my symptoms be connected in some way with the epilepsy and brain damage that the sister I never knew was born with? Have I perhaps inherited a gene with links to my mother's psychotic illness, but that has affected my nervous system in a different way, with physical symptoms, i.e. nerve sensitivity to pain, noise and constriction? I am not a doctor, so I cannot say.

Whilst half-listening to a radio programme recently I picked up on a comment that research has found that close contact with mother and child is very important between the ages of three to five for the development of serotonin in the brain. This is a neurotransmitter, which has a role in calming and sleep and is found especially in the intestinal mucosa. My contact with my mother between those years was certainly not constant, and my life was not settled. Perhaps lack of serotonin plays some role in my subsequent condition?

I was referred to a gastroenterologist after the unnecessary surgery I had years ago. Her first remarks were, 'No more procedures; no more tests'. She questioned me in detail about my life history, after which she told me that chronic bowel symptoms were often linked to early life experiences, and that childhood trauma, or loss of a parent, together with the consequent suppression of the emotions that should have been expressed at the time can be programmed into the personality and develop into physical (somatised) symptoms later in life – (*Perhaps caused by lack of serotonin? - My comment*) She gave her opinion quite forcefully that unconscious but early-learned coping mechanisms that are developed in childhood are reinforced later in life when other stressful events occur, which can then appear as physical symptoms.

This consultant did appear concerned about me, gave me a very long consultation and explained what she thought was the reason for my pain, but her recommended treatment of Prozac and psychotherapy did not help. Sadly, I couldn't tolerate the former and the latter was considered undesirable, but I greatly appreciate her concern and the time she gave me. I think the increase in female doctors and consultants in my lifetime is a very good societal change.

My mother certainly 'disappeared' on numerous occasions in my early childhood, but I cannot remember being distressed or feeling rejected at the time (but remember feeling alone and at times, I suppose, a bit desolate). I think I understood that I was not to be a nuisance to the various elderly folk who cared for me; children were often supposed to be 'seen but not heard' in those days. I also think that I didn't ask questions when I was a child. I kept a calm untroubled exterior during the various unsettling childhood experiences, which perhaps hid an unacknowledged turmoil, or sense of isolation, or, as this doctor suggested, desertion. Perhaps my mind blocked out disturbing events that may have surrounded my mother's early nervous breakdowns and enforced periods in hospital? Perhaps that's where I learned the coping mechanisms with which I 'keep going' now! These unidentified but possibly locked up feelings from long ago were thought by this consultant to have expressed themselves in the painful physical symptoms I have experienced for most of my adult life. Can any of this be true? Perhaps it is an easy answer for symptoms that cannot be understood, or that doctors can do little to help. Perhaps my family history suggests this opinion, and prevents them from considering alternative diagnoses. I cannot decide, but I have to admit that it was only when the consultant expressed this theory some years ago that I felt anyone had some understanding of the reality and severity of the physical pain that I have had for so long. Sadly she didn't have the answer, but I thank her for her kind concern. It seems tough that if you cope you then suffer!

I have read that bowel problems are apparently often related to emotional repression or rejection; psychologists consider that a young child subconsciously considers the disappearance of his or her mother as a rejection, and that this can be reinforced by events in later life, and the body is 'punished' in some subconscious way. I find it impossible to believe that the circumstances surrounding parts of my life, especially the early years' experiences that appeared normal to me at the time, could possibly precipitate the pain I have suffered so many years later.

The real meaning of the word 'psychosomatic' is not that 'it's all in the mind' as many people think, (implying that the patient's symptoms are imagined) but that the physical body has been affected in some way; the symptoms have been caused, or aggravated, by continued stress, or bottled-up feelings. If the hurts to the mind and emotions have been shut off, or the subconsciously perceived desertion, loneliness, or lack of affection, is not understood, is denied, or is in other ways repeated, the effects are considered likely to appear in physical symptoms with irritated or damaged nerve endings, but this is difficult to understand and hard to accept.

Many who have trodden a stony path in life will know the concrete reality of physical pain or mental agony, and its continual persistence, and have had to withstand many kinds of anguish. They often wear a mask of good humour in order to get through each day and find that there are very few who can share or understand the suffering that is hidden behind the mask. My mask is now wearing very thin.

I have read that there is evidence that schizophrenia used to be considered a bodily, and not a mental illness, but that the development of the antipsychotic drugs in the 1950s halted further research into *why* mental illness occurred. There grew a total dependence on treating the symptoms, and the efficacy of the new drugs.

I have read that damage to the lining of the gut has been found in autopsies of schizophrenic patients. Is there a link between schizophrenia and coeliac disease, or, perhaps between multiple food intolerances, irritable bowel syndrome and pelvic pain? Could my gut problems, which are apparently caused by irritated nerves, be genetically connected in some way to my mother's mental illness? It was traditionally held that the 'bowels were the seat of the emotions'. Should there be some research into links between food intolerances, the bowel, intractable pain and mental illness? Perhaps the psychiatrists, gastroenterologists and food allergy/intolerance specialists need to get together!

I wonder whether the theory that the mercury content in the nation's amalgam teeth fillings has been tested. Could the mercury in my 1958 tooth fillings have been the initial cause of my facial pain, revealed a few months' later after a stressful confinement? Could the replacement in about 1984 of four other amalgam fillings with ceramic ones have initiated my bowel irritation and caused the pelvic pain to begin in a little later? Both procedures were done without the special precautions that are now considered essential to prevent the ingestion of mercury vapour or minute fragments of the metal. This is thought by some dentists to cause damage to the nervous system, intractable pain or even diseases such as MS. If the doctors won't acknowledge the possibility of the truth of this theory they don't give themselves the opportunity to think about it, test them and evaluate it.

All these thoughts have occurred to me as I was writing this book. None of these ramblings of mine are likely to become fields of research, but I cling to the hope that clinical research will find the key to cure this abominable, relentless, constant torture. Expressions such as 'pain in the neck' (or elsewhere!) 'a bear with a sore head', 'a gut feeling' or 'it's getting on my nerves', must have originated with people who actually suffered these colourful descriptions of pain that applied to symptoms in the nerve endings of the head, neck, gut and elsewhere.

Nerves are actual, physical systems in our body, even though many seem to think they only refer to the nebulous, imaginary feelings of the weak-kneed or faint-hearted. Nobody could function without his or her autonomic and sympathetic nervous systems

I wish there was some kind of support group for people who suffer pain and bizarre symptoms in unmentionable areas. Am I such an oddity?

I have retained my Christian faith, but nowadays I find it hard to sing the joyful, triumphant, trusting hymns of earlier years. I can't sing the words of many of the hymns I grew up with, with the confidence and conviction that I used to have, so, as I now can't sing, I don't try! Some of the verses are just not true in my experience. I suppose my life is summed up in my, slightly altered, words of a very famous old hymn: '*She* who would valiant be 'gainst all disaster. Let *her* in constancy follow the Master. There's no discouragement shall make *me* once relent, *my* first avowed intent, to be a pilgrim'.

I cannot believe that this mortal life of pain has been ordained or planned for me by God. I have now suffered intense, constant pain for over fifty years, and I cannot see that a loving God would plan such a life to test me. I quite agree with the statement that I sometimes hear, that 'no one can be assured of an easy pathway through the years', but it is rather a glib remark, that doesn't consider that 'ease' seems to have given me the slip throughout most of my life. Nor can I agree with the kind (?) remark, 'Never mind! God has got His plan for you'. It makes me question the suitability, the love or the kindness of the plan. 'Never' mind? Of course I mind the troubled years I have had. You can't 'not mind' when pain has prevented one reaching, or enjoying, so many of the good, enjoyable, exciting and useful goals life offers.

I would have to reply that life isn't fixed; we are not programmed. We have been given brains – and common sense - to make wide choices, which are not of necessity 'bad' or 'wrong' or 'not in His will'. Many are not even choices; they just occur. Bad things happen regardless of one's will. I seem to have been denied the opportunity of doing many worthwhile and enjoyable things, and cannot see a useful, or positive, plan in my life when constant pain has denied me so much, and put a huge 'pain drain' on everything I do. What I have done and value – bringing up my sons, my brief teaching career, my share in the partnership of an (almost) fifty-five year marriage, and, indeed, in having two books published! – has been done to the accompaniment of severe, intrusive pain. It makes me sad to remember that my years of teaching were cut short when I felt I was making a contribution to the development of a few of the next generation.

I feel sure that one's genetic make-up, nerve responses, individual physical strengths or weaknesses, the strength of will, the accidents at birth, or during development before birth, one's upbringing, events, or circumstances that may occur in childhood or in later life, the experiences one goes through, and the life choices that are made, or are forced upon one through circumstance, shocks and stress, all link up (together with our DNA) to make the package that develops in every individual. It's not all fixed.

God doesn't plan a life of suffering, or a lack of relatives, or living in a danger zone or a war-torn country or extreme poverty – or extreme wealth, for that matter. Many children have grown up with a dearth of relatives, through war, or poverty or natural disaster. Their loneliness, their hunger, their brief lives, their pain or suffering... are not God's plan, but one of the nasty accidents, whims of life, or wickedness of others, inheritance together with the patterning of individual DNA., or just where they happen to have been born That can't be a personalised plan; it would be cruelty and so unfair.

 My life, as has many others, seems in many ways to have been a path of suffering. As my mother expressed it after her first, brain-damaged, baby was born, 'That's your lot; you've got to get on with it'. How sadly her 'lot' affected her, but this was not her 'destiny', nor could it possibly be God's plan for her before time began, but was the result of, shall I say, perhaps a mis-match of, or imbalance in, the ingredients in the 'recipe' of her life. (Inadequate food in WW1, or a consequence of being one of the survivors of the 1918 influenza epidemic, for example.) Nor can I believe that Peggy – whose short existence began nine months before she was born – was born to a pre-destined plan. There was no opportunity for her to make wrong decisions. How cruel it would have been for God's plan to affect her in such a disastrous way. My father's or my mother's, solitary or sad lives, were not paths planned specifically for them by God. I have only appreciated their great sadnesses since I have grown older. It is a mystery why some seem to have a stony, often lonely, pathway throughout their lives. Life is an enigma.

I find it somewhat puzzling when I compare the years of mental suffering my mother endured from the time of my birth, with the years of physical pain that I have experienced through most of my own adult life. I have now had severe pain for as many years as my mother was in a psychiatric hospital. Another comparison is the similarity between my father's loss of a parent when he was seven years old, and my loss (although not through death) of my mother when I was eight. This thought was often in my mind when bringing up my children. I was determined that I wouldn't allow a third generation in my family to grow up with only one parent. They were going to have a father and a mother, come what may. That wasn't circumstance or inheritance or, dare I say, a divine plan, but my persistence!

Nobody appeared to understand or explain what might be happening in my body, what might have caused the neuralgic pain and other symptoms, or why they were so bizarre. In some sense it has been somewhat similar to my childhood experience, when conversation about my mother appeared taboo, explanations were not given, and she was never discussed. Over the years I have been passed from one doctor or hospital department to another, in a similar way as in my early childhood I went from one home to another. It seems strange that so many of life's experiences seem to have repeated themselves in differing ways: I was an only child, with only one distantly-related cousin; I worked on my own in a basement office before I married, my marriage was to an only son, so no sisters or brothers-in-law. We are sometimes unaware at the time that we are going down an almost identical path in life's journey, - it's the same play but with different scenes.

It seems to be an irony of life that one can appear to overcome circumstances, in many senses be happy and fulfilled, but that the body, mind, nerves, emotions or spirit seem to demand a price if they have not been equally valued or nourished.   A 'breakdown' after traumatic circumstances could mean not only a nervous breakdown, but equally a breakdown of the immune system, the digestive system, or some other - perhaps a genetically weaker - part of the person. Struggling on and coping is perhaps not always the best way to recovery but it is often the only way for most sufferers, and is what society expects.

Is there a key to unlock this door of pain? I count my blessings - I really do, when I consider the other illnesses and afflictions that many suffer - but the satisfaction of the things I have achieved, the little good I hope I have done, the love and companionship I have shared, the adventure, the good times, the enrichment, the beauty I have experienced, and the fun and fulfilment I have otherwise enjoyed do not compensate for the persistent presence of pain.

As I come to the end of my story I realise that in my two books I have covered well over a century of a number of aspects of social history, not only personal narrative. I have written of many of the social, medical, educational and many other changes that have occurred during that long period. Although 'Child of the Thirties' was about my own childhood, I devoted a chapter to the early life of both my parents, and included a little about the grandparents that I never knew, so I have covered a period from becore the last decade of the nineteenth century to the end of the first decade of the twenty-first! I hope that my story has contained joy as well as distress. I hope the 'almonds and raisins' of life - the bitter and the sweet - have combined to make a homogenous mix.

Perhaps my long periods sitting on a typist's chair while typing my first two, unpublished, books in the 1980s were the initial cause of my present 'under-carriage' pain. I have since typed two further books sitting, I am sure, for far too long, but on a more supportive seat, so I think I will now stop typing, bring my story to a conclusion, shut down my computer for a while and get off my typist's chair.

Lightning Source UK Ltd.
Milton Keynes UK
09 December 2010

164108UK00001B/2/P